# Pediatric Dermatology

*Editor*

MOISE L. LEVY

# DERMATOLOGIC CLINICS

www.derm.theclinics.com

*Consulting Editor*
BRUCE H. THIERS

April 2013 • Volume 31 • Number 2

**ELSEVIER**

1600 John F. Kennedy Boulevard • Suite 1800 • Philadelphia, Pennsylvania, 19103-2899

http://www.theclinics.com

**DERMATOLOGIC CLINICS Volume 31, Number 2**
**April 2013 ISSN 0733-8635, ISBN-13: 978-1-4557-7082-3**

Editor: Stephanie Donley
Developmental Editor: Teia Stone

*Dermatologic Clinics* (ISSN 0733-8635) is published quarterly by Elsevier Inc., 360 Park Avenue South, New York, NY 10010-1710. Months of publication are January, April, July, and October. Business and editorial offices: 1600 John F. Kennedy Blvd., Suite 1800, Philadelphia, PA 19103-2899. Customer service office: 11830 Westline Drive, St. Louis, MO 63146. Periodicals postage paid at New York, NY, and additional mailing offices. Subscription prices are USD 346.00 per year for US individuals, USD 532.00 per year for US institutions, USD 404.00 per year for Canadian individuals, USD 636.00 per year for Canadian institutions, USD 473.00 per year for international individuals, USD 636.00 per year for international institutions, USD 159.00 per year for US students/residents, and USD 230.00 per year for Canadian and international students/residents. International air speed delivery is included in all *Clinics* subscription prices. All prices are subject to change without notice. **POSTMASTER:** Send address changes to *Dermatologic Clinics*, Elsevier Health Sciences Division, Subscription Customer Service, 3251 Riverport Lane, Maryland Heights, MO 63043. **Customer Service: 1-800-654-2452 (U.S. and Canada); 314-447-8871 (outside U.S. and Canada). Fax: 314-447-8029. E-mail: journalscustomerservice-usa@elsevier.com (for print support); journalsonlinesupport-usa@elsevier.com (for online support).**

*Reprints.* For copies of 100 or more, of articles in this publication, please contact the Commercial Reprints Department, Elsevier Inc., 360 Park Avenue South, New York, New York 10010-1710. Tel.: (212) 633-3813; Fax: (212) 462-1935; Email: repritns@elsevier.com.

The *Dermatologic Clinics* is covered in *MEDLINE/PubMed (Index Medicus), Current Contents/Clinical Medicine, Excerpta Medica, Chemical Abstracts,* and *ISI/BIOMED.*

Printed and bound by CPI Group (UK) Ltd, Croydon, CR0 4YY

Transferred to digital print 2012

# Contributors

## CONSULTING EDITOR

**BRUCE H. THIERS, MD**
Professor and Chairman, Department of
Dermatology and Dermatologic Surgery,
Medical University of South Carolina,
Charleston, South Carolina

## EDITOR

**MOISE L. LEVY, MD**
Chief, Pediatric Dermatology and Physician-in-
Chief, Dell Children's Medical Center, Austin;
Clinical Professor, Dermatology UT-
Southwestern Medical School, Dallas; Clinical
Professor, Dermatology and Pediatrics, Baylor
College of Medicine, Houston, Texas

## AUTHORS

**MUHAMMAD ALI, MD**
Department of Radiology, Boston Children's
Hospital, Boston, Massachusetts

**ANNA M. BENDER, MD**
Division of Pediatric Dermatology, Department
of Dermatology, Johns Hopkins University,
Baltimore, Maryland

**MEGAN M. BROWN, BS**
Department of Dermatology, University of
New Mexico School of Medicine, Albuquerque,
New Mexico

**JOHN C. BROWNING, MD, FAAD, FAAP**
Division of Dermatology and Cutaneous
Surgery; Pediatric Dermatology Section,
Department of Pediatrics, The University of
Texas Health Science Center at San Antonio,
San Antonio, Texas

**KRISTI CANTY, MD**
Assistant Professor of Pediatrics and
Dermatology, Section of Dermatology,

Department of Pediatrics, Children's Mercy
Hospital, Kansas City, Missouri

**SARAH L. CHAMLIN, MD**
Division of Dermatology, Ann & Robert H. Lurie
Children's Hospital of Chicago, Northwestern
University Feinberg School of Medicine,
Chicago, Illinois

**GULRAIZ CHAUDRY, MB, ChB**
Department of Radiology, Boston Children's
Hospital; Assistant Professor, Harvard Medical
School, Boston, Massachusetts

**KELLY M. CORDORO, MD**
Assistant Professor of Dermatology and
Pediatrics, Department of Dermatology,
University of California, San Francisco,
San Francisco, California

**BETH A. DROLET, MD**
Professor of Dermatology and Pediatrics,
Medical Director of Birthmarks and Vascular
Anomalies, Children's Hospital of Wisconsin;
Department of Dermatology, Medical College
of Wisconsin, Milwaukee, Wisconsin

**JONATHAN A. DYER, MD**
Assistant Professor of Dermatology and Child
Health, University of Missouri, Columbia,
Missouri

**ADELAIDE A. HEBERT, MD**
Department of Dermatology, The University
of Texas Medical School-Houston, Houston,
Texas

**KRISTEN E. HOLLAND, MD**
Associate Professor, Department of
Dermatology, Medical College of Wisconsin,
Milwaukee, Wisconsin

**NATALIA JAIMES, MD**
Dermatology Service, Universidad Pontificia
Bolivariana; Aurora Skin Cancer Center,
Medellín, Colombia

**DELMA Y. JARRETT, MD**
Department of Radiology, Boston Children's
Hospital; Clinical Instructor, Harvard Medical
School, Boston, Massachusetts

**MIRYAM KERNER, MD**
Department of Dermatology, Memorial
Sloan-Kettering Cancer Center, New York,
New York

**MOISE L. LEVY, MD**
Chief, Pediatric Dermatology and Physician-in-
Chief, Dell Children's Medical Center, Austin;
Clinical Professor, Dermatology UT-
Southwestern Medical School, Dallas; Clinical
Professor, Dermatology and Pediatrics, Baylor
College of Medicine, Houston, Texas

**ASHFAQ A. MARGHOOB, MD**
Department of Dermatology, Memorial
Sloan-Kettering Cancer Center, New York,
New York

**ANN L. MARQUELING, MD**
Clinical Assistant Professor of Dermatology
and Pediatrics, School of Medicine, Stanford
University, Stanford, California

**BRANDIE J. METZ, MD**
Pediatric Dermatology of Orange County,
Irvine, California

**OMAR PACHA, MD**
Department of Dermatology, The University
of Texas Medical School-Houston, Texas

**MICHAEL PERRY, MD**
Senior Medical Student, The University Texas
Medical Branch, Dallas, Texas

**ALON SCOPE, MD**
Department of Dermatology, Sheba
Medical Center, Sackler School of
Medicine, Tel Aviv University, Tel Aviv,
Israel; Department of Dermatology,
Memorial Sloan-Kettering Cancer Center,
New York, New York

**AIMEE C. SMIDT, MD**
Departments of Dermatology and Pediatrics,
University of New Mexico School of Medicine,
Albuquerque, New Mexico

**WILLIAM C. STREUSAND, MD**
Collaborative Care, Child, Adolescent,
and Adult Psychiatry; Adjunct Professor,
Department of Educational Psychology,
University of Texas at Austin; Executive and
Medical Director, CollaboraCare for Kids,
Austin, Texas

**ALLISON SWANSON, MD**
Assistant Professor of Pediatrics and
Dermatology, Section of Dermatology,
Department of Pediatrics, Children's Mercy
Hospital, Kansas City, Missouri

# Contents

Skin disease is highly prevalent in the United States, and it has been well-documented that patients with skin disease experience financial, psychological, social, and quality-of-life (QoL) burdens beyond those of the general population. Pediatric patients and their caregivers are particularly vulnerable to the burden of skin disease. Over the past decade disease-specific indices for QoL measurement in pediatric dermatology have been developed. Most of this research has focused on acne, atopic dermatitis, hemangiomas, ichythosis, psoriasis, and vitiligo. This article provides an overview of QoL assessment in pediatric dermatology for these six conditions.

Dermatitis is a frequent cause for referral to the pediatric dermatologist. In this article, a brief overview is given of common childhood dermatoses as well as some rarer dermatoses that may give the clinician cause for concern. Widespread scaling and erythema, described as erythroderma, are a cause of frustration for patients, families, and their physician(s). Both unusual and common skin disorders can present in this fashion. Just as recognizing common dermatoses is important, it is also important to recognize when a dermatitis fails to fit the common pattern and may prompt further investigation.

This article outlines the epidemiology, pathogenesis, clinical presentation, diagnosis, and treatment of childhood morphea. Also known as localized scleroderma, morphea is a fibrosing disorder of the skin and subcutaneous tissues. Morphea is differentiated from systemic sclerosis (scleroderma) based on the absence of sclerodactyly, Raynaud phenomenon, and nail-fold capillary changes. Confusion may occur because patients with morphea often have systemic symptoms such as malaise, fatigue, arthralgias, myalgias, and positive autoantibodies. Unlike morphea, systemic sclerosis has organ involvement, particularly gastrointestinal, pulmonary, and renal.

This article reviews some of the recent literature on therapeutic modalities and their efficacy in common pediatric skin conditions. Immunotherapy and laser therapy of warts and molluscum contagiosum show therapeutic promise. Bleach baths may help in eradicating *Staphylococcus aureus* carriage and in improving atopic dermatitis. Cephalexin continues to show efficacy even with increased incidence of community-acquired methicillin-resistant *Staphylococcus aureus*. More studies have looked at the use of systemic immunosuppressants for alopecia areata and vitiligo in children, although risks and benefits of therapy must be weighed. The excimer laser shows promise as a treatment modality for both alopecia areata and vitiligo.

# DERMATOLOGIC CLINICS

# Preface

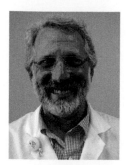

Moise L. Levy, MD
*Editor*

Pediatric Dermatology was last published in *Dermatologic Clinics* in 1998. Since that time, our specialty has grown dramatically in number and influence. The Society for Pediatric Dermatology is a robust group with international membership. Clinical and research activities in pediatric dermatology continue to flourish.

This volume is dedicated to Pediatric Dermatology. I have asked experienced and some newer "stars" in our specialty, as well as outstanding authorities in general dermatology and other areas of medicine, to discuss areas of interest to those clinicians who care for children and adolescents. The area of vascular birthmarks continues to evolve and presents challenges in the area of diagnosis and treatment. Dr Chaudry and colleagues have given us a current view of the approach to imaging of these lesions, while Drs Holland and Drolet review their approach to the infant with hemangioma. Difficulties in the care of the child with severe psoriasis are addressed by Drs Cordoro and Marqueling and a broad review of the topic of recalcitrant dermatitis is presented by Dr Bender. Other topics, such as photodermatoses, genodermatoses, morphea, procedural pediatric dermatology, dermoscopy, and a general

therapeutic update of selected pediatric dermatologic disorders, are reviewed. Finally, the importance of behavioral therapies pertaining to dermatologic care and the assessment of quality of life for patients dealing with pediatric skin disorders are covered.

We hope you enjoy this issue and that the topics prove to be a useful resource for you in the care of your patients.

Moise L. Levy, MD
UT-Southwestern Medical School
5323 Harry Hines Boulevard
Dallas, TX 75390, USA

Dermatology and Pediatrics
Baylor College of Medicine
1 Baylor Plaza
Houston, TX 77030, USA

Dell Children's Medical Center
Pediatric and Adolescent Dermatology
1301 Barbara Jordan Boulevard, Suite 200
Austin, TX 78723, USA

E-mail address:
mlevy@sfcaustin.com

Dermatol Clin 31 (2013) ix
http://dx.doi.org/10.1016/j.det.2013.02.001
0733-8635/13/$ – see front matter © 2013 Published by Elsevier Inc.

# Quality of Life in Pediatric Dermatology

Megan M. Brown, BS[a], Sarah L. Chamlin, MD[b],
Aimee C. Smidt, MD[c,d],*

## KEYWORDS

• Quality of life • Patient-focused care • Pediatric dermatology • Skin disease

## KEY POINTS

• Patients with skin disease experience financial, psychological, social, and quality-of-life burdens beyond those of the general population.
• Children and adolescents undergo rapid, formative stages of physical, intellectual, emotional, and social development, and are particularly vulnerable to disruptions, such as chronic skin disease.
• This article provides an overview of quality-of-life issues and assessment in pediatric dermatology, with a specific focus on acne, atopic dermatitis, hemangiomas, ichthyosis, psoriasis, and vitiligo.

## INTRODUCTION

Skin disease is highly prevalent in the United States, and it has been well-documented that patients with skin disease experience financial, psychological, social, and quality-of-life (QoL) burdens beyond those of the general population.[1–4] Pediatric patients and their parents are particularly vulnerable to the burden of skin disease.[5–8] Children and adolescents are unique in that they undergo rapid, formative stages of physical, intellectual, emotional, and social development, and are particularly vulnerable to disruptions, such as chronic diseases. Recent research has focused on describing and measuring the QoL impact (physical, psychological, and social) on children and adolescents affected by skin disorders.[9–13] For clinicians, an understanding of current research on the QoL burden of skin disease on pediatric patients helps to frame patient interactions and to guide interventions for affected children and their parents.

Chronic disease in childhood may negatively affect development and overall QoL.[6,8,14] Pediatric patients with skin disease are more likely to experience depression, low self-esteem, lack of sleep, bullying, poor social interactions, poor medical compliance, and poorer health outcomes as adults.[14–24] Furthermore, the burden of pediatric skin disease affects the family unit as a whole.

Various scales and indices have been developed to measure QoL in children and adolescents affected by skin disease. However, pediatric patients represent a unique challenge when measuring and describing QoL.[5–7,10,11,25,26] Multidimensional factors, such as patient age, communication ability, caregiver status, and socioeconomic status, must be taken into account.

This article provides a framework by which clinicians may understand QoL issues in six common

Disclosure: The authors/editors have no conflict of interest to disclose. No financial support was required for this manuscript.
[a] Department of Dermatology, University of New Mexico School of Medicine, 1021 Medical Arts Avenue Northeast, Albuquerque, NM 87131, USA; [b] Division of Dermatology, Ann & Robert H. Lurie Children's Hospital of Chicago, Northwestern University Feinberg School of Medicine, 225 East Chicago Avenue, Box 107, Chicago, IL 60611, USA; [c] Department of Dermatology, University of New Mexico School of Medicine, 1021 Medical Arts Avenue Northeast, Albuquerque, NM 87131, USA; [d] Department of Pediatrics, University of New Mexico School of Medicine, 1021 Medical Arts Avenue Northeast, Albuquerque, NM 87131, USA
* Corresponding author. 1021 Medical Arts Avenue Northeast, Albuquerque, NM 87131.
E-mail address: ASmidt@salud.unm.edu

pediatric dermatologic conditions and includes a summary of applicable QoL indices by diagnosis. **Box 1** represents common indices that have been used in pediatric dermatology, although others may be considered. We also suggest realistic strategies to translate this information into practical means to improve clinical practice and research.

## QOL MEASUREMENT IN PEDIATRIC DERMATOLOGY

Interest in QoL measurement in pediatric patients with skin disease has grown in recent years, and started with an increased recognition of the psychosocial burden experienced by young patients with disease and their families, and recognition of the importance of patient-focused care.[27] In 1995, Lewis-Jones and Finlay developed the Children's Dermatology Life Quality Index (CDLQI). This was the first tool designed to specifically assess the impact of skin disease on children[3,12] as a parallel to the Dermatology Life Quality Index (DLQI), the first dermatology-specific QoL index designed for adults.

The concept of patient-focused care takes into account the patients' (or caregivers') perceptions, knowledge, and concerns into the medical treatment plan. It is meant to merge patient and caregiver education with evidence-based medicine to achieve optimal medical management for a particular individual. Benefits of patient-focused care include improved patient-clinician communication, better monitoring of treatment progress, increased patient compliance, superior physician performance, and greater patient satisfaction. QoL measurement may facilitate patient-focused care, be useful in measuring clinical research outcomes, and provide the patient and the physician with an additional objective means to assess treatment.[2,15,27–30]

There are multiple indices validated to measure QoL in adults with skin disease. A few examples of adult QoL indices include the DLQI, Dermatology-Specific Quality of Life, Dermatology Quality of Life Scale, Skindex-29, and Skindex-16.

Currently, two QoL indices specific for pediatric dermatology exist: the CDLQI and Skindex-Teen. Other disease-specific indices used in pediatric dermatology to measure QoL are detailed later. Some of these tools measure parental response to disease as a proxy for their young children. The 10-item CDLQI has been validated and widely used, is available in many languages, and also has been expanded to include a young patient-accessible cartoon version. The CDLQI is designed for use in patients 5 to 16 years old. The

score range is 0 to 30, with a higher score representing greater QoL impairment.

Skindex-Teen, developed by our group, is a validated 22-item questionnaire that focuses on QoL in adolescents (ages 12–17 years) with skin disease. It includes subscales pertaining to physical symptoms and psychosocial functioning. The initial validation study of this index found that, in general, adolescents with skin disease are most often bothered by physical symptoms (especially itching and pain), appearance and impact on clothing choices, and effects on self-esteem and self-image. The score range is 0 to 84, with a higher score representing a greater QoL impairment.

Although few studies have used CDLQI and Skindex-Teen to measure QoL in general pediatric dermatology practices, over the past decade many disease-specific indices for QoL measurement have been developed. Most of this research has focused on acne, atopic dermatitis (AD), hemangiomas, ichthysis, psoriasis, and vitiligo.

## ACNE VULGARIS

Acne vulgaris is extremely prevalent in adolescents (ages 12–17 years): more than 90% of males and 80% of females experience this condition during their lifetime.[1,3] QoL issues have been well-studied in acne vulgaris. Adolescence is a critical time of development of self-worth, and there is much emphasis on body image during this period. Coexistent morbidities in many adolescent patients with acne vulgaris include low self-esteem, social isolation, and depression and suicidal ideation.[31–36] Of note, scarring related to acne vulgaris may lead to permanent physical morbidity, and decreased social functioning into adulthood.[37]

Adolescents with acne vulgaris have poorer mental health scores than peers with asthma, epilepsy, diabetes, coronary artery disease, back pain, or arthritis.[38,39] The Acne Disability Index (ADI), Cardiff Acne Disability Index (CADI), and the Acne-QoL index are validated indices for identifying and assessing adolescents with acne vulgaris who experience QoL impairment.[40]

The ADI is a validated 48-item acne QoL questionnaire that addresses the following categories: psychological, physical, recreational, employment, self-awareness, social reaction, skin care, and financial. A score is calculated by the sum of each category score, the total of which is then converted into the final percent score. This index is found to be somewhat cumbersome for use in routine clinical care. Simpler, more rapidly used, modified indices have been developed as alternatives to the ADI, including the CADI and Acne QoL

**Box 1**
**Commonly used QoL indices in pediatric dermatology literature[a,b]**

*Acne vulgaris*
- CDLQI
- Skindex-Teen
- CADI
- ADI
- Acne QoL Index

*Atopic dermatitis*
- CDLQI
- Skindex-Teen
- IDQOL
- CADIS
- QoLPCAD
- PIQoL
- DFI

*Hemangioma*
- CDLQI
- MHI
- Skindex-Teen
- TNO-AZL

*Ichthyosis*
- CDLQI
- DLQI
- HRQoL
- NHP
- SF-36
- Skindex-Teen

*Psoriasis*
- CDLQI
- PLSI
- SF-36
- Skindex-Teen

*Vitiligo*
- CDLQI
- Skindex-Teen
- Skindex-29
- SF-36
- DLQI
- Skin Discoloration Impact Questionnaire

*Abbreviations:* ADI, Acne Disability Index; CADI, Cardiff Acne Disability Index; CADIS, Child Atopic Dermatitis Impact Scale; CDLQI, Children's Dermatology Life Quality Index; DFI, Dermatitis Family Impact Questionnaire; DLQI, Dermatology Life Quality Index; HRQoL, Health-related Quality of Life; IDQOL, Infants' Dermatitis Quality of Life Index; MHI, Mental Health Inventory; NHP, Nottingham Health Profile; PIQoL, Parent's Index Atopic Dermatitis Quality of Life; PSLI, Psoriasis Stress Life Inventory; QoLPCAD, Quality of Life in Primary Caregivers with Atopic Dermatitis; SF-36, Short Form-36; TNO-AZL, TNO-AZL Quality of Life Questionnaire.

[a] For any skin condition the following global dermatologic QoL indices may be considered: CDLQI, DLQI, Skindex-29, Skindex-Teen, and SF-36.

[b] Many of these indices may be accessed at no cost through Cardiff University (www.dermatology.org.uk/quality/quality), the Patient-Reported Outcome and Quality of Life Instruments Database (www.proqolid.org), or TNO Innovation for Life (http://www.tno.nl/index.cfm).

index. The CADI is modeled after the ADI but contains only five questions, with a score range 0 to 15. A higher score indicates increased QoL impairment. Benefits include simplicity of use, adequate gauging of patient self-perception of acne vulgaris, and that it requires only minutes to complete.[40,41] The Acne QoL index is another validated 19-item questionnaire that addresses four categories: (1) self-perception, (2) role-emotional, (3) role-social, and (4) acne symptoms. The total score is the sum of category scores: a higher score indicates better QoL.[42,43] The CADI or Acne QoL indices offer validated, succinct measures of QoL impact on patients with acne.

Psychosocial impairment in adolescents with acne vulgaris can be quite significant.[19] Patients with more severe QoL impairment should raise consideration by the physician of more aggressive or systemic treatments.[4] In some cases, referral for an evaluation by a mental health specialist may be warranted.[44] Effective treatment successfully minimizes the QoL burden of this common disease.[39]

## ATOPIC DERMATITIS

AD affects up to 17% of children in the United States, most commonly infants and young children, and is characterized by recurrent, chronic flares of inflammation and pruritus. The psychological, financial, and social burdens of AD are substantial.[45,46]

Parents report that their children with AD experience sleep disturbance, and are more clingy, frustrated, and irritable.[17,47,48] Studies have found a correlation between AD and attention-deficit/hyperactivity disorder.[49–53] Infants with AD are also found to be at greater risk for development of mental health problems by age 10 years.[48]

The Infants' Dermatitis Quality of Life Index (IDQOL) is a validated 10-item questionnaire designed for parents of children younger than age 4 years. It addresses difficulty with mood, sleep, play, family activities, mealtime, treatment, dressing and bathing, and parental perception of their child's current dermatitis severity. Increased impairment is associated with higher score. Scores range from 0 to 30, with 30 being the maximum. A higher score represents greater QoL impairment.

The Childhood Atopic Dermatitis Development Impact Scale (CADIS) is a validated tool for children younger than 6 years of age. It includes 45 items in the following four subscale categories: (1) physical health, (2) emotional health, (3) physical functioning, and (4) social functioning. Both parent and child are evaluated in each of the four subscales. The score range is 0 to 180, with a higher score reflecting greater QoL impairment.

Other QoL assessment indices, including the Quality of Life in Primary Caregivers of Children with Atopic Dermatitis, Parents' Index of Quality of Life in Atopic Dermatitis, and the Dermatitis Family Impact Questionnaire (DFI), focus on qualifying the burden of AD on the family unit. These indices are useful because they may allow for greater clinical education focused on reducing the burden of AD on the family as a whole, or for support group referral (eg, the National Eczema Foundation).

The prevalence and burden of AD in teenagers is less well understood. Adolescents with AD are at significant risk of impaired QoL similar to that of acne vulgaris, including predisposition to depression, impaired social interaction with members of the opposite sex, and sexual functioning.[54] Using Skindex-Teen, adolescents with AD generally experienced similar impairment in QoL as those with acne.[22]

Indices to accurately measure QoL in pediatric patients with AD are highly relevant to clinical practice and research. To more completely gauge the comprehensive burden of disease, the clinician should aim to objectively review QoL and physical impairment.[55,56]

Patients with severe QoL impairment caused by AD may be in greater need of aggressive treatment strategies to minimize comorbidities and the long-term psychosocial effects of their disease. It is critical to involve both the caregiver and patient in these treatment strategies.

## INFANTILE HEMANGIOMAS

Infantile hemangiomas are found in 1% to 3% of all neonates and 10% of children within the first year of life.[57–59] They are a benign, yet often disfiguring or function-threatening, vascular tumor that most commonly arises in a visible region, such as the head or neck. They usually increase in size during the first year of life and most regress or involute by school age.[58,59] Of note, large facial hemangiomas and other large segmental hemangiomas can be associated with systemic findings (ie, PHACE syndrome, PELVIS syndrome, airway lesions), which may add to the emotional burden for the family.

Narrative data on QoL of children and caregivers of children with infantile hemangiomas is extensive. Patients and caregivers routinely experience social stigmatization, grief, guilt, sadness, and anxiety. Caregivers have been noted to undergo a predictable five-stage sequence of shock, denial, sadness, anger, and gradual acceptance of their child's condition.[58,60] Children, in particular, may experience decreased self-esteem and significantly reduced psychosocial functioning.[23] Caregivers are at additional risk of extreme distress because of unwarranted accusations of child abuse.[61]

Hoornweg and colleagues have designed a hemangioma-specific QoL questionnaire known as the TNO-AZL Quality of Life Questionnaire (TNO-AZL).[58,59] These acronyms are abbreviated titles for the Netherlands Organization for Applied Scientific Research (TNO) and the Dutch hospital where the questionnaire was developed (AZL). The preschool version (TAPQoL) is designed for children age 6 months to 6 years, whereas the child form (TACQoL-CF) is for ages 6 to 15 years. In their study of 236 children with hemangiomas, affected children had comparable or better QoL scores than age-matched healthy children in all domains except anxiety. There was no significant difference in scores based on lesion location or presence of complicated associated medical course. Domains where children with hemangioma had slightly better QoL than healthy children included physical symptoms, motor function, cognitive, and emotions. However, when mothers were surveyed with the TAPQoL and TACQoL-CF, they reported that their children (especially those with complicated hemangiomas) experienced more negative emotions than healthy children. The score range of both TNO-AZL forms (TAPQoL and TACQoL-CF) is 0 to 100. A higher score reflects better QoL.

This study warrants further investigation because there is a discrepancy in the extensive narrative data indicating impaired QoL and the findings of this study, which describe QoL equal or better than that of the age-matched healthy children. This may reflect a paradox in that children with hemangiomas typically receive increased parental and healthcare support, which may encourage a higher level of self-esteem and functioning.

Additionally, the findings in this study represent a population limited to Dutch patients in Amsterdam and may be caused by increased education and support through participation in the study.

The Mental Health Inventory has been used to collect data on parents of children with hemangiomas. When the Mental Health Inventory was used to study parental distress with infantile hemangiomas in a study involving six married couples, it was found that medical complications of the hemangioma were significantly associated with distress. Parental perception of surface area or visibility of the hemangioma was not significantly correlated with distress.[62] Current descriptive data and generic outcome scales support a notable psychosocial burden on families of infants with hemangiomas and further work is needed to specifically measure this outcome.

Parents and caregivers of children with infantile hemangiomas often require extensive education on the natural history and clinical outcomes and may benefit from support group referral and counseling. QoL measurement may aid in identifying the needs of individual patients and their families for these services. Bibliotherapy (a means of exploring feelings and experiences through fiction) has been cited as a method to reduce feelings of social isolation in children and caregivers.[61,63,64] Additional modes of intervention, such as interactive music therapy, may be considered.[65]

Support groups are useful resources for affected families because they provide easily accessible advice and information on advocacy, daily activities, and information on financial resources (**Table 1**). Additionally, clinician educators are excellent resources for children and caregivers of children with hemangiomas.[66]

## ICHTHYOSIS

The congenital ichthyoses are a diverse group of hereditary conditions of cornification characterized by dry skin, scale, erythema, hyperkeratosis, and often significant disfigurement. There are more than 20 subtypes of ichthyosis and multiple genetic mutations have been discovered for these

---

**Table 1**
**Educational sites and patient advocacy groups for children with skin disease**

| Disease | Organization[a] | Web Site |
|---|---|---|
| Acne vulgaris | Acne.org: Acne treatment and community | www.acne.org |
| | Acne Help | www.acnehelp.org.uk |
| Ichthyosis | Foundation for Ichthyosis and Related Skin Types | www.scalyskin.org |
| | Ichthyosis Support Group | www.ichthyosis.org.uk |
| | National Registry for Ichthyosis and Related Disorders | http://depts.washington.edu/ichreg/ichthyosis.registry/ |
| Infantile hemangioma | Hemangioma Investigator Group | www.hemangiomaeducation.org |
| Atopic dermatitis | National Eczema Association | www.nationaleczema.org |
| | National Eczema Society | www.eczema.org |
| Vascular anomalies | National Organization of Vascular Anomalies | www.novanews.org |
| | Vascular Birthmark Foundation | www.birthmark.org |
| Psoriasis | National Psoriasis Foundation | www.psoriasis.org |
| | The Psoriasis Association | www.psoriasis-association.org.uk |
| | Psoriasis Help Organization | www.psoriasis-help.org.uk |
| | Psoriasis and Psoriatic Arthritis Alliance | www.papaa.org |
| | Sparklestone Foundation | www.sparklestone.org/skinfire.org |
| Vascular birthmarks | Vascular Birthmarks Foundation | www.birthmark.org |
| Vitiligo | Vitiligo Support International | www.vitiligosupport.org |
| | Vitiligo Info | www.vitiligoinfo.org |
| | Vitiligo Society | www.vitiligosociety.org.uk |

[a] The authors of this manuscript have no affiliations to disclose regarding these organizations. This list is not meant to endorse a specific organization; rather, it is designed to provide an overview of available educational sites and advocacy groups.

chronic, lifelong disorders.[67] Ichthyosis vulgaris is the most common, with a prevalence of 1 in 300 births, and is inherited in an autosomal-dominant manner. X-linked recessive ichthyosis is the next most common and thought to occur in 1 in 3000 births.[67–69] Lamellar ichthyosis, nonbullous congenital ichthyosiform erythroderma, and bullous congenital ichthyosiform erythroderma are rarer, but not uncommonly encountered in pediatric dermatology.

Recently, there has been increased recognition of QoL issues in older adolescents and adults with ichthyosis. Studies have used the DLQI to measure impact on QoL of older adolescents (older than age 17) and adults with ichthyosis.[70,71] Other groups have used general health-related QoL indices, such as the HRQoL, Nottingham Health Profile (NHP), and Short Form-36 (SF-36).[69,72] Additionally, a small subset of adults surveyed with the NHP and focused interview sessions reported that ichthyosis had negatively affected their life and that childhood was the period of greatest impact.[73] NHP scores range from 0 to 100 with a higher score reflecting greater QoL impairment. Specific studies on QoL in children with ichthyosis are limited. In 2010, a study by Ganemo used the CDQLI to study 15 Swedish children (age 5–16) with various forms of congenital ichthyosis.[69] Results indicated that "itch, scratchy, or painful skin" received the highest symptom score.

QoL scores for patients with ichthyosis show DLQI scores similar to those of AD and psoriasis.[69–71] Overall, female patients report more impairment in the subscales of daily activities and treatment than do males.

Additionally, descriptive data do exist on QoL issues for children and caregivers of children with ichthyosis. Feelings of fear, anxiety, social isolation, low self-esteem, and depression are common themes for afflicted children. Caregivers and families are affected by the time-consuming and costly aspects of patient care.[67–72] Descriptive studies and QoL measurement in adult patients with congenital ichthyosis indicates a need for further research and development of a specific QoL index for children and adolescents with this condition.

Cost is of particular concern for children and adolescents with ichthyosis. A recent study by Styperek and colleagues found that direct healthcare costs (prescriptions, outpatient visits, emergency room visits, and hospital costs) and indirect healthcare costs (missed days from work) were substantial.[73] Many patients averaged up to five outpatient visits per year with multiple hydrating and retinoid agents prescribed. Annual personal (out-of-pocket) costs were found to be highest in children: $1182 versus $790 in adults. Of note, patients with insurance had higher annual costs.

Care for children and adolescents with ichthyosis most often focuses on traditional medical treatment strategies, such as emollients and keratolytic agents. However, support groups, such as the Foundation for Ichthyosis and Related Skin Types and Ichthyosis Support Group, can be hugely beneficial for such patients and their caregivers. Clinical education and genetic counseling play a large role in providing the multidimensional care that children with ichthyosis and their caregivers require.[68,69,74]

## PSORIASIS

Psoriasis is a common, chronic inflammatory skin disease that begins for many patients in childhood or adolescence with up to one-third of newly diagnosed cases presenting by age 15. The overall prevalence of psoriasis is thought to be 1.43%, with equal distribution between the genders, although girls are more often diagnosed during childhood.[75,76] Onset of psoriasis before the third or fourth decade of life is associated with greater likelihood of family history of the disease, increased severity of disease, and increased psychological morbidity compared with those diagnosed later in life.[77]

There is a growing body of knowledge on QoL assessment in children and adolescents with psoriasis. Children and adolescents with psoriasis are more likely to experience anxiety, depression, decreased sexual intimacy, joint pain, chronic itching, and decreased perception of social connectivity.[5,78–80]

Currently, there are no specific scales for QoL measurement in pediatric psoriasis. Studies using CDLQI in children and adolescents have found that patients with AD or psoriasis report a significant impairment of QoL. The IDQOL may also be useful in assessing QoL impact in children with psoriasis. When QoL is measured in children with various chronic diseases with the Children Life Quality Index and CDLQI, children with cerebral palsy experience the greatest impairment (38%), followed by AD and renal disease (33%), cystic fibrosis (31.7%), urticaria and asthma (27.8%), and psoriasis (26.6%).[5,79,81] In this case, the percent impairment was reported as a percentage of the total possible index score.

A recent Swedish study included children as young as 4 years of age and used the IDQOL and the DFI. Younger children (age 5–8 years) and those with joint pain had greater impairment of QoL than those age 9 to 16 or without joint pain.[79]

Adolescents with psoriasis experience considerable impairment in QoL, as quantified by SF-36, DLQI, Psoriasis Disability Index, or Psoriasis Life Stress Inventory.[79,80,82,83] Studies have shown that adolescents with psoriasis experience negative effects on social and recreational activities, and significant feelings of social disconnect; many suffer from depression and anxiety. Those with joint pain experience greatest impairment of QoL. Patients with psoriasis also tend to be more likely to be on Medicaid as adults, an indicator of lower eventual socioeconomic status and social disconnect.[80,81,84,85]

Clinical education and patient-focused care may be combined with formal support groups and online support communities, such as the National Psoriasis Foundation. Patients report excellent benefit from these resources.[86–88]

## VITILIGO

Vitiligo is an acquired autoimmune depigmenting disorder found in about 1% of the US population, with prevalence of up to 8% in certain populations worldwide.[89] It tends to affect both genders equally. The peak age of diagnosis is within the first or second decade of life, although it may present earlier or even at birth. Darker-skinned individuals are particularly vulnerable to the disfiguring effects of vitiligo.[89–91]

Many patients with vitiligo experience a profound psychosocial burden from disease. Historically, many cultures associate this condition with leprosy, sexually transmitted diseases, and ostracism.[89] In a global context, many women with vitiligo are not considered desirable or acceptable for marriage.[91,92] A QoL assessment tool specific to vitiligo has not yet been developed, although QoL impairment in vitiligo has been extensively studied.[21,36,89,92–94]

The SF-36, Skindex-29, Skindex-Teen, DLQI, and Skin Discoloration Impact Evaluation Questionnaire have been used in studies assessing QoL of patients with vitiligo. Most studies include patients ranging from age 12 years to young adulthood. To our knowledge, there have been no specific studies assessing QoL in young children or caregivers of children with vitiligo. Women especially experience QoL impairment, particularly with such affected areas as the feet, legs, and arms.[93,95,96] In general, patients with vitiligo experience low self-esteem, social stigmatization, shame, avoidance of intimacy, anxiety, depression, adjustment disorder, fear, suicidal ideation, and other psychiatric morbidity.[36,92]

One study used the SF-36 and Skindex-29, along with the generic Course of Life questionnaire, to evaluate the effects of childhood vitiligo through adulthood. Particularly in social domains, patients with vitiligo experienced QoL impairment greater than or similar to patients with psoriasis.[34,91,92,97,98] SF-36 scores range from 0 to 100. A higher score indicates better QoL. Skindex-29 scores range from 0 to 100, with a higher score reflecting greater QoL impairment.

A strong patient-focused approach with extensive clinical education is helpful for patients with vitiligo. Online communities, such as the National Vitiligo Foundation and Vitiligo Support International, may increase social support. Cognitive behavioral therapy is being studied as a method to improve self-esteem and overall QoL in patients with vitiligo.[99,100]

One study that addressed coping strategies and group support for patients with vitiligo noted that living with this disease is a "continuous" struggle and one that requires long-term support.[101]

## SUMMARY

Skin disease results in QoL impairment for many affected children and adolescents. QoL measurement scales are therefore valuable clinical and research aids for this population. The two validated child- and skin-specific QoL indices designed for pediatric dermatology include CDLQI (for ages 5–16 years) and Skindex-Teen (for ages 12–17 years). These indices have been validated and can be used in a wide array of skin conditions.

Acne vulgaris significantly impacts QoL. The CADI and Acne QoL are useful and specific QoL assessment indices for acne vulgaris. The profound psychosocial impact of acne vulgaris is well documented, and it is important for healthcare providers to consider this impact. QoL indices may be particularly helpful in providing a patient-focused approach to care, assisting in monitoring treatment progress, and in determining if consultation with a mental health specialist is warranted.

AD and the associated pruritus place a significant QoL burden on patients and their families. The CADIS may be used for younger children with AD dermatitis. Additionally, caregivers of infants and children with AD also face QoL impairment. Specific QoL assessment indices, such as the CADIS, DFI, IDQOL, and Parents' Index of Quality of Life in Atopic Dermatitis, have been validated to measure the impact of disease on families. These indices can be used to identify patients who might benefit from more aggressive treatment to reduce overall burden of disease. Their use may also increase patient compliance and satisfaction.

Infantile hemangiomas often create a complex psychosocial burden for patients and their caregivers. Descriptive data on hemangiomas is extensive with one hemangioma-specific QoL scale currently published. Clinical education and family support is warranted for burdened patients and their caregivers. Online support communities and novel forms of therapy may help reduce associated anxiety and social isolation.

The impact on QoL in patient with congenital ichthyosis has been increasingly studied, although there is no QoL index specific to ichthyosis. Not only is ichthyosis a disfiguring condition with associated poor QoL, it also has a significant economic burden. It is important for healthcare providers to take this into account, and to consider a multidisciplinary approach to care. Support groups for this condition may be particularly helpful for patients and their families.

Psoriasis is comparable with AD in terms of effects on QoL. The degree of QoL impairment in pediatric patients with psoriasis or AD has been found to be only slightly less than that of patients with cerebral palsy. The IDQLI, CDLQI, and SF-36 are validated QoL indices used but not specific for pediatric psoriasis. Clinical education and patient-focused care may be combined with formal support groups and online support communities.

Vitiligo can be associated with a profound impact on QoL. These patients are especially vulnerable to social stigmatization. The DLQI, Skindex-29, and Skindex-Teen can be used in adolescents with vitiligo. A strong patient-focused approach with extensive clinical education should be used for these patients.

It is important that dermatologists be aware of available QoL indices to aid in providing more complete, individualized, and patient-focused care, especially in pediatric and adolescent patients. Several of these QoL indices could be used in everyday clinical practice. Additionally, it is hoped that research in dermatology will increasingly include QoL measures as a measurement of treatment outcomes. We look forward to the future development of disease-specific QoL indices for the most common pediatric dermatologic conditions, including hemangiomas, congenital ichthyoses, and vitiligo.

## REFERENCES

1. Bickers DR, Lim HW, Margolis D, et al. The burden of skin diseases: 2004 a joint project of the American Academy of Dermatology Association and the Society for Investigative Dermatology. J Am Acad Dermatol 2006;55(3):490–500.
2. Chren MM, Weinstock MA. Conceptual issues in measuring the burden of skin diseases. J Investig Dermatol Symp Proc 2004;9(2):97–100.
3. Holme SA, Man I, Sharpe JL, et al. The children's dermatology life quality index: validation of the cartoon version. Br J Dermatol 2003;148(2):285–90.
4. Finlay AY. The burden of skin disease: quality of life, economic aspects and social issues. Clin Med 2009;9(6):592–4.
5. Beattie PE, Lewis-Jones MS. A comparative study of impairment of quality of life in children with skin disease and children with other chronic childhood diseases. Br J Dermatol 2006;155(1):145–51.
6. Wallander JL, Varni JW. Effects of pediatric chronic physical disorders on child and family adjustment. J Child Psychol Psychiatry 1998;39(1):29–46.
7. Wallander JL, Varni JW, Babani L, et al. Children with chronic physical disorders: maternal reports of their psychological adjustment. J Pediatr Psychol 1988;13(2):197–212.
8. Eiser C. Psychological effects of chronic disease. J Child Psychol Psychiatry 1990;31(1):85–98.
9. Chamlin SL, Cella D, Frieden IJ, et al. Development of the childhood atopic dermatitis impact scale: initial validation of a quality-of-life measure for young children with atopic dermatitis and their families. J Invest Dermatol 2005;125(6):1106–11.
10. Clarke SA, Eiser C. The measurement of health-related quality of life (QOL) in paediatric clinical trials: a systematic review. Health Qual Life Outcomes 2004;2:66.
11. Cremeens J, Eiser C, Blades M. Characteristics of health-related self-report measures for children aged three to eight years: a review of the literature. Qual Life Res 2006;15(4):739–54.
12. Lewis-Jones MS, Finlay AY. The children's dermatology life quality index (CDLQI): initial validation and practical use. Br J Dermatol 1995;132(6):942–9.
13. Lewis-Jones MS, Finlay AY, Dykes PJ. The infants' dermatitis quality of life index. Br J Dermatol 2001;144(1):104–10.
14. Garralda ME, Palanca MI. Psychiatric adjustment in children with chronic physical illness. Br J Hosp Med 1994;52(5):230–4.
15. Chren MM. Doctor's orders: rethinking compliance in dermatology. Arch Dermatol 2002;138(3):393–4.
16. Corkum P, Moldofsky H, Hogg-Johnson S, et al. Sleep problems in children with attention-deficit/hyperactivity disorder: impact of subtype, comorbidity, and stimulant medication. J Am Acad Child Adolesc Psychiatry 1999;38(10):1285–93.
17. Chamlin SL, Mattson CL, Frieden IJ, et al. The price of pruritus: sleep disturbance and cosleeping in atopic dermatitis. Arch Pediatr Adolesc Med 2005;159(8):745–50.

18. Daud LR, Garralda ME, David TJ. Psychosocial adjustment in preschool children with atopic eczema. Arch Dis Child 1993;69(6):670–6.

19. Golics CJ, Basra MK, Finlay AY, et al. Adolescents with skin disease have specific quality of life issues. Dermatology 2009;218(4):357–66.

20. Gupta MA, Gupta AK, Watteel GN. Perceived deprivation of social touch in psoriasis is associated with greater psychologic morbidity: an index of the stigma experience in dermatologic disorders. Cutis 1998;61(6):339–42.

21. Schwartz R, Sepulveda JE, Quintana T. Possible role of psychological and environmental factors in the genesis of childhood vitiligo. Rev Med Chil 2009;137(1):53–62.

22. Smidt AC, Lai JS, Cella D, et al. Development and validation of Skindex-teen, a quality-of-life instrument for adolescents with skin disease. Arch Dermatol 2010;146(8):865–9.

23. Williams EF III, Hochman M, Rodgers BJ, et al. A psychological profile of children with hemangiomas and their families. Arch Facial Plast Surg 2003;5(3):229–34.

24. Pittet I, Berchtold A, Akre C, et al. Are adolescents with chronic conditions particularly at risk for bullying? Arch Dis Child 2010;95(9):711–6.

25. Crossley J, Eiser C, Davies HA. Children and their parents assessing the doctor-patient interaction: a rating system for doctors' communication skills. Med Educ 2005;39(8):820–8.

26. Cremeens J, Eiser C, Blades M. Brief report: assessing the impact of rating scale type, types of items, and age on the measurement of school-age children's self-reported quality of life. J Pediatr Psychol 2007;32(2):132–8.

27. Irwin RS, Richardson ND. Patient-focused care: using the right tools. Chest 2006;130(Suppl 1): 73S–82S.

28. Chren MM. Interpretation of quality-of-life scores. J Invest Dermatol 2010;130(5):1207–9.

29. Salek MS, Khan GK, Finlay AY. Questionnaire techniques in assessing acne handicap: reliability and validity study. Qual Life Res 1996;5(1):131–8.

30. Irwin RS. Patient-focused care: the 2003 American College of Chest Physicians Convocation Speech. Chest 2004;125(5):1910–2.

31. Smithard A, Glazebrook C, Williams HC. Acne prevalence, knowledge about acne and psychological morbidity in mid-adolescence: a community-based study. Br J Dermatol 2001;145(2):274–9.

32. Krowchuk DP, Stancin T, Keskinen R, et al. The psychosocial effects of acne on adolescents. Pediatr Dermatol 1991;8(4):332–8.

33. Rapp DA, Brenes GA, Feldman SR, et al. Anger and acne: implications for quality of life, patient satisfaction and clinical care. Br J Dermatol 2004; 151(1):183–9.

34. Krejci-Manwaring J, Kerchner K, Feldman SR, et al. Social sensitivity and acne: the role of personality in negative social consequences and quality of life. Int J Psychiatry Med 2006;36(1):121–30.

35. Magin PJ, Pond CD, Smith WT, et al. Acne's relationship with psychiatric and psychological morbidity: results of a school-based cohort study of adolescents. J Eur Acad Dermatol Venereol 2010;24(1): 58–64.

36. Kiec-Swierczynska M, Dudek B, Krecisz B, et al. The role of psychological factors and psychiatric disorders in skin diseases. Med Pr 2006;57(6): 551–5 [in Polish].

37. Brown BC, McKenna SP, Siddhi K, et al. The hidden cost of skin scars: quality of life after skin scarring. J Plast Reconstr Aesthet Surg 2008;61(9):1049–58.

38. Mallon E, Newton JN, Klassen A, et al. The quality of life in acne: a comparison with general medical conditions using generic questionnaires. Br J Dermatol 1999;140(4):672–6.

39. Tan JK. Psychosocial impact of acne vulgaris: evaluating the evidence. Skin Therapy Lett 2004;9(7): 1–3, 9.

40. Walker N, Lewis-Jones MS. Quality of life and acne in Scottish adolescent schoolchildren: use of the Children's Dermatology Life Quality Index (CDLQI) and the Cardiff Acne Disability Index (CADI). J Eur Acad Dermatol Venereol 2006;20(1):45–50.

41. Motley RJ, Finlay AY. Practical use of a disability index in the routine management of acne. Clin Exp Dermatol 1992;17(1):1–3.

42. Girman CJ, Hartmaier S, Thiboutot D, et al. Evaluating health-related quality of life in patients with facial acne: development of a self-administered questionnaire for clinical trials. Qual Life Res 1996;5(5):481–90.

43. Gupta MA, Johnson AM, Gupta AK. The development of an acne quality of life scale: reliability, validity, and relation to subjective acne severity in mild to moderate acne vulgaris. Acta Derm Venereol 1998;78(6):451–6.

44. Gupta MA, Gupta AK. Antidepressant drugs in dermatology. Skin Therapy Lett 2001;6(8):3–5.

45. Laughter D, Istvan JA, Tofte SJ, et al. The prevalence of atopic dermatitis in Oregon schoolchildren. J Am Acad Dermatol 2000;43(4):649–55.

46. Mancini AJ, Kaulback K, Chamlin SL. The socioeconomic impact of atopic dermatitis in the United States: a systematic review. Pediatr Dermatol 2008; 25(1):1–6.

47. Chamlin SL, Frieden IJ, Williams ML, et al. Effects of atopic dermatitis on young American children and their families. Pediatrics 2004;114(3):607–11.

48. Schmitt J, Chen CM, Apfelbacher C, et al. Infant eczema, infant sleeping problems, and mental health at 10 years of age: the prospective birth cohort study LISAplus. Allergy 2011;66(3):404–11.

49. Romanos M, Gerlach M, Warnke A, et al. Association of attention-deficit/hyperactivity disorder and atopic eczema modified by sleep disturbance in a large population-based sample. J Epidemiol Community Health 2010;64(3):269–73.

50. Schmitt J, Romanos M. Lack of studies investigating the association of childhood eczema, sleeping problems, and attention-deficit/hyperactivity disorder. Pediatr Allergy Immunol 2009;20(3):299–300 [author reply: 301].

51. Harari M, Dreiher J, Czarnowicki T, et al. SCORAD 75: a new metric for assessing treatment outcomes in atopic dermatitis. J Eur Acad Dermatol Venereol 2012;26:1510–5.

52. Oranje AP. Practical issues on interpretation of scoring atopic dermatitis: SCORAD index, objective SCORAD, patient-oriented SCORAD and three-item severity score. Curr Probl Dermatol 2011;41: 149–55.

53. Schram ME, Spuls PI, Leeflang MM, et al. EASI, (objective) SCORAD and POEM for atopic eczema: responsiveness and minimal clinically important difference. Allergy 2012;67:99–106.

54. Magin P, Heading G, Adams J, et al. Sex and the skin: a qualitative study of patients with acne, psoriasis and atopic eczema. Psychol Health Med 2010;15(4):454–62.

55. Charman CR, Venn AJ, Williams H. Measuring atopic eczema severity visually: which variables are most important to patients? Arch Dermatol 2005;141(9):1146–51 [discussion: 1151].

56. Charman C, Chambers C, Williams H. Measuring atopic dermatitis severity in randomized controlled clinical trials: what exactly are we measuring? J Invest Dermatol 2003;120(6):932–41.

57. Chang LC, Haggstrom AN, Drolet BA, et al. Growth characteristics of infantile hemangiomas: implications for management. Pediatrics 2008;122(2): 360–7.

58. Hoornweg MJ, Grootenhuis MA, van der Horst CM. Health-related quality of life and impact of haemangiomas on children and their parents. J Plast Reconstr Aesthet Surg 2009;62(10):1265–71.

59. Hoornweg MJ, Smeulders MJ, van der Horst CM. Prevalence and characteristics of haemangiomas in young children. Ned Tijdschr Geneeskd 2005; 149(44):2455–8.

60. Dieterich-Miller CA, Safford PL. Psychosocial development of children with hemangiomas: home, school, health care collaboration. Child Health Care 1992;21(2):84–9.

61. Weinstein JM, Chamlin SL. Quality of life in vascular anomalies. Lymphat Res Biol 2005;3(4):256–9.

62. Kunkel EJ, Zager R, Hausman C, et al. An interdisciplinary group for parents of children with hemangiomas. Psychosomatics 1994;36:524–32.

63. Blechinger T, Klosinski G. The meaning of bibliotherapy and expressive writing in child and adolescent psychiatry. Prax Kinderpsychol Kinderpsychiatr 2011;60(2):109–24.

64. Thomas Editor SP. Bibliotherapy: new evidence of effectiveness. Issues Ment Health Nurs 2011; 32(4):191.

65. Barrera ME, Rykov MH, Doyle SL. The effects of interactive music therapy on hospitalized children with cancer: a pilot study. Psychooncology 2002; 11(5):379–88.

66. Cohen SG. Hemangiomas in infancy and childhood: psychosocial issues require close attention. Adv Nurse Pract 2005;13(11):41–4.

67. Shwayder T, Ott F. All about ichthyosis. Pediatr Clin North Am 1991;38(4):835–57.

68. DiGiovanna JJ, Robinson-Bostom L. Ichthyosis: etiology, diagnosis, and management. Am J Clin Dermatol 2003;4(2):81–95.

69. Ganemo A, Sjoden PO, Johansson E, et al. Health-related quality of life among patients with ichthyosis. Eur J Dermatol 2004;14(1):61–6.

70. Mazereeuw-Hautier J, Dreyfus I, Barbarot S, et al. Factors influencing quality of life of inherited ichthyosis: a qualitative study in adult using focus groups. Br J Dermatol 2012;166:646–8.

71. Ganemo A, Lindholm C, Lindberg M, et al. Quality of life in adults with congenital ichthyosis. J Adv Nurs 2003;44(4):412–9.

72. Lundberg L, Johannesson M, Silverdahl M, et al. Health-related quality of life in patients with psoriasis and atopic dermatitis measured with SF-36, DLQI and a subjective measure of disease activity. Acta Derm Venereol 2000;80(6):430–4.

73. Styperek AR, Rice ZP, Kamalpour L, et al. Annual direct and indirect health costs of the congenital ichthyoses. Pediatr Dermatol 2010;27(4):325–36.

74. Kamalpour L, Gammon B, Chen KH, et al. Resource utilization and quality of life associated with congenital ichthyoses. Pediatr Dermatol 2011;28(5):512–8.

75. Rogers M. Childhood psoriasis. Curr Opin Pediatr 2002;14(4):404–9.

76. Nevitt GJ, Hutchinson PE. Psoriasis in the community: prevalence, severity and patients' beliefs and attitudes towards the disease. Br J Dermatol 1996; 135(4):533–7.

77. Gupta MA, Gupta AK, Watteel GN. Early onset (< 40 years age) psoriasis is comorbid with greater psychopathology than late onset psoriasis: a study of 137 patients. Acta Derm Venereol 1996;76(6): 464–6.

78. Lundberg L, Johannesson M, Silverdahl M, et al. Quality of life, health-state utilities and willingness to pay in patients with psoriasis and atopic eczema. Br J Dermatol 1999;141(6):1067–75.

79. Ganemo A, Wahlgren CF, Svensson A. Quality of life and clinical features in Swedish children with psoriasis. Pediatr Dermatol 2011;28(4):375–9.

80. Seidler EM, Kimball AB. Socioeconomic disability in psoriasis. Br J Dermatol 2009;161(6):1410–2.

81. Gupta MA, Gupta AK. Depression and suicidal ideation in dermatology patients with acne, alopecia areata, atopic dermatitis and psoriasis. Br J Dermatol 1998;139(5):846–50.

82. Sampogna F, Chren MM, Melchi CF, et al. Age, gender, quality of life and psychological distress in patients hospitalized with psoriasis. Br J Dermatol 2006;154(2):325–31.

83. Ferrandiz C, Pujol RM, Garcia-Patos V, et al. Psoriasis of early and late onset: a clinical and epidemiologic study from Spain. J Am Acad Dermatol 2002;46(6):867–73.

84. de Jager ME, de Jong EM, van de Kerkhof PC, et al. An intrapatient comparison of quality of life in psoriasis in childhood and adulthood. J Eur Acad Dermatol Venereol 2011;25(7):828–31.

85. Gupta MA, Gupta AK. Depression modulates pruritus perception. A study of pruritus in psoriasis, atopic dermatitis and chronic idiopathic urticaria. Ann N Y Acad Sci 1999;885:394–5.

86. Nijsten T, Rolstad T, Feldman SR, et al. Members of the national psoriasis foundation: more extensive disease and better informed about treatment options. Arch Dermatol 2005;141(1):19–26.

87. Nijsten T, Margolis DJ, Feldman SR, et al. Traditional systemic treatments have not fully met the needs of psoriasis patients: results from a national survey. J Am Acad Dermatol 2005;52(3 Pt 1):434–44.

88. Abel EA, Moore US, Glathe JP. Psoriasis patient support group and self-care efficacy as an adjunct to day care center treatment. Int J Dermatol 1990; 29(9):640–3.

89. Alikhan A, Felsten LM, Daly M, et al. Vitiligo: a comprehensive overview part I. Introduction, epidemiology, quality of life, diagnosis, differential diagnosis, associations, histopathology, etiology, and work-up. J Am Acad Dermatol 2011;65(3): 473–91.

90. Taylor A, Pawaskar M, Taylor SL, et al. Prevalence of pigmentary disorders and their impact on quality of life: a prospective cohort study. J Cosmet Dermatol 2008;7(3):164–8.

91. Linthorst Homan MW, Spuls PI, de Korte J, et al. The burden of vitiligo: patient characteristics associated with quality of life. J Am Acad Dermatol 2009;61(3):411–20.

92. Linthorst Homan MW, Sprangers MA, de Korte J, et al. Characteristics of patients with universal vitiligo and health-related quality of life. Arch Dermatol 2008;144(8):1062–4.

93. Sampogna F, Raskovic D, Guerra L, et al. Identification of categories at risk for high quality of life impairment in patients with vitiligo. Br J Dermatol 2008;159(2):351–9.

94. Kent G, al-Abadie M. Factors affecting responses on dermatology life quality index items among vitiligo sufferers. Clin Exp Dermatol 1996;21(5):330–3.

95. Pope AW, Ward J. Self-perceived facial appearance and psychosocial adjustment in preadolescents with craniofacial anomalies. Cleft Palate Craniofac J 1997;34(5):396–401.

96. Radtke MA, Schafer I, Gajur A, et al. Willingness-to-pay and quality of life in patients with vitiligo. Br J Dermatol 2009;161(1):134–9.

97. Linthorst Homan MW, de Korte J, Grootenhuis MA, et al. Impact of childhood vitiligo on adult life. Br J Dermatol 2008;159(4):915–20.

98. Sampogna F, Picardi A, Chren MM, et al. Association between poorer quality of life and psychiatric morbidity in patients with different dermatological conditions. Psychosom Med 2004;66(4):620–4.

99. Shenefelt PD. Biofeedback, cognitive-behavioral methods, and hypnosis in dermatology: is it all in your mind? Dermatol Ther 2003;16(2):114–22.

100. Papadopoulos L, Bor R, Legg C. Coping with the disfiguring effects of vitiligo: a preliminary investigation into the effects of cognitive-behavioural therapy. Br J Med Psychol 1999;72(Pt 3):385–96.

101. Thompson AR, Kent G, Smith JA. Living with vitiligo: dealing with difference. Br J Health Psychol 2002;7(Pt 2):213–25.

# The Child with Recalcitrant Dermatitis: When to Worry?

Anna M. Bender, MD[a], Moise L. Levy, MD[b,c,d],*

## KEYWORDS

- Recalcitrant dermatitis • Children • Dermatoses • Erythroderma

## KEY POINTS

- Dermatitis may be localized to the diaper area or to periorificial areas in children, giving possible clues to the cause.
- The more common causes of widespread dermatitis include atopic dermatitis, infantile seborrheic dermatitis, and psoriasis.
- Rarer causes of widespread recalcitrant dermatitis are many and include ichthyoses, immunodeficiency, metabolic, and neoplastic disorders.
- Recalcitrant dermatitis may be difficult to treat and may be a harbinger of an alternative and more worrisome diagnosis prompting further workup.

Dermatitis is a frequent cause for referral to the pediatric dermatologist (**Box 1**). In this article, a brief overview is given of common childhood dermatoses, as well as some rarer dermatoses that may give the clinician cause for concern. Widespread scaling and erythema, described as erythroderma, are a cause for frustration for patients, families, and their physician(s). Both unusual and common skin disorders can present in this fashion. Just as recognizing common dermatoses is important, it is also important to recognize when a dermatitis fails to fit the common pattern and may prompt further investigation.

## LOCALIZED DERMATITIS

Dermatitis may be localized to the diaper area or to periorificial areas in children, giving possible clues to the cause, including both common and rarer skin manifestations. Sometimes, the dermatitis may be more generalized. Seborrheic dermatitis may be more marked in skin folds and areas occluded by the diaper in infants. This condition is often confused with psoriasis. Whereas atopic dermatitis typically spares the diaper area, seborrheic dermatitis is commonly seen in the diaper area. Seborrheic dermatitis often presents in the first months of life with scaly red patches, often involving the flexural skin folds as well as the diaper area along with thick, greasy scale on the scalp. The condition can often present in a generalized fashion, in addition to the more common distribution (**Fig. 1**). In contrast to atopic dermatitis, which is almost invariably pruritic, infantile seborrheic dermatitis is usually asymptomatic. Most cases of infantile seborrheic dermatitis clear easily with topical therapy such as low-potency topical corticosteroid. This condition should improve and resolve over the first several months of age.

Contact dermatitis is also on the differential of common dermatoses of childhood. Typical of "outside jobs" caused by external skin contact with allergic substances, a patterned eruption is often seen. Often, a high index of suspicion is needed to make such a diagnosis. Such is the case with so-called Lucky Luke diaper dermatitis.[1] Irritant contact dermatitis is the most common

a Division of Pediatric Dermatology, Department of Dermatology, Johns Hopkins University, 200 North Wolfe Street, Suite 2107, Baltimore, MD 21287, USA; b Pediatric/Adolescent Dermatology, Dell Children's Medical Center, 4900 Mueller Boulevard, Austin, TX 78723, USA; c UT Southwestern Medical School, 5323 Harry Hines Boulevard, Dallas, TX 75390, USA; d Dermatology and Pediatrics, Baylor College of Medicine, 1 Baylor Plaza, Houston, TX 77030, USA
* Corresponding author. 1301 Barbara Jordan Boulevard, Suite 200, Austin, TX 78723, USA.
*E-mail address:* mllevy@seton.org

Dermatol Clin 31 (2013) 223–228
http://dx.doi.org/10.1016/j.det.2012.12.001
0733-8635/13/$ – see front matter © 2013 Published by Elsevier Inc.

> **Box 1**
> **Causes of pediatric dermatitis**
>
> - Atopic dermatitis
> - Seborrheic dermatitis
> - Psoriasis
> - Contact dermatitis
> - Infectious diseases
> - Drug eruptions
> - Inherited disorders

localized rash occurring in the diaper area. It often presents as well-demarcated eczematous patches, more marked on the convex surfaces of the buttocks and usually sparing the skin folds. Allergic contact dermatitis may also occur in childhood caused by dyes or other components of the diaper, although it is less common compared with irritant contact dermatitis in infants and young children.

In contrast to contact dermatitis, psoriatic diaper dermatitis often presents with well-demarcated brightly erythematous plaques involving the diaper area, including the skin folds (**Fig. 2**). Psoriasis involving the diaper area may respond poorly to low-dose topical corticosteroids used to treat common irritant diaper dermatitis. A family history of psoriasis can be helpful in making this diagnosis in infancy or early childhood. Keeping in mind the diaper area as a common location for psoriasis is also helpful when evaluating a confluent patch of scaling and erythema in this location.

In addition to diagnosing primary inflammatory dermatoses occurring in the diaper area, the possibility of infection should also be considered. Common infections may include candidiasis, bullous impetigo secondary to *Staphylococcus aureus*, and perianal streptococcal infection. Such infections should be included in the differential diagnosis of rashes in the diaper area,

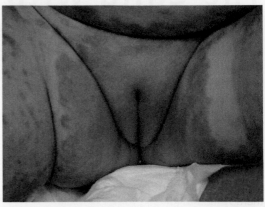

**Fig. 2.** Confluent erythematous plaque involving the diaper area in psoriasis.

especially ones that do not respond to topical corticosteroids alone.

Infantile candidiasis should be suspected when a child presents with an erythematous patch or plaque (which may often be moist) involving folds in the diaper area; axillary skin can be involved as well. Patients may have surrounding scaling erythematous papules or pustules, often described as satellites. Potassium hydroxide smears or fungal culture should be diagnostic. In the healthy patient, topical azole antifungals are curative.

Staphylococcal diaper dermatitis usually presents as a superficial vesiculobullous process; often, patients present with well-circumscribed superficially eroded areas of skin, with minimal or no surrounding erythema (**Fig. 3**). As with candidiasis in healthy infants, topical antibiotics can be useful. Staphylococcal scalded skin syndrome can be seen in patients of all ages. Tender and diffuse erythema is usually seen, with sparing of mucous membranes. As a result of the involvement of desmoglein 1, keratinized skin is the

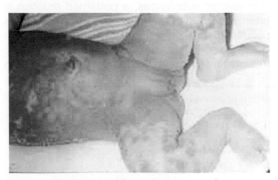

**Fig. 1.** Diffuse plaque like and scaling erythema on an infant with seborrheic dermatitis.

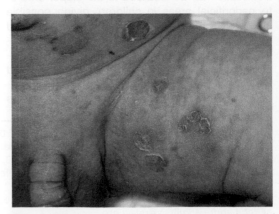

**Fig. 3.** Discrete superficial erosions with mild erythema typical of staphylococcal diaper dermatitis.

clinical target rather than mucous membranes in this toxin-mediated illness.[2] The evolution is rapid, although, once the condition is diagnosed, appropriate antibiotic therapy results in prompt resolution.

Streptococcal disease can occur in the setting of group A beta-hemolytic streptococcal infections with typical facial erythema and circumoral pallor or as streptococcal diaper dermatitis. Characteristically, streptococcal diaper dermatitis is seen in a perianal distribution. Rather than purely epidermal erythema, psoriatic-appearing scale can be seen. Appropriate cultures and antibiotic therapy lead to (often) prompt resolution.

Rarer causes of diaper dermatitis that fail to respond to typical therapies include metabolic and nutritional deficiencies. Multiple nutritional deficiencies such as zinc deficiency, essential fatty acid deficiency, and malabsorption syndromes such as cystic fibrosis (CF) may also present with recalcitrant diaper, as well as more diffuse dermatitis (**Fig. 4**). Zinc deficiency may occur secondary to acrodermatitis enteropathica, which is an autosomal-recessive genetic disorder that may occur sporadically because of nutritional zinc deficiencies. It typically presents with diarrhea, periorificial and acral dermatitis, and alopecia approximately 1 to 2 weeks after weaning from breast milk. It may progress to failure to thrive if not treated. The eruption and symptoms quickly resolve with zinc supplementation. Such patients classically present with a periorificial scaling dermatitis. Many have periungual involvement, with erythema and pustules. Pure zinc deficiency is usually associated with decreased levels of serum alkaline phosphatase because this enzyme requires zinc for its function. Essential fatty acid and biotin deficiencies can also resemble zinc deficiency clinically. Acrodermatitis enteropathica-like eruptions have also been reported in patients with

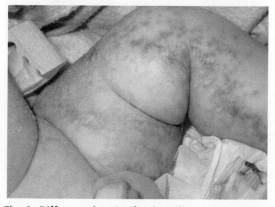

**Fig. 4.** Diffuse and periorificial erythema on a patient with CF.

malabsorption syndromes such as CF and in patients with other metabolic disorders such as organic acidurias. In CF, the same general pattern of erythema is seen. Clues to the diagnosis of CF in this setting can include larger than usual stools, often with mucus.

Testing for zinc and alkaline phosphatase, as well as serum amino and urine organic acids might be indicated, depending on the more likely diagnosis. Serum $CO_2$ is helpful to assess acid/base status, because many organic acidemias present with systemic acidosis.

Rarely, a persistent diaper dermatitis that does not respond to standard anticandidal therapies or topical steroids may be a sign of Langerhans cell histiocytosis (LCH). LCH is a rare disorder involving histiocyte infiltration of the skin plus possible infiltration of other organs, which can be fatal. Classically, it may present with purpuric macules or papules with hemorrhagic crusts in the diaper area, axillae, and scalp. Erosive areas on the gingivae can be seen in infants. The skin findings of LCH are most commonly misdiagnosed as seborrheic dermatitis or irritant diaper dermatitis in infants. Therefore, it is important to consider this diagnosis in diaper rashes that fail to improve after standard therapies. Extracutaneous manifestations such as lymphadenopathy, hepatomegaly, and bony lesions may be present. Diagnosis is based on a high index of suspicion leading to a biopsy that shows a Langerhans cell infiltrate with CD1a+ positivity on immunohistochemistry. A complete evaluation should include investigation of organ function and assessment of bones for possible involvement.

## GENERALIZED DERMATITIS AND ERYTHRODERMA

As mentioned earlier, the term erythroderma describes a diffuse, often scaling, erythematous skin eruption. Although not diagnostic of the primary cause of the skin findings, the most common cause of generalized dermatitis in children is atopic dermatitis. Epidemiologic studies suggest that an atopic diathesis may exist in more than 20% of the population[3] and atopic dermatitis may affect more than 15% of school children.[4] Atopic dermatitis commonly develops in the first year of life in approximately 60% of cases, often presenting with erythematous scaly patches on the cheeks beginning around 2 months of life. The infantile pattern also typically involves the extensor extremities. The distribution of rash in childhood atopic dermatitis after age 2 years changes to involve the popliteal and antecubital fossae primarily and may consist of more lichenified plaques. If the condition is severe and uncontrolled, patients may present with extensive erythroderma.

Severe generalized dermatitis may present as exfoliative erythroderma and is a cause for concern. Severe exfoliative erythroderma that is improperly managed can lead to electrolyte and fluid imbalances, sepsis secondary to a defective skin barrier, high-output cardiac failure, and even death. In addition to treating the skin and preventing secondary infection in erythrodermic patients, it is of equal importance to evaluate the cause of the erythroderma in order to tailor therapy toward the underlying cause. The more common causes of erythroderma in infants and children include skin disorders such as severe atopic dermatitis, infantile seborrheic dermatitis, and psoriasis. The rarer causes of erythroderma in infants and children include ichthyosiform erythrodermas, immunodeficiency syndromes, cutaneous T-cell lymphoma, and medication reactions.[5] Infectious diseases, such as staphylococcal or streptococcal toxic shock syndromes, can present with erythroderma, although in an acute manner.[6]

Multiple ichthyoses can be associated with erythroderma. These ichthyoses include lamellar ichthyosis (LI), bullous (epidermolytic ichthyosis/ EI) and nonbullous congenital ichthyosis, Sjögren-Larsson syndrome, neutral lipid syndrome, trichothiodystrophy, and Netherton syndrome.[7] LI often presents with a collodion membrane at birth. Later, patients develop coarse dark scales, palmoplantar hyperkeratosis, alopecia, and prominent flexural involvement. Complications include ectropion and eclabion. Nonbullous congenital ichthyosiform erythroderma (NBCIE) may or may not be associated with a collodion membrane at birth. The rash presents with fine scaling overlying generalized erythroderma, along with palmoplantar keratoderma. Hair and nails may also be affected. LI and NBCIE, both autosomal-recessive in inheritance, are two forms of ichthyosis now grouped under the heading of autosomal-recessive congenital ichthyosis (ARCI). Sjögren-Larsson syndrome may present with a pruritic ichthyosis in infancy along with mental retardation and development of spasticity. Neutral lipid storage diseases may also present with fine scaling overlying erythroderma. Histology shows lipid-laden vacuoles in keratinocytes and granulocytes. Trichothiodystrophy also known as PIBIDS or Tay syndrome presents with photosensitivity, ichthyosis, brittle hair, intellectual impairment, decreased fertility, and short stature. Patients show low cysteine content in their hair, and polarized microscopy of their hairs shows tiger-tail alternating light and dark bands. Netherton syndrome is an autosomal-recessive disorder caused by mutations in SPINK5 that encodes the serine protease inhibitor, LEKT1. Patients present with atopy, generalized erythroderma, failure to thrive, trichorrhexis invaginata (bamboo hair with a ball-and-socket morphology), and later, ichthyosis linearis circumflexa (showing classic double-edged scale) (Fig. 5).[8,9] In addition to genetic testing, immunohistochemical analysis can be performed on biopsy specimens to confirm the diagnosis of Netherton syndrome by showing lack of LEKT1 antibody staining.[10]

Widespread dermatitis may also be a sign of a primary immunodeficiency disorder. Primary immunodeficiency syndromes commonly associated with dermatitis include Wiskott-Aldrich syndrome, hyper-IgE syndrome, and severe combined immunodeficiency (SCID) syndromes, including Omenn syndrome. A history of atopic dermatitis-like rash and multiple, recurrent, severe, or unusual cutaneous or systemic infections along with failure to thrive and other systemic signs may signal the clinician to further assess for possible underlying immunodeficiency syndromes.[11,12]

Wiskott-Aldrich syndrome is an X-linked recessive disorder usually seen in males. It presents with a rash appearing identical to atopic dermatitis in the first few months of life. This dermatitis is often recalcitrant and shows characteristic petechiae and purpura. Patients show evidence of thrombocytopenia and are susceptible to recurrent sinopulmonary bacterial infections. Spontaneous hemorrhage can occur. Additional features include hepatosplenomegaly and lymphadenopathy. There is an increased incidence of leukemia and lymphoma occurring in 13% to 22% of

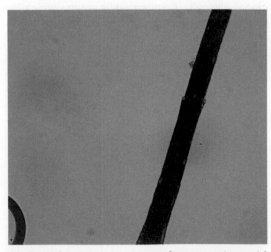

Fig. 5. Trichorrhexis invaginata from a patient with Netherton syndrome.

patients.[13] Because this syndrome is clinically progressive and has a high mortality as a result of infection, hemorrhage, and malignancy, it is important to identify this disorder early in its course. HIES, also known as Job syndrome, is a disorder associated with immunodeficiency and recurrent infections in the setting of (atopic) dermatitis, which is often persistent. Infections include cold abscesses, bronchitis, lung abscesses, pneumonia, otitis media, and sinusitis. Patients show coarsening of facial features and a broad nasal bridge. Delayed eruption and retention of primary teeth are observed. Skeletal anomalies, osteoporosis, and predisposition to bony fractures are other features of hyper-IgE syndrome. When a child with atopic dermatitis develops multiple recurrent cutaneous and sinopulmonary infections, it is important to check levels of polyclonal IgE to evaluate for the possibility of HIES. The presence of mutation in the gene encoding signal transducer and activator of transcription 3 (STAT3) which is seen in most patients with autosomal-dominant HIES, may be used to help differentiate HIES from atopic dermatitis.[14] In the setting of persistent viral or fungal diseases, the autosomal-recessive form of HIES caused by DOCK 8 mutations must be considered.[14,15] Omenn syndrome is a type of SCID that typically presents with widespread dermatitis. Patients may also show hepatomegaly, lymphadenopathy, alopecia, marked eosinophilia, and high serum IgE levels. Because of their deficiency of T lymphocytes, neonates may develop a generalized skin eruption as a result of an acute graft-versus-host response to maternal T-cell engraftment. Patients develop recurrent infections, failure to thrive, and diarrhea. They are also predisposed to severe candidal infections and pneumonia. Laboratory tests include T-cell and B-cell clonal analysis, which shows evidence of defects in V(D)J recombination.

Several signs should signal the clinician to evaluate for possible underlying primary immunodeficiencies.[9] Common signs include failure to thrive, malabsorption, chronic diarrhea, and multiple recurrent infections (Box 2). The infections may be unusually severe or chronic, recalcitrant to standard therapies, or involve unusual organisms. The type of infection (eg, extracellular bacterial, intracellular bacterial, viral, or fungal) may also give the clinician clue as to which part of the immune system may be impaired, resulting in humoral, cellular, or phagocytic defects.[16] A family history of consanguinity may be found if the disorder is autosomal or X-linked recessive.

A screening laboratory workup for evaluation for a possible primary immunodeficiency should be based on clinical findings and include a complete

---

**Box 2**
**Recalcitrant dermatitis: when to consider immunodeficiency**

- Four or more new ear infections/y
- Two or more pneumonias/y
- Failure to thrive
- Chronic diarrhea
- Recurrent deep skin/organ abscesses
- Persistent mucocutaneous candidiasis
- Need for intravenous antibiotics to clear infection

---

blood count with differential and smear, quantitative immunoglobulins, hair shaft evaluation, total complement levels, flow cytometry analysis of T and B cells if appropriate, and specific mutational studies (Box 3). If screening tests are abnormal, the patient should be referred for immediate assessment by a clinical immunologist.[13]

Skin biopsy might be needed for diagnosis of LCH or of graft-versus-host disease in the appropriate settings. One group of investigators found 58.5% sensitivity and 98.5% specificity for the diagnosis of immunodeficiency based on typical histopathology of either graft-versus-host disease or Omenn syndrome. The same study noted sensitivity and specificity of 100% for Netherton syndrome when staining skin biopsies for LEKTI antibody.[8] The investigators also looked at atopic dermatitis, psoriasis, and ichthyosis. Metabolic assays might also be indicated in some patients with recalcitrant dermatoses, as noted earlier.

---

**Box 3**
**Recalcitrant dermatitis: evaluation**

- Cultures (bacterial, fungal, viral)
- Complete blood count with differential
- Serum chemistries, including liver function tests, alkaline phosphatase, albumin, electrolytes
- Zinc, biotinidase, serum amino acids, urine organic acids
- Basic immune evaluation; quantitative immunoglobulins, IgE, complement levels
- Skin biopsy; immunohistochemistry
- Sweat chloride testing
- Hair shaft evaluation
- Specific immune testing (eg, flow cytometry analysis of T and B cells if indicated)
- Genetic testing

Attention to the metabolic needs of patients with diffuse dermatitis is key as well. The dermatologist should remain aware of this important facet of therapy in managing such patients.

Localized dermatoses and more widespread dermatoses may be seen in a host of common childhood skin disorders. It is important to remember the rarer causes of localized and generalized dermatitis in children, because such diseases may be associated with specific morbidity or necessitate a specific workup and therapy. Although dermatitis is common in children, recalcitrant dermatitis may be difficult to treat and may be a harbinger of an alternative and more worrisome diagnosis.

## REFERENCES

1. Roul S, Ducombs G, Leaute-Labreze C, et al. 'Lucky Luke' contact dermatitis due to rubber components of diapers. Contact Derm 1998;38:363–4.

2. Stanley JR, Amagai M. Pemphigus, bullous impetigo, and the staphylococcal scalded-skin syndrome. N Engl J Med 2006;355:1800–10.

3. Diepgen TL, Fartasch M. Recent epidemiological and genetic studies in atopic dermatitis. Acta Derm Venereol Suppl (Stockh) 1992;176:13–8.

4. Laughter D, Istvan JA, Tofte SJ, et al. The prevalence of atopic dermatitis in Oregon schoolchildren. J Am Acad Dermatol 2000;43(4):649–55.

5. Al-Dhalimi MA. Neonatal and infantile erythroderma: a clinical and follow-up study of 42 cases. J Dermatol 2007;34(5):302–7.

6. Bachur RG, Byer RL. Clinical deterioration among patients with fever and erythroderma. Pediatrics 2006;118:2450–60.

7. Oji V, Tadini G, Akiyama M, et al. Revised nomenclature and classification of inherited ichthyoses: results of the First Ichthyosis Consensus Conference in Soreze 2009. J Am Acad Dermatol 2010;63(4): 607–41.

8. DiGiovanna JJ, Robinson-Bostom L. Ichthyosis: etiology, diagnosis, and management. Am J Clin Dermatol 2003;4(2):81–95.

9. Sun JD, Linden KG. Netherton syndrome: a case report and review of the literature. Int J Dermatol 2006;45(6):693–7.

10. Leclerc-Mercier S, Bodemer C, Bourdon-Lanoy E, et al. Early skin biopsy is helpful for the diagnosis and management of neonatal and infantile erythrodermas. J Cutan Pathol 2010;37(2):249–55.

11. Slatter MA, Gennery AR. Clinical immunology review series: an approach to the patient with recurrent infections in childhood. Clin Exp Immunol 2008; 152(3):389–96.

12. Sewell WA, Khan S, Dore PC. Early indicators of immunodeficiency in adults and children: protocols for screening for primary immunological defects. Clin Exp Immunol 2006;145(2):201–3.

13. Filipovich AH, Mathur A, Kamat D, et al. Lymphoproliferative disorders and other tumors complicating immunodeficiencies. Immunodeficiency 1994;5(2): 91–112.

14. Schimke LF, Sawalle-Belohradsky J, Roesler J, et al. Diagnostic approach to the hyper-IgE syndromes: immunologic and clinical key findings to differentiate hyper-IgE syndromes from atopic dermatitis. J Allergy Clin Immunol 2010;126(3): 611–617.e1.

15. Chu EY, Freeman AF, Jing H, et al. Cutaneous manifestations of DOCK8 deficiency syndrome. Arch Dermatol 2012;148:79–84.

16. de Vries E, Clinical Working Party of the European Society for Immunodeficiencies (ESID). Patient-centred screening for primary immunodeficiency: a multi-stage diagnostic protocol designed for non-immunologists. Clin Exp Immunol 2006;145(2): 204–14.

# Pediatric Morphea

John C. Browning, MD[a,b,*]

## KEYWORDS

- Morphea • Systemic sclerosis • Localized scleroderma • Pediatric morphea

## KEY POINTS

- Morphea is a fibrosing disorder of the skin and subcutaneous tissues.
- The absence of sclerodactyly, Raynaud phenomenon, and nail-fold capillary changes distinguishes morphea from systemic sclerosis (scleroderma).

## BACKGROUND

Morphea, also known as localized scleroderma, is a fibrosing disorder of the skin and subcutaneous tissues. Morphea is differentiated from systemic sclerosis (scleroderma) based on the absence of sclerodactyly, Raynaud phenomenon, and nail-fold capillary changes.[1] Confusion may occur because patients with morphea often have systemic symptoms such as malaise, fatigue, arthralgias, myalgias, and positive autoantibodies.[2] Unlike morphea, systemic sclerosis has organ involvement, particularly gastrointestinal, pulmonary, and renal.

## EPIDEMIOLOGY

The incidence of morphea is estimated at 0.4 to 2.7 per 100,000 population.[3,4] A population-based study looked at morphea occurrence (adults and children) in Olmsted County, Minnesota, from 1960 to 1993, and estimated an annual incidence (age and sex adjusted) of 2.7 per 100,000 and a prevalence of 50 per 100,000.[3]

Morphea is more common in whites and women, with a female to male ratio ranging from 2.4:1 to 4.2:1.[2,5] Linear morphea, however, has an equal sex distribution.[3] Morphea has a bimodal age presentation and is equally common in adults and children. Ninety percent of children present between 2 and 14 years of age.[1] The mean age for adults presenting with morphea is in the mid-40s.[1]

Plaque-type morphea is the most common type affecting adults[3]; linear morphea is most common in children.[2,4,5] There is often a family history of other autoimmune diseases.[6] Rarely there is a family history of morphea (**Fig. 1**).[7]

## PATHOGENESIS

The pathogenesis of morphea is not fully understood. Imbalance of collagen production and destruction[1] is thought to be an important factor. Inflammation and vascular changes are also important. Mononuclear cells infiltrate the skin and surrounding blood vessels in early morphea[8]; this leads to functional and structural changes to the microvascular system.[8] Involvement is limited to tissues derived from the mesoderm.

Morphea plaques slowly soften over a period of 3 to 5 years when left untreated, but patients often develop new areas of involvement over their lifetime.[1] Trauma and radiation have been reported before the onset of morphea.[2,5,9,10] Morphea

Conflicts of Interest: None.
[a] Division of Dermatology and Cutaneous Surgery, The University of Texas Health Science Center at San Antonio, 7703 Floyd Curl Drive, San Antonio, TX 78229-3900, USA; [b] Pediatric Dermatology Section, Department of Pediatrics, The University of Texas Health Science Center at San Antonio, 7703 Floyd Curl Drive, MSC 7808, San Antonio, TX 78229-3900, USA
* Pediatric Dermatology Section, The University of Texas Health Science Center at San Antonio, 7703 Floyd Curl Drive, MSC 7808, San Antonio, TX 78229-3900.
E-mail address: browningj3@uthscsa.edu

Dermatol Clin 31 (2013) 229–237
http://dx.doi.org/10.1016/j.det.2012.12.002
0733-8635/13/$ – see front matter © 2013 Elsevier Inc. All rights reserved.

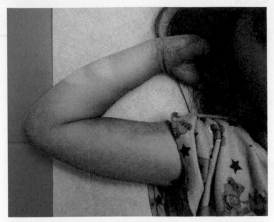

Fig. 1. Morphea and vitiligo in the same patient. Depigmented patches on the forearm and indurated plaque on the upper arm.

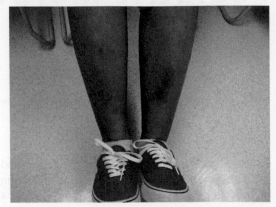

Fig. 2. Anterior shins of an adolescent female patient, where morphea occurred at sites of trauma.

following vaccination has also been reported.[11] A dental extraction has been reported before onset of ipsilateral progressive hemifacial atrophy.[10]

Elevated cytokines, soluble cell adhesion molecules, positive antinuclear antibodies (ANAs), and activated T lymphocytes have suggested autoimmunity as an important factor in the development of morphea.[8] Certain medications, such as bisoprolol, bleomycin, peplomycin, D-penicillamine, bromocriptine, L-5-hydroxytryptophane in combination with carbidopa, pentazocine, and balicatib, have been associated with development of morphea.[1] Borrelia has been implicated as a possible infectious cause of morphea, but other studies have refuted the association.[12–14] Vascular injury has also been proposed as a cause of morphea,[1] as supported by reduced capillaries and damaged endothelial cells.[13] Long stretches of disease remission are common, but most patients with morphea will develop new lesions over their lifetime (Fig. 2).[2]

## CLINICAL PRESENTATION

Peterson, in 1995, recommended the following classification system.[15]

Five subgroups:

- Circumscribed (plaque) morphea
- Generalized morphea
- Bullous morphea
- Linear morphea (includes en coup de sabre and progressive hemifacial atrophy)
- Deep morphea (includes subcutaneous morphea, morphea profunda, disabling pansclerotic morphea, and eosinophilic fasciitis)[15]

The classification system is controversial because it does not include the mixed types of morphea that can occur, and includes eosinophilic fasciitis as a subtype of morphea,[10] which some clinicians consider a separate entity.

The initial inflammatory stage of morphea is characterized by erythematous or violaceous patches or plaques; the central region becomes white and sclerotic while the active borders remain red.[1] Over time the active stage subsides, leaving behind sclerotic plaques that can be white or hyperpigmented. The overabundant collagen deposition destroys adnexal structures and hair follicles.[1]

- Circumscribed morphea: fewer than 3 indurated discrete plaques (Fig. 3)
  - Can be superficial or deep
  - Deep variant (morphea profunda) affects the dermis and subcutaneous tissues
  - Can involve the underlying fascia and muscle[1]
  - Often areas of pressure such as hips, waists, bra line[1]

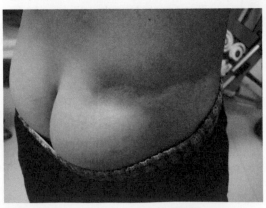

Fig. 3. Atrophic plaque on the buttock.

- o Breasts are commonly involved in women with sparing of the nipples[1]
- Generalized morphea: greater than 4 indurated plaques larger than 3 cm and/or involving 2 or more body sites but sparing the face and hands (**Figs. 4–7**)[1]
  - o Rare variant, 7% to 9% of those affected with morphea[2,5]
  - o More likely to have positive autoantibodies, especially ANAs
  - o Can have systemic symptoms such as myalgias, arthralgias, and fatigue
  - o Often confused with scleroderma
  - o Differentiated from systemic sclerosis by the absence of Raynaud phenomenon, nail-fold capillary changes, and sclerodactyly[1]
  - o Usually limited to the dermis, and rarely involves subcutaneous tissues
- Bullous morphea
  - o Presents as tense subepidermal bullae that occur within affected sclerodermoid plaques[16]
  - o Rare variant, no known trigger[16]
- Linear morphea (**Figs. 8 and 9**)
  - o Most common type in children
  - o Involves the lines of Blaschko, suggesting genetic mosaicism[17]
  - o Three variants include en coup de sabre, progressive hemifacial atrophy, and linear limb morphea
  - o Associated with underlying tissue atrophy
  - o En coup de sabre
    - Usually occurs on the paramedian forehead
    - Can be associated with underlying ocular and central nervous system (CNS) involvement, including headaches and seizures

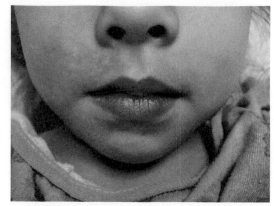

**Fig. 5.** Atrophic areas on the face of a child with generalized morphea.

- Typically follows Blaschko lines
- Can be associated with alopecia[18]
- Can present (less commonly) with more than 1 lesion[18]
- o Progressive hemifacial atrophy (also known as Parry-Romberg syndrome) (**Fig. 10**)
  - Minimal cutaneous changes with significant atrophy of the subcutaneous tissues
  - Can have overlap with en coup de sabre; thought to be different ends of the same condition
  - May have underlying seizures[19]
  - Mean age of onset of 13.6 years[19]
- o Linear limb morphea
  - Associated with muscle atrophy, limb-length discrepancies, and joint contractures
  - Usually unilateral
- o Most likely to have extracutaneous manifestations with linear morphea

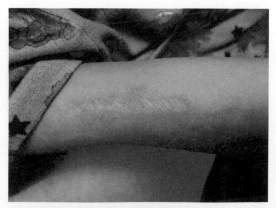

**Fig. 4.** Morphea on the arm of a child with generalized morphea. Note the indurated plaque next to an atrophic area.

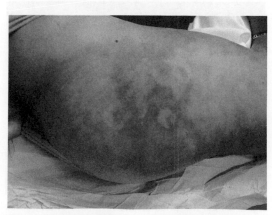

**Fig. 6.** Indurated plaques involving the hips and back in this child with generalized morphea.

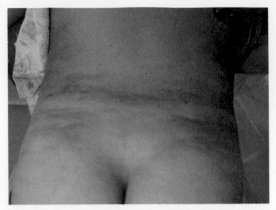

Fig. 7. Indurated plaques involving the hips and back in this child with generalized morphea.

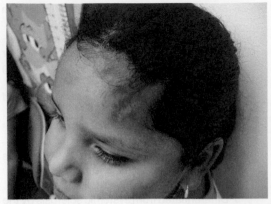

Fig. 9. Linea morphea in a female patient. Note the central white "burned-out" sclerotic area, with red advancing borders.

- One study[5] looked at 750 children with linear morphea and found the following complications:
  - Articular disease (47.2%), neurologic (17.1%), vascular (9.3%), ocular (8.3%), gastrointestinal (6.2%), respiratory (2.6%), cardiac (1%), and renal (1%)
- Deep morphea
  - Can affect the deep dermis, panniculus, fascia, or superficial muscle[16]
  - Patients present with taut, bound-down sclerotic skin
  - Diffuse, rather than linear lesions[18]
  - Can lead to significant functional disability
  - Variants include eosinophilic fasciitis, subcutaneous morphea, and morphea profunda
    - In morphea profunda patients present with diffuse, taut, bound-down sclerosis

of the skin with all layers involved, including a dense inflammatory infiltrate in the subcutaneous tissue[18]
- Eosinophilic fasciitis is characterized by symmetric, painful induration of the skin of the extremities with sparing of the hands and feet[18]
  - The skin often feels normal because the inflammation is deep, with sparing of the superficial layers
  - A linear depression along the courses of superficial veins is often seen; this is known as the "groove sign" and occurs because of relative sparing of the perivascular areas[18]
  - Joint contractures are common
  - Eosinophilia, hypergammaglobulinemia, increased sedimentation rate, and occasionally thrombocytopenia or hemolytic anemia can occur[18]

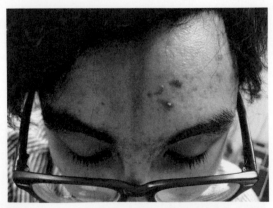

Fig. 8. Linear morphea on the forehead of an adolescent male patient. Note the violaceous hue in this active plaque.

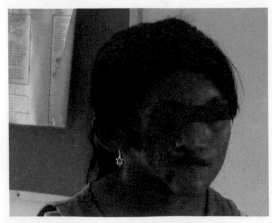

Fig. 10. Progressive hemifacial atrophy.

- Various hematologic malignancies have been reported with eosinophilic fasciitis[18]
- Pansclerotic morphea
  - Debilitating, affects subcutaneous tissues, including bone at times
  - Can affect the trunk, face, and extremities with sparing of the fingertips and toes[18]
  - Characterized by muscle atrophy, joint contractures, and nonhealing ulcers[1]
  - Increased risk for squamous cell carcinoma of the skin caused by chronic wounds (Table 1)[20]

## DIAGNOSIS

Diagnosis of morphea can usually be done by history and physical examination alone; however, skin biopsy may be helpful when the diagnosis is in question. Histology is characterized by perivascular infiltrate of lymphocytes, admixed with rare eosinophils and plasma cells in the reticular dermis; thickened collagen bundles; and late stages characterized by absent inflammatory cells, thickened collagen bundles with atrophic eccrine glands, diminished number of blood vessels, and trapped fat in the dermis.[1] Morphea and systemic sclerosis can look identical histologically,[18] so histology is not helpful in differentiating between them.

Thermograms can be performed, which will demonstrate a higher temperature in lesions of active morphea.[10] However, this may not be available in most clinical settings. Laser Doppler imaging and laser Doppler flowmetry can also be helpful in the assessment of morphea,[10] when available. Clinical evaluation and correlation is essential and cannot be replaced by diagnostic tests.

## COMPLICATIONS

Myalgias, arthralgias, and fatigue can occur (most commonly in generalized morphea). Neurologic manifestations, more commonly with en coup de sabre or progressive hemifacial atrophy, can include seizures, headaches, peripheral neuropathy, vascular malformations, and CNS vasculitis.[5] Ocular complications can occur with en coup de sabre morphea, and include sclerosis of the adnexal structures, anterior segment inflammation, and anterior uveitis.[1] Eyelid lesions, exophthalmos, uveitis, episcleritis, xerophthalmia, papilledema, and glaucoma can occur in up to 15% of cases.[21]

**Table 1**
**Different types of morphea**

| Morphea Type | Distribution | Systemic Symptoms |
|---|---|---|
| Circumscribed | <3 discrete plaques Superficial or deep Can involve fascia or muscle Often affects pressure areas | None |
| Generalized | >4 plaques Usually limited to dermis | Myalgias, arthralgias, fatigue No sclerodactyly, nail-fold changes, or Raynaud phenomenon |
| Bullous | Tense subepidermal bulla within a sclerodermoid plaque | None |
| Linear Morphea | | |
| En coup de sabre | Face, usually forehead | Headaches; central nervous system or vision changes |
| Linear limb | Unilateral arms or legs, can have muscle atrophy | Limb-length discrepancy Joint contracture |
| Progressive hemifacial atrophy | Minimal cutaneous change significant atrophy of muscle and bone | Seizures |
| Deep | Deep dermis, fat, fascia, or muscle | Joint contracture Functional disability |
| Pansclerotic | Subcutaneous tissues, including bone | Muscle atrophy Joint contracture Nonhealing ulcers Increased risk of squamous cell carcinoma |

Depression and anxiety are more common in patients with morphea.[1] Associated autoimmune diseases (vitiligo, type 1 diabetes, Hashimoto thyroiditis, Graves disease, and ulcerative colitis) have been reported in 2% to 5% of children with morphea.[1,22] Positive autoantibodies often occur in patients with morphea: homogenous ANA, anti–single-stranded DNA, antihistone antibodies, anti–topoisomerase II, and rheumatoid factor.[1,16] Beltramelli and colleagues[10] found that 19 of 26 patients (73%) had positive ANA.

## DIFFERENTIAL DIAGNOSIS

Systemic sclerosis is often a consideration when first evaluating a morphea patient. However, morphea is easily differentiated from systemic sclerosis based on the absence of sclerodactyly, Raynaud phenomenon, and nail-fold capillary changes.[1]

- All patients with Raynaud phenomenon should be examined for nail-fold capillary changes.
  - Primary Raynaud: isolated phenomenon, onset during second decade of life, no nail-fold capillary changes, does not cause necrosis; can affect up to 22% of the general population[1]
  - Secondary Raynaud: associated with an underlying autoimmune process, onset usually after 30 years of age, presence of nail-fold capillary changes (dilated vessels, hemorrhage, and eventual loss)[1]

Patients with systemic sclerosis often go on to develop calcinosis, which does not occur with morphea.[16] The anticentromere antibody is most closely associated with limited cutaneous systemic sclerosis, and the anti-Scl70 antibody is seen more often with diffuse cutaneous systemic sclerosis.[16] Another author has quoted the presence of ANAs (46%–80%), anti–single-stranded DNA antibodies (50%), and antihistone antibodies (47%).[23]

Systemic sclerosis and morphea likely share some common pathogenic mechanisms, but it is rare for morphea to evolve into systemic sclerosis.[16] An incorrect diagnosis of acquired port-wine stain can be mistaken in cases of early morphea (**Table 2**).[24]

## TREATMENT

Morphea lesions tend to regress spontaneously over 3 to 5 years, often leaving residual pigmentary or atrophic changes.[15,18] Therefore, treatment should be focused on treating active areas of involvement, characterized by a violaceous or erythematous margin. Important factors to consider include:

- Physical therapy to prevent contractures is important when linear scleroderma involves the limbs.[18]
- Ocular examination should be performed regularly in cases of en coup de sabre.
- Methotrexate, systemic corticosteroids, cyclosporine, and mycophenolate mofetil have all been reported as effective therapies in small retrospective or prospective studies.[25] There is a paucity of true evidence-based studies concerning treatment.
  - Topical corticosteroids
    - High-potency topical steroids can be applied once or twice daily to affected areas; lower-potency steroids should be used on the face or folds; care should be taken to prevent atrophy of the uninvolved skin. Systemic absorption should be a concern if large areas are involved. There is a lack of controlled studies looking at the use of topical steroids for morphea.
  - Topical vitamin D analogues
    - Calcipotriene ointment 0.005% under occlusion twice a day has been used, with good results.[26] Oral calcitriol has also been given to patients, with good success.[27]
  - Topical corticosteroid/calcipotriene ointment can also be used in place of separate applications.
  - Topical calcineurin inhibitors
    - Tacrolimus ointment 0.1% is another effective topical treatment. The benefit over topical corticosteroids is that atrophy of normal skin is not a concern.[13]
  - Several studies have shown benefit in using imiquimod cream.[13]
  - Intralesional corticosteroids
    - Triamcinolone, 5 mg/mL can be injected intralesionally once a month for 3 months.[13]
  - Oral corticosteroids
    - Oral corticosteroids can be helpful in rapidly progressive cases of morphea. However, caution is advised when using for longer than 1 month owing to side effects of long-term steroid use.
  - Methotrexate
    - Methotrexate can be given at 0.5 mg/kg weekly. It might be helpful to initiate a 1- to 2-month course of oral corticosteroids at the same time because of the slow onset of action for methotrexate.

**Table 2**
**Differentiating morphea from scleroderma**

| | Systemic Symptoms | Raynaud Phenomenon | Sclerodactyly | Nail-Fold Changes | Autoantibodies (Gupta % Fiorentino) |
|---|---|---|---|---|---|
| Systemic sclerosis (scleroderma) | + | + | + | + | Anticentromere (20%–30%) Anti-Scl70 (9%–20%) Anti–RNA polymerase (20%) |
| Morphea | ± | − | − | − | Antihistone (47%) Anti–single-stranded DNA (50%) Anti–topoisomerase II-$\alpha$ (76%) |

Concurrent folic acid can help with nausea and gastrointestinal upset. In some cases of persistent nausea, it may be helpful to divide the weekly methotrexate into 3 doses separated by 12 hours each or to try intramuscular administration. Beltramelli and colleagues[10] found methotrexate to either improve or stabilize morphea. Relapse following treatment with methotrexate has been reported.[28]

○ Methotrexate and intravenous pulsed methylprednisolone
  ■ One study showed significant improvement using methotrexate, 0.3 to 0.6 mg/kg per week and intravenous methylprednisolone, 30 mg/kg/d for 3 days per month for 3 months.[29]

○ Phototherapy
  ■ One study showed a good response in 75% of patients exposed to low-dose ultraviolet A (UVA) (340–400 nm, 20 J/cm$^2$).[30]
  ■ A more recent study showed benefit in using medium-dose UVA.[31]
  ■ It is thought that UVA therapy decreases COL I, COL III, and TGBF gene expression, and increases expression of IFNG.[32]
  ■ Narrow-band ultraviolet B (UVB) is helpful but is not as effective as medium-dose UVA1.[33]
  ■ Other studies have also shown phototherapy to be useful. UVA is more useful than UVB because of deeper penetration by the longer wavelength of light into the dermis.

**Table 3**
**Therapies often used in the treatment of morphea**

| Treatment | Evidence | Regimen |
|---|---|---|
| Topical corticosteroids | Anecdotal | Medium to high potency applied nightly Mon–Fri as long as needed |
| Oral corticosteroids | 36 | 0.5–1 mg/kg/d for 1–7 mo |
| Intralesional corticosteroids | Anecdotal | 5–10 mg/mL intralesionally every 1–2 mo as needed |
| Topical tacrolimus | 37,38 | 0.1% ointment twice daily |
| Topical calcipotriene | 39 | 0.005% ointment twice daily under occlusion × 3 mo |
| Oral calcitriol | 40 | 0.75 µg/d |
| High-dose UVA | 41 | 130 J/cm$^2$ 3 times weekly for 10 wk |
| Broadband UVA | 42 | 20 J/cm$^2$ 3 times weekly for 7 wk |
| Methotrexate | 43 | 0.3–0.6 mg/kg/wk; 25 mg maximum |
| Methotrexate and pulse steroids | 29 | 0.3–0.6 mg/wk plus methylprednisolone |
| Imatinib mesylate | 35 | 400 mg daily for adults |

○ Imatinib mesylate
  ▪ Imatinib mesylate is a tyrosine kinase inhibitor that is most commonly used to treat certain types of leukemia. It interferes with transforming growth factor β signaling via c-Abl and by blocking extracellular matrix synthesis.[34] Imatinib is also approved by the Food and Drug Administration (FDA) for treating mastocytosis and hypereosinophilic syndrome, other conditions marked by dysregulation of tyrosine kinase activity.[35] Side effects reported most frequently with imatinib include nausea, vomiting, edema, and muscle cramps.[35] Fluid accumulation, including ascites, pleural effusion, pericardial effusion, and pulmonary edema, has been reported in 1% to 2% of patients.[35] Although not FDA-approved for morphea, the ease of once-daily oral administration (400 mg/d for adults) makes imatinib mesylate a promising new treatment (Table 3).

## SUMMARY

Morphea, particularly linear morphea, can often affect children. Early diagnosis and management are crucial for good outcomes.

## REFERENCES

1. Fett N, Werth VP. Update on morphea: part I. Epidemiology, clinical presentation, and pathogenesis. J Am Acad Dermatol 2011;64(2):217–28 [quiz: 229–30].
2. Christen-Zaech S, Hakim MD, Afsar FS, et al. Pediatric morphea (localized scleroderma): review of 136 patients. J Am Acad Dermatol 2008;59(3): 385–96.
3. Peterson L, Nelson AM, Su WP, et al. The epidemiology of morphea (localized scleroderma) in Olmsted County 1960-1993. J Rheumatol 1997;24: 73–80.
4. Murray KJ, Laxer RM. Scleroderma in children and adolescents. Rheum Dis Clin North Am 2002;28(3): 603–24.
5. Zulian F, Athreya BH, Laxer R, et al. Juvenile localized scleroderma: clinical and epidemiological features in 750 children. An international study. Rheumatology (Oxford) 2006;45:614–20.
6. Leitenberger JJ, Cayce RL, Haley RW, et al. Distinct autoimmune syndromes in morphea: a review of 245 adult and pediatric cases. Arch Dermatol 2009; 145(5):545–50.
7. Pham CM, Browning JC. Morphea affecting a father and son. Pediatr Dermatol 2010;27(5):536–7.
8. Badea I, Taylor M, Rosenberg A, et al. Pathogenesis and therapeutic approaches for improved topical treatment in localized scleroderma and systemic sclerosis. Rheumatology (Oxford) 2009;48(3): 213–21.
9. Herrmann T, Günther C, Csere P. Localized morphea—a rare but significant secondary complication following breast cancer radiotherapy. Case report and review of the literature on radiation reaction among patients with scleroderma/morphea. Strahlenther Onkol 2009;185(9):603–7.
10. Beltramelli M, Vercellesi P, Frasin A, et al. Localized severe scleroderma: a retrospective study of 26 pediatric patients. Pediatr Dermatol 2010;27(5):476–80. http://dx.doi.org/10.1111/j.1525-1470.2010.01258.x.
11. Torrelo A, Suárez J, Colmenero I, et al. Deep morphea after vaccination in two young children. Pediatr Dermatol 2006;23(5):484–7.
12. Eisendle K, Grabner T, Zelger B. Morphoea: a manifestation of infection with Borrelia species? Br J Dermatol 2007;157(6):1189–98.
13. Colomé-Grimmer MI, Payne DA, Tyring SK, et al. Borrelia burgdorferi DNA and Borrelia hermsii DNA are not associated with morphea or lichen sclerosus et atrophicus in the southwestern United States. Arch Dermatol 1997;133(9):1174.
14. Vilela FA, Carneiro S, Ramos-e-Silva M. Treatment of morphea or localized scleroderma: review of the literature. J Drugs Dermatol 2010;9(10):1213–9.
15. Peterson LS, Nelson AM, Su WP. Classification of morphea (localized scleroderma). Mayo Clin Proc 1995;70:1068–76.
16. Gupta RA, Fiorentino D. Localized scleroderma and systemic sclerosis: is there a connection? Best Pract Res Clin Rheumatol 2007;21(6):1025–36.
17. Weibel L, Harper JI. Linear morphoea follows Blaschko's lines. Br J Dermatol 2008;159(1): 175–81.
18. Chung L, Lin J, Furst DE, et al. Systemic and localized scleroderma [review]. Clin Dermatol 2006; 24(5):374–92.
19. Tollefson MM, Witman PM. En coup de sabre morphea and Parry-Romberg syndrome: a retrospective review of 54 patients. J Am Acad Dermatol 2007;56: 257–63.
20. Wollina U, Buslau M, Heinig B, et al. Disabling pansclerotic morphea of childhood poses a high risk of chronic ulceration of the skin and squamous cell carcinoma. Int J Low Extrem Wounds 2007;6(4): 291–8.
21. Zulian F. Systemic manifestations in localized scleroderma. Curr Rheumatol Rep 2004;6:417–24.
22. Zulian F, Vallongo C, Woo P, et al. Localized scleroderma in childhood is not just a skin disease. Arthritis Rheum 2005;52(9):2873–81.

23. Takehara K, Sato S. Localized scleroderma is an autoimmune disorder. Rheumatology 2005;44: 274–9.

24. Nijhawan RI, Bard S, Blyumin M, et al. Early localized morphea mimicking an acquired port-wine stain. J Am Acad Dermatol 2011;64(4):779–82.

25. Fett N, Werth VP. Update on morphea: part II. Outcome measures and treatment. J Am Acad Dermatol 2011;64(2):231–42 [quiz: 243–4].

26. Cunningham BB, Landells ID, Langman C, et al. Topical calcipotriene for morphea/linear scleroderma. J Am Acad Dermatol 1998;92:211–5.

27. Elst EF, Van Suijlekom-Smit LW, Oranje AP. Treatment of linear scleroderma with oral 1,25-dihydroxy-vitamin D3 (calcitriol) in seven children. Pediatr Dermatol 1999;16:53–8.

28. Mirsky L, Chakkittakandiyil A, Laxer RM, et al. Relapse after systemic treatment in paediatric morphoea. Br J Dermatol 2012;166(2):443–5.

29. Uziel Y, Feldman BM, Krafchik BR, et al. Methotrexate and corticosteroid therapy for pediatric localized scleroderma. J Pediatr 2000;136:91–5.

30. Kerscher M, Volkenandt M, Gruss C, et al. Low-dose phototherapy for treatment of localized scleroderma. J Am Acad Dermatol 1998;38(1):21–6.

31. Andres C, Kollmar A, Mempel M, et al. Successful ultraviolet A1 phototherapy in the treatment of localized scleroderma: a retrospective and prospective study. Br J Dermatol 2010;162(2):445–7.

32. El-Mofty M, Mostafa W, Esmat S, et al. Suggested mechanism of action of UVA phototherapy in morphea: a molecular study. Photodermatol Photoimmunol Photomed 2004;20:93–100.

33. Kreuter A, Hyun J, Stucker M, et al. A randomized controlled study of low-dose UVA1, medium dose UVA1, and narrowband UVB phototherapy in the treatment of localized scleroderma. J Am Acad Dermatol 2006;54(3):440–7.

34. Distiler JH, Jungel A, Huber LC, et al. Imatinib mesylate reduces production of extracellular matrix and prevents development of experimental dermal fibrosis. Arthritis Rheum 2006;54:1298–308.

35. Bibi Y, Gottlieb AB. A potential role for imatinib and other small molecule tyrosine kinase inhibitors in the treatment of systemic and localized sclerosis. J Am Acad Dermatol 2008;59(4):654–8.

36. Joly P, Bamberger N, Crickx B, et al. Treatment of severe forms of localized scleroderma with oral corticosteroids: follow-up study on 17 patients. Arch Dermatol 1994;130(5):663–4.

37. Kroft EB, Groeneveld TJ, Seyger MM, et al. Efficacy of topical tacrolimus 0.1% in active plaque morphea: randomized, double-blind, emollient-controlled pilot study. Am J Clin Dermatol 2009;10(3):181–7.

38. Stefanaki C, Stefanaki K, Kontochristopoulos G, et al. Topical tacrolimus 0.1% ointment in the treatment of localized scleroderma. An open label clinical and histological study. J Dermatol 2008;35(11): 712–8.

39. Tay YK. Topical calcipotriol ointment in the treatment of morphea. J Dermatolog Treat 2003;14(4):219–21.

40. Hulshof MM, Bouwes Bavinck JN, Bergman W, et al. Double-blind, placebo-controlled study of oral calcitriol for the treatment of localized and systemic scleroderma. J Am Acad Dermatol 2000;43(6): 1017–23.

41. Stege H, Berneburg M, Humke S, et al. High-dose UVA1 radiation therapy for localized scleroderma. J Am Acad Dermatol 1997;36(6 Pt 1):938–44.

42. El-Mofty M, Zaher H, Bosseila M, et al. Low-dose broad-band UVA in morphea using a new method for evaluation. Photodermatol Photoimmunol Photomed 2000;16(2):43–9.

43. Fitch PG, Rettig P, Burnham JM, et al. Treatment of pediatric localized scleroderma with methotrexate. J Rheumatol 2006;33(3):609–14.

# Common Pediatric Skin Conditions with Protracted Courses: A Therapeutic Update

Allison Swanson, MD*, Kristi Canty, MD

## KEYWORDS

- Warts • Molluscum contagiosum • Bacterial skin infections • Impetiginized atopic dermatitis
- Alopecia areata • Vitiligo

## KEY POINTS

- Immune-based therapies, such as intralesional Candida, show promise and good efficacy in treatment of molluscum and warts in children.
- Clindamycin seems to be the treatment of choice in purulent skin and soft tissue infections (SSTIs) versus trimethoprim-sulfamethoxazole (TMP-SMX) and β-lactam antibiotics; however, clindamycin and β-lactam antibiotics show equal efficacy in nonpurulent SSTIs and are both superior to TMP-SMX.
- Dilute bleach baths help reduce *Staphylococcus aureus* colonization and improve eczema severity.
- Localized phototherapy with the excimer laser shows promise as a safe treatment modality for vitiligo and alopecia areata.

Common pediatric skin disorders can often be difficult to manage and studies of new treatment modalities in children are often lagging. This therapeutic update highlights some of the new literature on common infectious pediatric skin conditions (molluscum contagiosum [MC], warts, bacterial skin infections, and impetiginized atopic dermatitis) as well as 2 skin diseases that are often resistant to standard therapies (severe alopecia areata and vitiligo).

## MOLLUSCUM CONTAGIOSUM

MC is a poxvirus, which frequently affects children and is a common cause for visits to primary care doctors and dermatologists. Self-resolution of MC is the rule, but resolution can occasionally take many years. Parents often seek treatment for their children due to presence of concomitant dermatitis triggered or exacerbated by MC, risk of spread to other children, and social stigmata associated with visible lesions. Although there is still no Food and Drug Administration (FDA)-approved treatment for MC, different treatment modalities have been used by practitioners to speed clearance of the infection. In a survey of pediatric dermatologists performed by Coloe and Morrell,[1] the most common treatment modality used was topical Cantharadin. Other treatments in descending order of frequency included topical imiquimod, active nonintervention, curettage, cryotherapy, retinoids (oral and topical), cimetidine, salicylic acid, duct tape, Candida antigen, potassium hydroxide, and cidofovir. Few published data are available on efficacy of these treatments though. Ideally, treatment of molluscum is painless yet effective with few side effects, given the young age group it commonly affects.

Immunotherapy has become a more popular treatment choice of pediatric dermatologists, given signs of good efficacy with fewer side effects than destructive methods in the recent literature.

---

The authors have no disclosures or conflicts of interest.
Section of Dermatology, Department of Pediatrics, Children's Mercy Hospital, 2401 Gillham Road, Kansas City, MO, USA
* Corresponding author.
E-mail address: amswanson@cmh.edu

Dermatol Clin 31 (2013) 239–249
http://dx.doi.org/10.1016/j.det.2012.12.003
0733-8635/13/$ – see front matter © 2013 Elsevier Inc. All rights reserved.

One common form of immunotherapy is intralesional Candida antigen injection. For MC, the technique involves injection of no more than 0.3 mL of Candida antigen into 1 to 3 molluscum intralesionally at each visit at 4-week intervals until clearance of infection is achieved (**Fig. 1**). In a recent retrospective study by Enns and Evans,[2] 29 children with MC were treated with Candida antigen. Total number of treatments ranged from 1 to 6. Complete clearance was seen in 16 (55.2%) patients after an average of 2.5 total treatments. Partial clearance was seen in 11 (37.9%) after an average of 3.3 treatments, for a total treatment response rate of 93%. Only 2 patients did not respond and the average number of treatments was only 1.5 in these 2 patients, which the investigators hypothesize as a possible reason for lack of response. Pain was the only reported side effect in 4 patients in this study. In a similar retrospective study by Maronn and colleagues,[3] 47 patients with MC were treated with intralesional Candida antigen. Only 25 of these patients had follow-up, of whom 14 (56%) had complete clearance after an average of 3 treatments, 7 (28%) had partial clearance after an average of 4 treatments, and 4 (16%) had no improvement after an average of 3.33 treatments. No serious side effects were reported with use of the Candida antigen but most patients reported discomfort at the time of injection. Based on these 2 recent studies and anecdotal reports of success, intralesional Candida antigen injection offers a promising treatment of MC with few side effects. In the authors' opinion, Candida injection is a good option in patients who have many molluscum or concomitant dermatitis where destructive modalities may be irritating to the skin.

Imiquimod 5% cream is another attractive treatment of cutaneous viral infections, given the ability

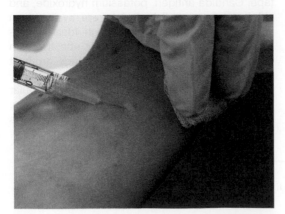

**Fig. 1.** Intralesional injection technique for Candida antigen into molluscum contagiosum. (*Courtesy of* University of Colorado Dermatology Department.)

for home application and lack of pain with application. Imiquimod exhibits antiviral and antitumor effects through activation of the innate immunity and up-regulation of cytokines, such as interferon-$\alpha$. In a small pharmacokinetic and safety study of imiquimod 5% cream in children with MC, when applied 3 times weekly for 4 weeks, low systemic drug levels were found and there were no serious adverse events, although application site reactions were reported in more than half of the participants.[4] Although clinical efficacy was not an endpoint of this study, no subjects had complete clearance of their MC in the short 4-week treatment time. In other recent studies, longer-duration imiquimod use has shown promise as an effective treatment of MC. In a prospective study by Al-Mutairi and colleagues,[5] the investigators compared the efficacy, safety, and acceptability of imiquimod 5% cream versus cryotherapy for MC. Imiquimod cream was applied 5 times weekly for up to 16 weeks in group A (37 patients) and cryotherapy was performed with liquid nitrogen for 2 10-second to 20-second cycles in group B (37 patients) at initial visit and 1 week later if needed. The investigators found more rapid clearance in the cryotherapy group with 100% clearance by 6 weeks, whereas the imiquimod group only had complete clearance in 22 (approximately 60%) by 6 weeks. By 12 weeks, however, no statistical difference was seen in MC clearance rates between the 2 groups, with approximately 92% complete clearance in the imiquimod group and 100% clearance in the cryotherapy group. At the 6-month follow-up, the cosmetic outcome was superior in the imiquimod-treated group, with only 2 patients having residual hypopigmentation versus 15 patients in the cryotherapy group with residual pigmentary alterations and 8 patients with scarring or atrophy, which was statistically significant. Relapse was seen in 3 patients in the cryotherapy group at 6 months and no relapse was seen in the imiquimod group, possibly due to the broader immune up-regulation seen with imiquimod versus destructive modalities. Imiquimod seems to have promise as an effective treatment of MC, especially for multiple small papules and in sensitive areas, such as the face and anogenital region; however, families should be educated on the potential high cost of the medication, long duration of treatment often needed, and the likelihood of erythema or other application site reaction with use.

No discussion of MC treatment is complete without an update on destructive modalities, which are still the most commonly used treatments by practitioners, including cantharadin and curettage as the most commonly used methods. Both cantharadin and curettage are effective, but past studies have shown that multiple treatments are necessary with frequent relapse and side effects, including severe blistering reactions as well as pain.[6,7] The limitation of these 2 modalities is their relative contraindication for facial molluscum. Other treatment options for facial molluscum include topical 20% to 35% trichloroacetic acid. This technique was reported by Bard and colleagues,[8] using the pointed edge of a broken cotton tip applicator with a small amount of tri-chloroacetic acid to the molluscum until a white frost appeared. They report minimal irritation and good efficacy with this technique. Another destructive modality with promise for practitioners with access to a pulsed dye laser (PDL) has been reported by Chatproedprai and colleagues.[9] In this prospective study of 20 children, 81% of patients treated with the 585-nm PDL with 1 or 2 total treatments had clearance of their mollus-cum versus 23% spontaneous clearance of mol-luscum in control patients.

## WARTS

Along the same lines as MC, warts (including common warts, flat warts, palmoplantar warts, and genital warts) occur frequently in children, affecting teenagers more commonly, and are a frequent cause of dermatology visits. Treatment options of warts are similar to those of MC, including topical salicylic acid, cryotherapy, can-tharadin, duct tape, PDL, retinoids, podophyllin, and immunotherapies, such as cimetidine, zinc, squaric acid dibutylester (SADBE) and diphency-prone (DPC), Candida antigen, and imiquimod. More-aggressive treatments include intralesional bleomycin, intralesional or topical 5-fluorouracil (5-FU), and interferon.[10] Imiquimod is the only medication with FDA approval for warts (genital warts only) in children 12 years or older.

Few new data are available on novel or estab-lished wart treatments. Intralesional Candida antigen was initially used for the treatment of warts before its recent reported use in MC. Candida antigen is an excellent treatment option when multiple warts are present. In a retrospective study, Maronn and colleagues[3] treated 170 wart patients with Candida antigen injections. The technique involved 0.3 mL injected into 1 or 2 warts at monthly intervals. Unfortunately, they had a low follow-up rate in this study, but complete clearance was seen in 48/55 (87%) of patients with follow-up after an average of 3.5 treatments. Only 4/55 (7%) had no improvement after an average of 3.75 treat-ments. Along the same immunotherapy line, both SADBE and DPC have been reported recently as

effective in treatment-resistant warts. Both of these agents require sensitization followed by application to warts once weekly up to nightly. In a recent study by Choi and colleagues,[11] they found that DPC and cryotherapy had equal initial complete clearance rates (62.5% vs 50.8%, respectively); however, at 12 months' follow-up, of those with complete clear-ance, the DPC group had 93% sustained clearance versus 76% in the cryotherapy group. The investi-gators hypothesized that DPC induced long-term immunity to human papilloma virus. A recent case report also demonstrated efficacy of SADBE in an immunosuppressed patient in multiple modality treatment-resistant warts.[12]

Oral zinc supplementation has recently been re-ported as a promising new immune modulating treatment for warts. A randomized, placebo-controlled study by Yaghoobi and colleagues[13] treated 32 children and young adults with zinc sulfate (10 mg/kg/d, maximum 600 mg daily) for up to 2 months' duration and 23 patients received placebo. Complete clearance of all warts was seen in 25/32 (78%) patients receiving zinc and 3/23 (13%) placebo patients, with no recur-rence of warts at 6-months' follow-up. The investigators found that patients whose warts re-sponded well to zinc treatment had dramatic increases in serum zinc levels, whereas nonre-sponders' serum levels only increased a small amount. The investigators did not discuss any side effects associated with oral zinc treatment. In another small study by Stefani and colleagues,[14] 9 patients were given high-dose zinc sulfate (10 mg/kg/d) and 9 patients were given oral cimet-idine (35 mg/kg/d) for 3 months. Five of 9 patients in the zinc sulfate group had complete clearance versus no complete clearance of warts in the cimetidine group. In this study, 5 of 9 patients in the zinc treatment group reported nausea, causing 1 6-year-old patient to drop out of the study. The investigators recommend dividing the zinc into 3 daily doses with meals to attenuate nausea. In a larger study of zinc versus placebo for recalci-trant warts, 20 of 23 patients in the zinc group had complete clearance of warts versus 0 of 20 in the placebo group after 2 months of treatment. All of the patients in the zinc-treated group re-ported nausea. The study also had a 46% dropout rate, which may have skewed results.[15] In the authors' opinion, zinc seems potentially a great treatment option for recalcitrant warts in children because it is painless and can be administered at home. Good preliminary efficacy results have been shown; however, the nausea may limit actual long-term use.

Topical 5-FU is a chemotherapeutic agent frequently used for nonmelanoma skin cancers and warts in adults. In a study by Gladsjo and colleagues,[16] 5-FU was studied with once-daily and twice-daily dosing in children with at least 2 common hand warts for 6 weeks under occlusion. Of the 39 total subjects (19 once-daily and 20 twice-daily dosing), there was no significant difference in improvement between the treatment protocols. Only 13% showed complete clearance of all warts at the end of the 6-week treatment period, although at least some improvement was seen in size or thickness of 88% of all treated warts. 5-FU levels were not measurable in 38 of the 39 subjects and no changes in complete blood count or liver function tests were observed in any subject. Although results from this study are not staggering in efficacy, the data are reassuring that the 5-FU may provide a well-tolerated, safe treatment of warts in children; however, over-the-counter salicylic acid treatments have more proved efficacy at a lower price point.[17]

Laser treatment of warts is increasing, with reports of efficacy of the PDL predominantly in the past. Recently, a large series of 348 patients using the long-pulsed Nd:YAG laser in children and adults with warts showed an impressive overall complete clearance rate of 96%. Laser treatments were performed every 4 weeks for a maximum of 4 treatments. The investigators found that more than 72% of common warts cleared after 1 laser treatment, whereas periungual and deep palmoplantar warts were slower to respond (64% and 44% clearance after one laser treatment, respectively). Pain was the reported by most patients when just topical anesthesia was used; therefore, lidocaine injections were recommended for the pain accompanying the laser procedure, which may be prohibitory in some children. Otherwise, side effects reported were very low, including bullae formation, dyspigmentation, and nail dystrophy.[18] For dermatologists with access to lasers, this promising treatment can be used.

## BACTERIAL SKIN INFECTIONS

Uncomplicated SSTIs, presenting as impetigo, abscesses, or cellulitis, are on the rise, especially with the increasing prevalence of community-acquired methicillin-resistant S aureus (CA-MRSA). Given the lack of commercially available rapid-detection tests for CA-MRSA, empiric antibiotic choices have moved away from previously more used β-lactam antibiotics to clindamycin and TMP-SMX.[19] Clinical trials on prevention of SSTIs and efficacy of different antibiotic treatments have recently been published. In a retrospective cohort study of more than 47,000 children with SSTIs treated with clindamycin, TMP-SMX, or a β-lactam

antibiotic, Williams and colleagues[19] found that clindamycin-treated patients were less likely to have treatment failure than the β-lactam–treated and TMP-SMX–treated children. They further divided these groups into children who had a drainage procedure (suggesting abscess type of skin infection) performed versus those who did not (suggesting impetigo type of skin infection). Of the 6407 children undergoing a drainage procedure, treatment failure was seen in 4.7% of clindamycin users, 11.2% of TMP-SMX users, and 11.1% of β-lactam users. In children without drainage procedures, treatment failure was seen in 4.9% of clindamycin users, 8.8% of TMP-SMX users, and 5.3% of β-lactam users. This study was performed in Tennessee where the prevalence of CA-MRSA is between 75% and 80%; however, this study did not compare treatment failures with bacterial culture results. A potential reason for treatment failure in the TMP-SMX cohort could include concurrent infection with Streptococcus pyogenes, in which TMP-SMX is ineffective. The investigators concluded that clindamycin should be considered first-line treatment of purulent SSTIs versus TMP-SMX and that in nonpurulent SSTIs β-lactam antibiotics may still be effective, even in CA-MRSA endogenous areas. Along similar lines, a recent prospective randomized controlled trial of cephalexin versus clindamycin for uncomplicated SSTIs (ie, not requiring hospitalization) in children was reported by Chen and colleagues.[20] Two hundred patients were enrolled and 97 subjects completed the study in each arm. Children were prescribed either cephalexin (40 mg/kg/d) or clindamycin (20 mg/kg/d), both given 3 times daily for 7 total days. Of the 200 specimens, 137 (69%) grew CA-MRSA. There was no difference in improvement or resolution of infection in the cephalexin arm versus the clindamycin arm at 48 to 72 hours after antibiotic initiation. Even in the CA-MRSA positive subgroup, the infection only worsened in 9% of cephalexin-treated patients versus 3% of clindamycin-treated patients, which did not reach statistical significance. At 7 days after initiation of antibiotic treatment, 97% of cephalexin-treated patients and 94% of clindamycin-treated patients had clinical resolution of infection, and when looking at only the CA-MRSA subgroup, 100% and 94% of patients had resolution of disease in the cephalexin versus clindamycin arms, respectively. A 3-month follow-up found an 18% recurrence of SSTIs but the risk of recurrence did not differ based on initial isolation of CA-MRSA versus methicillin-sensitive S aureus (MSSA) or based on antibiotic assignment. The majority of subjects did undergo spontaneous drainage or a drainage procedure for the infection. The investigators concluded that cephalexin and clindamycin are both viable empiric treatment options for uncomplicated SSTIs, even in CA-MRSA endemic areas, as long as management already includes drainage if needed and close follow-up of patients.

Eradication of S aureus carriage has become a large target for reducing frequency of SSTIs as well as adjuvant treatment of chronic skin disease, such as atopic dermatitis, which has a known propensity for superinfection. In a 4-arm study by Fritz and colleagues,[21] they compared the effectiveness of hygiene education only (control), intranasal mupirocin ointment twice daily for 5 days, intranasal mupirocin plus daily 4% chlorhexidine body washes for 5 days, and intranasal mupirocin plus daily dilute bleach baths (1/4 cup of 6% sodium hypochlorite in tub of water) for 5 days. The primary endpoint of the study was S aureus eradication (defined as absence of S aureus from the cultures areas in the nares, axillae, and inguinal folds) at 1-month and 4-month follow-ups. All 4 groups received hygiene education, which included instructions to discard emollients in jars; not to share personal hygiene items, such as razors, brushes, or towels; washing towels daily after each use; and washing bed linens once weekly. Three hundred total patients were enrolled (64% children), 75 in each arm. At 1-month follow-up, each treatment arm had statistically significant greater eradication than the control arm (38% in control group, 56% in intranasal mupirocin only group, 55% in mupirocin plus chlorhexidine group, and 63% in mupirocin plus bleach bath group). At 4-months' follow-up with no further intervention, only the intranasal mupirocin plus bleach bath group showed statistically significant reduction in S aureus colonization. The study is encouraging given the low cost and accessibility of bleach. Also, in this study, the interventions were only performed for 5 days total. More long-term use of these preventive measures may help to further decrease S aureus carriage and subsequent clinical infection. This study did see recurrent SSTIs in all 4 arms of the study, suggesting that endogenous colonization is not the only risk factor for infection, but environmental factors and person-to-person transmission also play a role.

When looking at disease severity in atopic dermatitis, treatment of S aureus colonization by way of intranasal mupirocin and dilute bleach baths has been found to improve patient eczema. In a small prospective randomized study by Huang and colleagues,[22] patients with moderate to severe atopic dermatitis were given dilute bleach baths (0.005% concentration) twice weekly for 5 to 10 minutes and intranasal mupirocin twice daily for 5 consecutive days each month for 3 total

months versus plain water and petrolatum in the same fashion (control group). Of the 25 patients who returned for follow-up, significant improvement in Eczema Area and Severity Index (EASI) scores were seen at 1-month and 3-months' follow-up, especially in bath-submerged skin sites. No significant difference was seen in EASI scores from the head and neck between the placebo and treatment groups, suggesting the importance of the bleach baths in treatment efficacy. Skin and nares cultures continued to grow S aureus in this study despite use of mupirocin and bleach baths and quantitative bacterial assays were not performed to see if suppression (but not clearance) of S aureus colonies was occurring or if bleach baths can improve eczema severity through other mechanisms.

To round out the therapeutic update on treatment of bacterial skin infections, specifically in children with atopic dermatitis, a recent study by Travers and colleagues[23] looked at the role of oral antibiotics in impetiginized eczema. It has been well documented that the occurrence of CA-MRSA infection in children with atopic dermatitis is much lower than in the general population, even in CA-MRSA prevalent areas.[22,24] In this prospective study, 59 children with clinically impetiginized eczema had bacterial cultures performed from their skin and then were treated with topical corticosteroids (triamcinolone 0.1% ointment for body and desonide ointment for face or intertriginous areas), oral antihistamines (hydroxyzine or doxepin), and cephalexin (25–50 mg/kg/d) for a total of 2 weeks. At follow-up repeat cultures were performed and EASI score assessments were repeated as well as levels of bacterial products and cytokines measured from affected skin samples. Of the staphylococcal isolates, only 15% were MRSA, which was consistent with previous studies reporting lower prevalence of CA-MRSA infection in atopic patients.[22,24] The 9 patients with MRSA all had improvement in EASI score with the prescribed regimen and 48 of 50 of patients with MSSA had improvement in EASI scores. Seven of 9 MRSA isolates showed lower colony-forming units (4 of 7 had unmeasurable levels) and 47 of 50 MSSA isolates showed lower colony-forming units with the treatment. Defensin levels were higher in all treated skin and interleukin-4 and interleukin-13 levels were lower in treated skin. The investigators hypothesize that the combined treatment regimen with topical steroids, oral antihistamines, and oral cephalexin, regardless of antibiotic susceptibility, improves impetiginized atopic dermatitis skin lesions by reversing antimicrobial peptide deficiencies, normalizing barrier function, and suppressing Th2 cytokines. Although a complex study, the overall take-home message from this and the other cited studies is that cephalexin may still be a good empiric treatment choice for SSTIs and impetiginized eczema and is often better tolerated with fewer side effects than clindamycin and TMP-SMX. In addition, dilute bleach baths seem to be a promising adjuvant treatment to help reduce the frequency of SSTIs and improve eczema severity.

## ALOPECIA AREATA

Alopecia areata is the most common form of non-scarring hair loss in children. Most patients with patchy alopecia enter remission within a year, but there is a subset of patients who have a progressive course that is recalcitrant to many treatments and difficult to manage. Currently, there are no FDA-approved drugs for the treatment of this disease and there are few evidence-based treatment options for this age group.

A recent review by Alkhalifah and colleagues[25] looked at newly recognized treatments of alopecia areata and provided a treatment algorithm based on age. For children less than 10 years of age, the suggested first-line treatment is a combination of 5% minoxidil solution twice daily along with a midpotency topical corticosteroid. If patients do not respond to minoxidil and steroids within 6 months, then short-contact therapy with anthralin may be helpful. For patients 10 years and older with less than 50% scalp involvement, intralesional injections of triamcinolone acetinoide is suggested as first-line therapy. If these patients do not respond to intralesional injections within 6 months, then other therapeutic options can be offered, such as 5% minoxidil, potent topical corticosteroids under occlusion at night, and short-contact therapy with anthralin. For patients over the age of 10 years who also have greater than 50% scalp involvement, suggested therapies include topical immunotherapy with DPC alone or in conjunction with intralesional triamcinolone acetonide for recalcitrant patches. If these patients remain nonresponders after a 6-month trial, then other treatment options include 5% minoxidil solution, topical clobetasol propionate under occlusion, or short-contact anthralin.

Despite the many modalities available, many patients with alopecia areata continue to have a progressive, relapsing, and chronic course of disease. Because no one therapeutic intervention has been found curative or preventative, research continues to look at other treatment options.

Retrospective studies of adults with severe alopecia areata have been shown to have significant hair regrowth with the combination of methotrexate and low dose corticosteroids.[26,27] There is limited information, however, on the benefits of methotrexate use in children with severe alopecia areata. A retrospective study looked at 14 children between the ages of 8 and 18 years with greater than 50% scalp involvement and a mean duration of alopecia for 5.7 years who were treated with once weekly methotrexate (dose range 15–25 mg) for a mean duration of 14.2 months. Methotrexate was considered successful (area of regrowth 50%–74% or better and maximum relapse of 1%–24% of the area) in 5 of the 13 children studied with no serious side effects reported. Of note, 4 of the 5 responders initially received concurrent short-term corticosteroids, which were used in the past as monotherapy without previous improvement. The investigators of this study concluded that methotrexate should be considered cautiously for severe and resistant childhood alopecia areata.[28]

Oral corticosteroids have been shown to induce hair regrowth initially, but in patients with more severe forms of alopecia areata, there is often relapse. In addition, studies often exclude children due to the potential side effects with long-term use of oral corticosteroids. Intravenous methylprednisolone is thought to have a more potent effect on lymphocytes compared with oral steroids and thus may be a better treatment. Myung and colleagues[29] looked at the efficacy, tolerability, relapse rate, and prognostic indicators in patients treated with methylprednisolone. Seventy patients ranging in age from 5 to 58 years old with severe alopecia areata with a bald surface area of greater than 50%, alopecia totalis, and alopecia universalis were treated with IV methylprednisolone (25 mg/kg per day, maximum dose of 1000 mg, twice daily on 3 consecutive days); 70% of patients showed terminal hair growth and 41% showed complete response (more than 90% of terminal hair regrowth). At 12 months' postinfusion, 72% of the patients who had achieved complete response were still in remission. Investigators found that duration before treatment and type of alopecia were prognostic factors. All types of alopecia areata responded best if treated within 3 months. Severe alopecia with greater than 50% scalp involvement also responded to pulsed methylprednisolone if treated within 6 months. Overall, only 28.6% of patients experienced minor side effects, such as headache/dizziness and gastrointestinal discomfort. Thus, this study suggests that pulsed methylprednisolone is well tolerated and effective in all types of alopecia areata. The type of alopecia areata and the duration of disease should factor into the decision to treat with pulsed methylprednisolone. This study opens the door for use of pulsed methylprednisolone in the treatment of severe alopecia; however, further studies are necessary to determine the long-term safety and efficacy in pediatric patients.

The safety and efficacy of combining cyclosporine and methylprednisolone for the treatment of severe alopecia areata (greater than 50% loss of scalp hair or greater than 10 patches scattered over the scalp and body), including alopecia totalis and universalis, was investigated recently. This study looked at 46 pediatric and adult patients (10 under the age of 18 years). Cyclosporine (dose of 200 mg per day orally) was initially given and methylprednisolone was dosed at 12 mg twice daily orally. The dose of methylprednisolone was reduced by 4 mg per day per week and the dose of cyclosporine was tapered by 50 mg per day weekly or every 2 weeks after stopping methylprednisolone. The duration of treatment for children was 7 to 11 weeks. Complete remission (total regrowth of hair during treatment) and partial remission (a patch or incomplete hair regrowth) were used to define improvement. Three patients (one less than 18 years old) discontinued the study due to side effects (facial hypertrichosis and irregular menstruation). Of the 43 remaining patients, 88.4% had improvements, of which 76.6% were complete remissions. Failure of regrowth was seen in 11.6%. Side effects were noted in 56.5% of patients with gastrointestinal disturbance the most common and none of which was serious enough to warrant discontinuation.[30] This study shows the combination of cyclosporine and methylprednisolone can be successful in treating all forms of severe alopecia. The investigators of this study suggested, however, the potential for serious side effects and the unknown long-term efficacy of this combination warrant further evaluation.

In 1998, Goddard and colleagues[31] published a case report of a patient with Crohn disease and alopecia totalis who, after receiving azathioprine, subsequently had complete resolution of alopecia. Since that time, no further investigations have looked at this medication as a possible treatment of alopecia areata, possibly due to the risk of myelosuppression, delayed onset of action, and reported cases of inducing alopecia. Recently, Farshi and colleagues[32] looked at azathioprine as a possible treatment in patients with alopecia areata after this group met another patient with Crohn disease and a history of alopecia universalis, which resolved during treatment on azathioprine. An open pilot study treated 20 patients ranging in age from 8 to 57 years with moderate to severe alopecia areata (20% or greater of scalp area involvement), alopecia totalis, and alopecia universalis, with the duration of disease ranging from 12 to 84 months who were treated with azathioprine (2 mg/kg daily for 6 months). This study demonstrated a statistical significant difference in the mean hair loss percentage and the mean hair loss score after treatment. Overall, azathioprine was generally well tolerated. One patient in this study withdrew, however, due to elevation of liver enzymes. Although this medication can induce hair loss, this particular study demonstrates a possible role for azathioprine in the treatment of severe alopecia.

The 308-nm excimer laser has been used to treat diseases, such as vitiligo, psoriasis, and atopic dermatitis in children. In recent years, this laser has also been reported in the literature as a possible treatment modality for alopecia areata.[33–35] It is speculated to cause induction of T-cell apoptosis and thus result in hair regrowth.[33] Recently, the efficacy of this laser was investigated in 11 children between the ages of 4 and 14 years, 9 of whom had recalcitrant alopecia areata and 2 had alopecia totalis. Each patient had at least 1 additional area of alopecia that was equivalent in size (size range from 2–5 cm) to act as the control. All medications were discontinued 6 weeks prior to starting the treatments, and patients were then treated with the laser twice weekly for 12 weeks. Of the 22 lesions on the scalp, 63% showed complete regrowth and 18% (including the 2 patients with totalis) had no regrowth at 12 weeks. Of the lesions that responded, the respective control lesion showed no response. None of the lesions treated on the extremities responded. Four of the patients with patchy alopecia of the scalp who responded to treatment had hair loss in the treated area at the 6-month follow-up visit. No major adverse events were noted and, overall, the therapy was well tolerated.[36] This study demonstrated the 308-nm excimer laser may be a valid treatment modality for selective cases of patchy alopecia in children.

## VITILIGO

Vitiligo is a commonly acquired depigmentation disorder of the skin that presents before age 20 in approximately half of affected patients. As with alopecia areata, this condition can be frustrating to treat. There is no cure and complete repigmentation is rare with current treatment modalities. There is no FDA-approved treatment for vitiligo in children and many of the therapeutic regimens for children are extrapolated from studies conducted in adults. Recently published pediatric-specific reviews and new treatment-based studies that take into account children with vitiligo are discussed.

Tamesis and Morelli[37] reviewed studies looking at various treatment modalities in childhood vitiligo and recommended a treatment algorithm for children. For patients with less than 20% body surface area involvement, first-line treatment recommendations include topical therapies alone (potent corticosteroids for the body and calcineurin inhibitors in patients over age 2 years for involvement of the face, neck, and genital areas) or in combination with calcipotriol. Suggested treatments for patients with greater than 20% body surface area involvement include phototherapy favoring narrowband UV-B over psoralen–UV-A. Excimer laser is also a consideration, although only small areas can be treated at one time. The investigators note that topical therapies can be added to phototherapy but comparable studies are limited in children. If a surgical approach is desired, transplantation of suction blisters is the favored modality.

The 308-nm excimer laser can be used to treat vitiligo in all ages; however, studies looking at the efficacy of this modality in children are largely lacking. A retrospective study of 30 patients with 40 vitiligo patches looked at the efficacy of this laser in the pediatric population. Greater than 50% repigmentation was seen in 56.7% of patients, and repigmentation was greater than 75% in 12.5% of patients. The neck, face, and trunk tended to respond best.[38] The addition of topical therapies used in combination with this laser has produced promising results in mainly adult studies.[39,40] A single-blinded, randomized comparative study looked at 49 children (6–14 years) with symmetric lesions bilaterally distributed on the face, trunk, and hands who were treated twice weekly with the 308-nm excimer laser alone or in combination with topical 1% pimecrolimus. Of the 48 patients evaluated after 30 weeks of treatment, 71% of the patients who received the combination treatment achieved 51% or greater repigmentation compared with 50% who received monotherapy. Combination therapy was found statistically better than excimer therapy alone. In addition, this study demonstrated the excimer laser was safe and effective with minimal side effects when used in the pediatric population.[41] Because this laser provides localized ultraviolet radiation to areas of vitiligo, caution should be used when combining this modality with calcineurin inhibitors because this class of medication bears a black box warning that suggest it may cause skin cancers.

With better understanding of the underlying pathogenesis in vitiligo, not only are new modalities of treatment being attempted but also even common medications that are used to treat other disease processes are being tried as well. One recent theory of the possible pathogenesis of vitiligo includes epidermal oxidative stress that is believed to play a role in melanocyte degeneration.[42] Recently, several studies have been published that look at medications and supplements with antioxidant properties. Minocycline was attempted to treat patients with vitiligo due to the drug's anti-inflammatory, immunomodulatory, and antioxidant properties. Thirty-two patients, ranging in age from 14 to 52 years, with slow, progressive vitiligo were treated with minocycline (100 mg/d for 3 months). Patients were monitored for new areas of depigmentation, increasing size of existing lesions, and signs of repigmentation. In 29 patients, the progression of disease was halted, 7 patients showed marked repigmentation, and only 3 patients showed development of new lesions or enlargement of current lesions.[43] Overall, the new use of this medication shows promise, but further controlled studies are needed.

*Ginkgo biloba*, like minocycline, is known to have anti-inflammatory, immunomodulatory, and antioxidant properties. A prospective, open-label, nonrandomized feasibility trail was conducted with 12 patients aged 12 to 35 years with vitiligo who were treated with *Ginkgo biloba* (60 mg twice daily for 12 weeks). A significant improvement in total Vitiligo Area Scoring Index measurements and Vitiligo European Task Force spread and a trend toward improvement on Vitiligo European Task Force measurements of vitiligo area was found.[44] Again, this supplement shows some promise, but larger, randomized, double-blinded studies are needed.

Surgical treatments have been found effective interventions for the treatment of vitiligo in adults.[45] Surgery is invasive and not without risks; therefore, it is used less often in children. Due to the limitations in currently accepted therapeutics for children and the promising results seen with the use of surgery in adults, more studies are looking at surgical treatments as an option in stable and recalcitrant childhood vitiligo. Transplanted autologous cultured pure melanocytes are a well-established treatment option in stable and recalcitrant vitiligo in adults. Recently, the efficacy of transplanted autologous cultured pure melanocytes was looked at in children and adolescents compared with adults. Melanocytes were isolated from the roof of a suction blister and cultured and then the suspension was transplanted to laser-denuded skin in 12 children (8–12 years) and 20 adolescents (13–17 years) and compared with 70 adults. Satisfactory (repigmentation of 50% or more) results of repigmentation in the treated areas were comparable in children and adolescents to those seen in adults. This study suggests transplanted autologous cultured pure melanocytes may be considered in children and adolescents with stable or recalcitrant disease.[46]

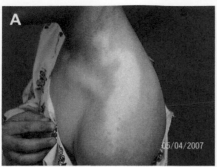 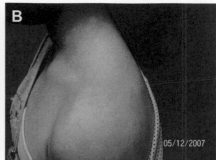

Fig. 2. (*A*) A 7-year-old girl with segmental vitiligo on the left shoulder before grafting. (*B*) Complete repigmentation 9 months after grafting. (*Courtesy of* Dr Sanjeev V. Mulekar.)

Another new and effective surgical technique used for stable vitiligo in adults is grafting using a noncultured epidermal suspension. Recently, 2 studies have implored this technique in children with some promising results. Both studies looked at the safety and efficacy of this procedure. The first study retrospectively looked at the long-term results of 25 children (ages ranged from 4–16 years) with stable (at least 6 months) segmental and focal vitiligo, which was treated with autologous noncultured cellular grafting. Of the patients with segmental lesions, 62% showed excellent repigmentation (95%–100% repigmentation), 15% showed good response (65%–94% repigmentation), 8% had a fair response (25%–64% repigmentation), and 15% had a poor response (0%–24% repigmentation) (**Fig. 2**). Seventy-five percent of focal lesions had an excellent response, 8% had a good response, 8% had a fair response, and 8% had a poor response. All patients who developed repigmentation retained the pigmentation until the conclusion of the follow-up (9–54 months).[47] The second study was a clinical trial in children and adolescents (8–17 years) with all types of vitiligo. Thirteen patients with a total of 19 lesions of stable vitiligo (generalized, segmental, and focal) for at least a year were transplanted and followed for a year postgrafting. Of the 19 lesions, 79% had greater than 90% repigmentation and the remaining 21% had 75% to 90% repigmentation after a year. No major adverse effects were noted. Only 1 recipient site infection occurred in this study.[48] Both studies obtained donor grafts using a split-graft technique with graft sizes one-third to one-tenth the size of the recipient site. In both studies, the procedures were well tolerated. A concern with using a split-thickness graft is the possibility of an unsightly scar at the donor site. In these studies, hyperpigmentation was the main finding at the donor sites, which improved over time. Overall, surgical treatments for vitiligo in children are promising but are not without risk. Candidates

should be those patients who have failed nonsurgical therapies, have stable disease, and do not demonstrate the Koebner phenomenon.

In conclusion, more clinical trials on treatment efficacy of common pediatric skin conditions have become available, although most studies have small sample sizes and further studies need to be done. Immunotherapy and laser-based therapies show promise for treatment of warts and MC as well as vitiligo and alopecia areata. Bleach baths, clindamycin, and β-lactam antibiotics seem logical empiric choices for treatment of superficial skin infections and impetiginized atopic dermatitis, even with increasing MRSA incidence. More work on systemic immunosuppressant therapies in vitiligo and alopecia areata needs to be done.

## REFERENCES

1. Coloe J, Morrell D. Cantharidin use among pediatric dermatologists in treatment of molluscum contagiosum. Pediatr Dermatol 2009;26:405–8.
2. Enns LL, Evans MS. Intralesional immunotherapy with Candida antigen for the treatment of molluscum contagiosum in children. Pediatr Dermatol 2011;28:254–8.
3. Maronn M, Salm C, Lyon V, et al. One-year experience with Candida antigen immunotherapy for warts and molluscum. Pediatr Dermatol 2008;25:189–92.
4. Myhre PE, Levy ML, Eichenfield LF, et al. Pharmacokinetics and safety of imiquimod 5% cream in the treatment of molluscum contagiosum in children. Pediatr Dermatol 2008;25:88–95.
5. Al-Mutairi N, Al-Doukhi A, Al-Faraq S, et al. Comparative study of the efficacy, safety, and acceptability of imiquimod 5% cream versus cryotherapy for molluscum contagiosum in children. Pediatr Dermatol 2010;27:388–94.
6. Simonart T, Maertelaer VD. Curettage treatment for molluscum contagiosum: a follow-up survey study. Br J Dermatol 2008;159:1144–7.

7. Hanna D, Hatami A, Powell J, et al. A prospective randomized trial comaring the efficacy and adverse effects of four recognized treatments of molluscum contagiosum in children. Pediatr Dermatol 2006;23:574–9.

8. Bard S, Shiman MI, Bellman B, et al. Treatment of facial molluscum contagiosum with trichloroacetic acid. Pediatr Dermatol 2009;26:425–6.

9. Chatproedprai S, Suwannakarn K, Wananukul S, et al. Efficacy of pulsed dyed laser (585 nm) in the treatment of molluscum contagiosum subtype 1. Southeast Asian J Trop Med Public Health 2007;38:849–54.

10. Boull C, Groth D. Update: treatment of cutaneous viral warts in children. Pediatr Dermatol 2011;28:217–29.

11. Choi MH, Seo SH, Kim IH, et al. Comparative study on the sustained efficacy of diphencyprone immunotherapy versus cryotherapy in viral warts. Pediatr Dermatol 2008;25:398–9.

12. Huang W, Morrell D. Successful treatment of recalcitrant warts with topical squaric acid in immunosuppressed child. Pediatr Dermatol 2008;25:275–6.

13. Yaghoobi R, Sadighha A, Baktash D. Evaluation of oral zinc sulfate effect on recalcitrant multiple viral warts: a randomized placebo-controlled clinical trial. J Am Acad Dermatol 2009;60:706–8.

14. Stefani M, Bottino G, Fontenelle E, et al. Efficacy comparison between cimetidine and zinc suphate in the treatment of multiple and recalcitrant warts. An Bras Dermatol 2009;84:23–9.

15. Yaghoobi R, Sadighha A, Baktash D. Oral zinc sulfate in the treatment of recalcitrant viral warts: randomized placebo-controlled clinical trial. Br J Dermatol 2002;146:423–31.

16. Gladsjo JA, Saenz AB, Bergman J, et al. 5% 5-Fluorouracil cream for treatment of verruca vulgaris in children. Pediatr Dermatol 2009;26:279–85.

17. Kwok CS, Holland R, Gibbs S. Efficacy of topical treatments for cutaneous warts: a meta-analysis and pooled analysis of randomized controlled trials. Br J Dermatol 2011;165:233–46.

18. Han TY, Lee JH, Lee CK, et al. Long-pulsed Nd:YAG laser treatment of warts: report on a series of 369 cases. J Korean Med Sci 2009;24:889–93.

19. Williams DJ, Cooper WO, Kaltenbach LA, et al. Comparative effectiveness of antibiotic treatment strategies for pediatric skin and soft-tissue infections. Pediatrics 2011;128:e479–87.

20. Chen AE, Carroll KC, Diener-West M, et al. Randomized controlled trial of cephalexin versus clindamycin for uncomplicated pediatric skin infections. Pediatrics 2011;127:e573–80.

21. Fritz SA, Camins BC, Eisenstein KA, et al. Effectiveness of measures to eradicate Staphylococcus aureus carriage in patients with community-associated skin and soft-tissue infections:

a randomized trial. Infect Control Hosp Epidemiol 2011;32:872–80.

22. Huang JT, Abrams M, Tlougan B, et al. Treatment of Staphylococcus aureus colonization in atopic dermatitis decreases disease severity. Pediatrics 2009;123:e808–14.

23. Travers JB, Kozman A, Yao Y, et al. Treatment outcomes of secondarily impetiginized pediatric atopic dermatitis lesions and the role of oral antibiotics. Pediatr Dermatol 2011;29:289–96.

24. Matiz C, Tom WL, Eichenfield LF, et al. Children with atopic dermatitis appear less likely to be infected with community acquired methicillin-resistant Staphylococcus aureus: the San Diego experience. Pediatr Dermatol 2011;28:6–11.

25. Alkhalifah A, Alsantali A, Wang E, et al. Alopecia areata update part II treatment. J Am Acad Dermatol 2010;62:191–202.

26. Joly P. The use of methotrexate alone or in combination with low dose oral corticosteroids in the treatment of alopecia totalis or universalis. J Am Acad Dermatol 2006;55:632–6.

27. Chartaux E, Joly P. Long-term follow-up of the efficacy of methotrexate alone or in combination with low doses of oral cortiscosteroids in the treatment of alopecia areat totalis or universalis. Ann Dermatol Venereol 2010;137:507–13.

28. Royer M, Bodemer C, Vabres P, et al. Efficacy and tolerability of methotrexate in severe childhood alopecia areata. Br J Dermatol 2011;165:407–10.

29. Myung IM, Lee SS, Lee Y. Prognostic factors in methylprednisolone pulse therapy for alopecia areata. J Dermatol 2011;38:767–72.

30. Kim BJ, Min SU, Park KY, et al. Combination therapy of cyclosporine and methylprednisolone on severe alopecia areata. J Dermatolog Treat 2008;19:216–20.

31. Goddard CJ, August PJ, Whorwell PJ. Alopecia totalis in a patient with Crohn's disease and its treatment with azathioprine. Postgrad Med J 1989;65:188–9.

32. Farshi S, Mansouri P, Safar F, et al. Could azathioprime be considered as a therapeutic alternative in the treatment of alopecia areata? A pilot study. Int J Dermatol 2010;49:1188–93.

33. Gundogan C, Greve B, Raulin C. Treatment of alopecia areata with the 308-nm xenon chloride excimer laser: case report of two successful treatments with the excimer laser. Lasers Surg Med 2004;34:86–90.

34. Zakaria W, Passeron T, Ostovari N, et al. 308-nm excimer laser therapy in alopecia areata. J Am Acad Dermatol 2004;51:837–8.

35. Raulin C, Gundogan C, Greve B, et al. Excimer laser therapy of alopecia areata—side-by-side evaluation of a representative area. J Dtsch Dermatol Ges 2005;3:524–6 [in German].

36. Al-Mutairi N. 308-nm excimer laser for the treatment of alopecia areata in children. Pediatr Dermatol 2009;26:547–50.

37. Tamesis ME, Morelli JG. Vitiligo treatment in childhood: a state of art review. Pediatr Dermatol 2010; 27:437–45.

38. Cho S, Zheng Z, Park YK, et al. The 308-nm excimer laser: a promising device for the treatment of childhood vitiligo. Photodermatol Photoimmunol Photomed 2011;27:24–9.

39. Passeron T, Ostovari N, Zakaria W, et al. Topical Tacrolimus and the 308-nm excimer laser: a synergistic combination for the treatment of vitiligo. Arch Dermatol 2004;140:1065–9.

40. Patel N, O'Haver J, Hansen R. Vitiligo therapy in children: a case for considering excimer laser treatment. Clin Pediatr 2010;49:823–9.

41. Hui-Lan Y, xiaio-Yan H, Jian-Yong F, et al. Combination of the 308-nm excimer laser with topical picrolimus for the treatment of childhood vitiligo. Pediatr Dermatol 2009;26:354–6.

42. Passi S, Gradinetti M, Maggio F, et al. Eperidermal oxidative stress in vitiligo. Arch Dermatol 1998;11:81–5.

43. Parsad D, Kanwar A. Oral minocycline in the treatment of vitiligo—a preliminary study. Dermatol Ther 2010;23:305–7.

44. Szczurko O, Shear N, Taddio A, et al. Ginkgo biloba for the treatment of vitiligo vulgaris: an open label pilot clinical trial. BMC Complement Altern Med 2011;11:21.

45. Gawkrodger DJ, Ormerod AD, Shaw L, et al. Guideline for the diagnosis and management of vitiligo. Br J Dermatol 2008;159:1051–76.

46. Hong WS, Hu DN, Qian GP, et al. Treatment of vitiligo in children and adolescents by autologous cultured pure melanocytes transplantation with comparison of efficacy to results in adults. J Eur Acad Dermatol Venereol 2011;25:538–43.

47. Mulekar SV, Al eisa A, Delvi MB, et al. Childhood vitiligo: a long-term study of localized vitiligo treated by noncultured cellular grafting. Pediatr Dermatol 2010; 27:132–6.

48. Shni K, Parsad D, Kanwar AJ. Noncultured epidermal suspension transplantation for the treatment of stable vitiligo in children and adolescents. Clin Exp Dermatol 2011;36:607–12.

# Imaging of Vascular Anomalies

Delma Y. Jarrett, MD*, Muhammad Ali, MD,
Gulraiz Chaudry, MB, ChB

## KEYWORDS

- Vascular anomalies • Vascular malformation • Hemangioma • Imaging

## KEY POINTS

- Vascular anomalies can be divided into two groups, tumors and malformations, on the basis of biologic behavior.
- Types of vascular tumors include infantile hemangioma and kaposiform hemangioendothelioma. Infantile hemangioma is seen as a well-defined mass with fast flow, whereas kaposiform hemangioendothelioma has poorly defined, infiltrative margins and is strongly associated with Kasabach-Merritt phenomenon.
- Low-flow malformations include venous and lymphatic malformations. LM can be subdivided into macrocystic, which demonstrate peripheral and septal enhancement, and microcystic, which appear more solid.
- Fast-flow vascular malformations include arteriovenous fistula and arteriovenous malformation. In arteriovenous fistula, there is a direct connection between the artery and vein, whereas in arteriovenous malformation, an intervening nidus is seen. Neither has an associated mass.

## INTRODUCTION

Vascular anomalies comprise a diverse group of conditions in the pediatric and adult age group. The subject is often complicated by the use of improper descriptive terminology. Although the biologic classification proposed by Mulliken and Glowacki in 1982[1] and later adopted by the International Society for the Study of Vascular Anomalies[2] substantially helped to resolve this dilemma, vague terminology continues to be used in the clinical setting and medical literature. Accurate characterization of vascular anomalies is crucial in predicting the clinical course, prognosis, and need for intervention. It is therefore important to adhere to a standard classification system in clinical assessment and radiologic characterization.

Mulliken and Glowacki divided vascular anomalies into two groups: hemangiomas and malformations, with the first category later expanded to include multiple vascular tumors in addition to hemangiomas. This distinction is based on

endothelial cell characteristics. Vascular tumors consist of proliferating cells with increased mitotic activity. Malformations arise from abnormal vascular channels in the absence of abnormally proliferating endothelium.[1,3]

Infantile hemangiomas (IH) are the most common type of vascular tumor; however, they must be distinguished from other vascular tumors including rapidly involuting congenital hemangiomas (RICH), noninvoluting congenital hemangiomas (NICH), kaposiform hemangioendothelioma (KHE), and tufted angioma.

Vascular malformations can be further divided into slow-flow, fast-flow, and mixed lesions. Slow-flow lesions include capillary, venous, and lymphatic malformations (LM). Fast-flow lesions are arteriovenous malformations (AVM) and arteriovenous fistulas (AVF).

## IMAGING

Although the diagnosis can sometimes be made clinically, radiologic assessment is often helpful

Harvard Medical School, Department of Radiology, Boston Children's Hospital, 300 Longwood Avenue, Boston, MA 02115, USA
* Corresponding author.
E-mail address: delma.jarrett@childrens.harvard.edu

Dermatol Clin 31 (2013) 251–266
http://dx.doi.org/10.1016/j.det.2012.12.004
0733-8635/13/$ – see front matter © 2013 Elsevier Inc. All rights reserved.

in the management of vascular anomalies, particularly for atypical or deep lesions, and is important for treatment planning. Ultrasound (US) and magnetic resonance imaging (MRI) are the mainstay of imaging vascular anomalies, with limited roles for radiography and computed tomography (CT).

US is a relatively accessible, noninvasive modality that can be performed in the often young patient population without sedation or ionizing radiation. With gray-scale imaging, the vascular anomaly can be characterized as cystic, composed of channels, or as a solid mass with well or poorly defined margins. Calcifications can be identified as echogenic foci with posterior shadowing. With Doppler imaging, one can assess for the presence and distribution of blood flow to the lesion. Spectral waveforms can determine if the flow is arterial or venous, and assess for the presence of shunting. Skin lesions should be imaged with a high-frequency linear transducer, although deeper lesions necessitate lower-frequency transducers.

MRI is superior to US in evaluating the extent of the lesion, including the tissue planes and adjacent structures involved. Routine sequences include short time inversion recovery (STIR)/T2-weighted images with fat saturation (FS), which for most vascular anomalies provide sharp contrast between the lesion and normal tissue. Depending on the appearance of these fluid-sensitive sequences, T1-weighted FS postcontrast images may be useful to assess perfusion to the anomaly. MR angiography (MRA) is sometimes helpful in the assessment of fast-flow vascular anomalies. Techniques include noncontrast imaging angiography using two-dimensional time-of-flight or phase-contrast imaging, or dynamic imaging with gadolinium-enhanced time resolved MRA, which allows the arterial and venous phases to be imaged separately, demonstrating feeding arteries, draining veins, and location of shunts. Large vessels can be imaged using spin echo (SE) sequences, where they appear as signal voids, or gradient recall echo (GRE) sequences, where vessels are bright. GRE images also demonstrate calcification and blood products, either from bleeding of the anomaly or from thrombus.

Radiographs may be used to assess the bony changes associated with vascular anomalies. These are almost always related to malformations rather than hemangiomas and include periosteal reaction, well-defined lucent lesions in the bone, leg length discrepancy, and overgrowth of the affected side.[4] CT is largely reserved for accurate evaluation of bone destruction.

# VASCULAR TUMORS
## Infantile Hemangiomas

### Background and clinical presentation

IH are the most common tumors of infancy, with risk factors including fair skin, prematurity, and female gender.[5] They are most commonly found in the head and neck region, followed by the trunk, then the extremities. Subtle skin findings are sometimes present at birth, although in most cases the diagnosis is made at 2 to 4 weeks of age. IH then typically undergo a 6- to 8-month period of rapid growth in neonatal life, plateauing at 10 to 12 months, followed by a period of involution lasting 1 to 7 years.[3]

The cutaneous manifestation depends on the depth of the tumor, with superficial lesions appearing raised and red ("strawberry appearance"), whereas the overlying skin can be normal with deeper lesions.[6]

### Radiologic imaging

**Ultrasound** The US appearance of IH depends on whether it is in the proliferating to plateau phase or the involuting phase. In the earlier phases, it appears as an echogenic, well-circumscribed soft tissue mass. Gray-scale imaging can occasionally demonstrate anechoic channels, corresponding to the high-flow vessels. Color Doppler imaging is better at demonstrating the vascularity, with high vessel density seen (five or more vessels in a square centimeter), and arterial and venous waveforms obtained (**Fig. 1**A, B).[6,7] Involuting IH are rarely imaged because they are unlikely to present a diagnostic dilemma at that stage, but have been described as isoechoic, difficult to differentiate from adjacent soft tissues, and with no demonstrable blood flow.[7]

**Magnetic resonance imaging** The MRI appearance of IH also depends on its stage of growth. During the proliferative and plateau phase, they are seen as focal, lobulated soft tissue masses that are isointense to muscle on T1-weighted images, hyperintense on T2-weighted images, and demonstrate homogeneous enhancement (see **Fig. 1**C–F).[8,9] SE and GRE sequences demonstrate enlarged high-flow vessels within the mass, although intralesional flow voids may be difficult to discern in early infancy. These features can help to distinguish IH from other tumors, such as sarcomas, which tend to enhance heterogeneously, and have a more random distribution of vessels.[8]

Histologically, involuting IH are replaced by fibrofatty tissue. This is reflected in their MRI appearance, where they follow the signal intensity of the surrounding fat. There is also a decrease in enhancement and visualized vessels.[8]

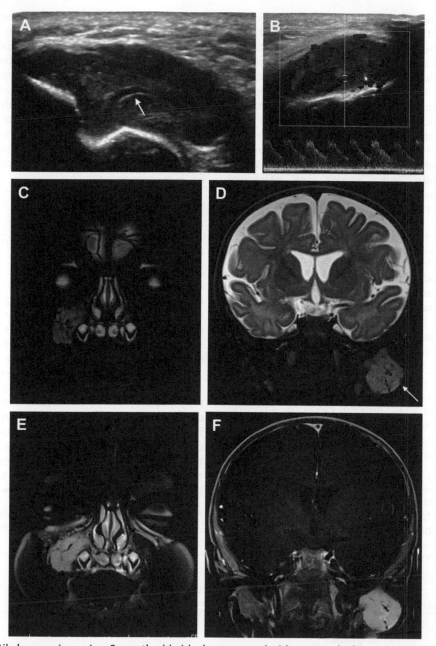

**Fig. 1.** Infantile hemangiomas in a 3-month-old girl who presented with mass under her right eye. (*A*) Ultrasound image of the right face lesion demonstrates a well-defined mass in the subcutaneous tissues, abutting the underlying bone, with hypoechoic channels corresponding to vessels (*arrow*). (*B*) Color Doppler image confirms that the mass is hypervascular, with low-resistance arterial waveforms. MRI was performed at 4 months of age. Coronal STIR images again show the mass below the right eye (*C*) and a second IH involving the left parotid gland (*D, arrow*). Both are hyperintense on fluid-weighted sequence with dark flow voids corresponding to vessels. After intravenous contrast administration the IH of the right face (*E*) and left parotid (*F*) demonstrate homogenous enhancement.

**Angiography** Angiographically, IH appear as well-circumscribed masses, with a lobular pattern of intense tissue staining. They are supplied by slightly enlarged but otherwise normal branches of systemic arteries, demonstrate a distinct tumor blush, and are drained by small veins that communicate with dilated but otherwise normal local veins. Typically, no direct AV shunting is seen within the mass.[10]

**Imaging associations** In certain cases, additional imaging is required to screen for other potential anomalies. The presence of five or more cutaneous hemangiomas raises suspicion for the presence of visceral, particularly liver, hemangiomas. These infants should be screened by US or MRI.[3] Large cervicofacial hemangiomas in a "beard" distribution are associated with subglottic airway hemangiomas, which in addition to direct imaging by endoscopy can be imaged MRI, CT, and high-resolution US.[11–13] Large facial hemangiomas are associated with PHACE syndrome.[13,14] Those in the lumbosacral region are associated with spinal anomalies including tethered cord, spinal lipoma, and intraspinal hemangioma, and with SACRAL and LUMBAR syndromes (**Table 1**).[15–17]

### Treatment and complications
Because IH spontaneously involute, most do not require treatment. However, medical therapy may be indicated if the location of the hemangioma compromises vision or the airway. Currently, the first line of treatment is oral administration of propranolol or steroids. In addition, if multifocal hepatic hemangiomas are identified, thyroid-function testing should be performed as soon as possible. The triiodothyronine deiodinase produced by these tumors peripherally deactivates T3 and these infants often require large doses of thyroid hormone replacement for correction.[18] Intralesional injections, embolization, and resection are generally reserved for a small minority of hemangiomas causing significant cosmetic deformity or cardiac failure.

## Congenital Hemangiomas

### Clinical presentation
In contrast to IH, CH reach their maximum size at the time of birth and can sometimes be diagnosed prenatally. Unlike IH, there is no gender predilection and the tumors do not test positive for glucose transported protein 1.[19] CH demonstrate two patterns of clinical progression. Most undergo rapid postnatal involution, resolving by 14 months of age, as a RICH. Alternatively, the CH never regresses and continues to grow proportionally with the child, and is called NICH.[20] Some of the lesions demonstrate initial rapid decrease in size and then plateau and remain unchanged. Therefore, it is possible that NICH represents a later stage of RICH in some patients.[19]

CH are usually solitary and often involve the head or the limbs near a joint.[20,21] The involved skin is usually blue or violaceous, with telengiectasias; a pale peripheral halo is more characteristic of NICH than RICH.[22]

### Radiologic imaging
**Ultrasound** The sonographic findings in CH are often similar to IH, with a fast-flow soft tissue mass seen in both cases (**Fig. 2**). Features more suggestive of CH are heterogeneity, calcifications, and increased conspicuity of intralesional vessels.[21]

RICH and NICH cannot initially be easily distinguished from each other by US. However, as they involute, RICH are characterized by tortuous compressible channels demonstrating venous flow. These correspond to the histologic finding of thin-walled drainage channels separated by fibrous tissue.[23] NICH are more likely to demonstrate microshunting,[21] manifested as increased turbulence or pulsatility in the venous waveforms.

**Magnetic resonance imaging** CH are isointense on T1- and hyperintense on T2-weighted images,

---

**Table 1**
**Syndromes associated with infantile hemangiomas**

| Syndrome | | IH Distribution |
|---|---|---|
| PHACE | Posterior fossa brain malformation<br>Hemangiomas<br>Arterial anomalies<br>Coarctation of the aorta and cardiac defects<br>Eye abnormalities | Large, facial |
| LUMBAR | Lower body IH and other skin defects<br>Urogenital anomalies and ulceration<br>Myelopathy<br>Bony deformities<br>Anoretal malformations, Arterial anomalies<br>Renal anomalies | Extensive of lower half of body, often involving entire limb |
| SACRAL | Spinal dysraphism<br>Anogenital<br>Cutaneous<br>Renal and urologic anomalies, associated with an<br>    angioma of lumbosacral localization | Perineal |

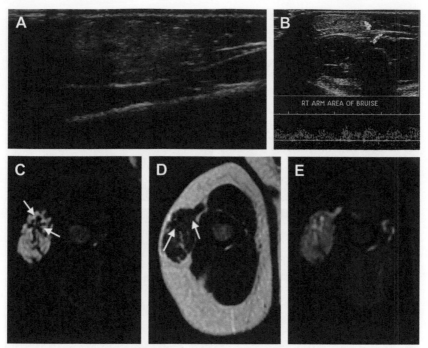

**Fig. 2.** RICH in 6-month-old boy with multiple vascular birthmarks, which rapidly regressed in the first yew years of life. (*A*) Sagittal ultrasound image of a right arm lesion shows a hyperechoic mass in the subcutaneous tissues. (*B*) Transversely oriented ultrasound image of the mass with color Doppler shows internal vascularity, with low-resistance arterial waveforms. MRI was performed at 8 months of age. Axial STIR (*C*) and axial T1 images (*D*) through the right arm lesion show a lesion that is hyperintense on the fluid-weighted sequence with prominent flow voids related to intralesional vessels (*arrows*). (*E*) On T1 FS image, after administration of intravenous gadolinium, there is homogeneous enhancement.

with intense enhancement after contrast administration. They are more likely to have heterogeneous enhancement and poorly defined borders than IH, although they still lack surrounding edema, which can be seen in more aggressive lesions (**Fig. 3**).[21] On SE and GRE sequences, feeding and draining vessels can be seen.

**Angiography** NICH demonstrate arterial feeding vessels, with tumor-like capillary blush. They have dilated draining veins as can be seen with AVF or AVM (**Fig. 3**). However, unlike these entities, NICH do not demonstrate early venous drainage.[20]

Because of their natural history, RICH are less likely to be assessed angiographically, but do demonstrate inhomogenous parenchymal staining; large, irregular, and disorganized feeding arteries; direct AV shunts; and intravascular thrombi.[24]

### Complications and treatment
Because of the rapid involution in most RICH cases, no treatment is required. In a few cases, there is redundant skin after involution with central fissuring and ulceration, which necessitates surgical resection.[22] NICH are surgically resected.

### Kaposiform Hemangioendothelioma
#### Background and clinical presentation
KHE is a rare vascular lesion that can be congenital, with 50% presenting at birth in one series,[25] but can also present later in childhood.[26] They grow rapidly, and are locally aggressive, but have been seen to spontaneously regress.[25,27,28] There is no gender preference. They often involve the trunk, extremities, retroperitoneum, and rarely the cervical/facial region. The overlying skin is red to purple in color with a rim of ecchymosis, and is warm and edematous to palpation.[25] Importantly, there is a frequent association with Kasabach Merritt phenomenon (KMP), a consumptive coagulopathy,[25] with 90% of cases of KMP occurring secondary to KHE.[26]

#### Ultrasound
On US, KHE has variable echogenicity. The margins are ill defined, a major distinguishing characteristic from IH (**Fig. 4**A, B). They may also contain foci of calcification, a feature not seen in IH. Although there have been reports of decreased vessel density compared with IH, color Doppler imaging characteristics cannot reliably differentiate the two lesions.[28]

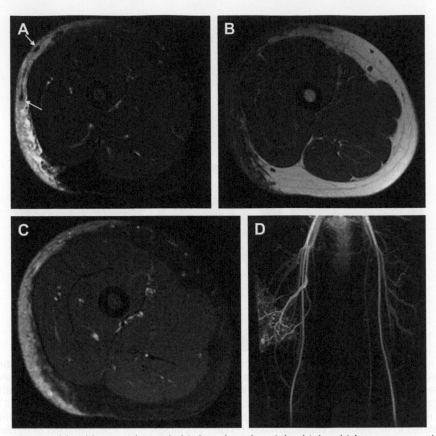

**Fig. 3.** NICH in 8-year-old girl born with purple birthmark on her right thigh, which grew proportionately with her. (*A*) Axial T2 FS image through the right thigh shows mass in the anterior subcutaneous tissues with poorly defined margins. It contains flow voids from prominent intralesional vessels (*arrows*). The mass is hypointense on T1 image (*B*) and demonstrates diffuse enhancement on T1 FS postcontrast image (*C*). (*D*) MR angiogram shows numerous prominent feeding arteries, draining veins, and tumor-like blush of the mass.

On MRI, KHE are seen as soft tissue masses that are hypointense to isointense to muscle on T1-weighted images, and heterogeneously hyperintense on T2-weighted images. They are infiltrative, extending to involve multiple tissue planes, with ill-defined borders, stranding in the subcutaneous tissues, and overlying skin thickening. On postgadolinium T1-weighted images, the tumor demonstrates a strong reticular enhancement pattern, corresponding to the same pattern seen on T2-weighted images (**Fig. 4**C–E). Associated prominent vascular channels are seen either on postcontrast images or as flow voids on SE sequences.[25,29] Compared with IH where the size of the feeding and draining vessels is proportional to the size of the tumor, the vessels of KHE are small relative to tumor size. KHE may contain hemosiderin, blood products, or fibrosis,[25] which are best demonstrated on GRE images.

### Complications and treatment

There is significant mortality associated with KHE, ranging from 10% to 30%, with the rate higher for retroperitoneal tumors.[25–27] This is caused by the sequela of local invasion and the high association with KMP. The mainstay of treatment is medical therapy with agents including vincristine, corticosteroids, ticlopindine, interferon-$\alpha$,[30] and propranolol.[27] Surgical resection may be possible in localized cases.

## SLOW-FLOW VASCULAR MALFORMATIONS
### Venous Malformation

#### Background and clinical presentation

VM are congenital malformations characterized by dilated venous channels deficient in smooth muscle. These channels also lack normal valves and have stagnant flow.[31] VM may take many different forms, ranging from varicosities and ectasias to complex channels and localized spongiform masses.[3]

Like all vascular malformations, they are present at birth. VM do not regress and grow proportionately with the patient, with periods of enlargement during puberty and pregnancy because of hormonal influence. On physical examination, VM

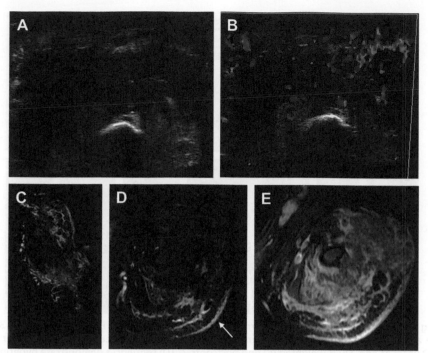

**Fig. 4.** KHE in the upper left arm of an 11-month-old boy. (*A*) Transverse US mage shows poorly defined heterogeneous soft tissue mass of the arm. (*B*) Color Doppler demonstrates hypervascularity. Coronal (*C*) and axial (*D*) T2 FS images demonstrate an infiltrative hyperintense lesion involving multiple tissue planes, with areas of skin thickening (*arrow*). (*E*) Axial T1 FS postcontrast images show heterogeneous enhancement.

are soft, compressible, and nonpulsatile. The overlying skin may be normal or have a bluish tinge. Maneuvers that increase venous pressure (dependant position, crying, Valsalva) cause them to increase in size.[32,33] VM most commonly involve the head and neck, followed by the extremities, with truncal involvement less frequently seen. Although skin involvement is common, VM can extend to or have isolated involvement of muscle, bone, and abdominal organs.[34]

### Radiographic imaging

**Ultrasound** There is a varied US appearance of VM that reflects the different morphologies of this entity, ranging from the hypoechoic or heterogeneous spongiform appearance of localized cavernous spaces, to anechoic vascular channels of dysplastic veins (**Fig. 5**).[7,33,35] When Doppler flow is present, it is monophasic, low-velocity flow.[33] Twenty percent of VM show no flow on Doppler imaging because of either undetectably slow flow or true lack of flow secondary to thrombosis.[34] In this case, the lack of cystic cavities can help distinguish them from LM.[33] Phleboliths can be seen as hyperechoic, shadowing foci.

**Magnetic resonance imaging** STIR or T2 FS sequences are the most useful to assess the extent of the lesion, which can often be underestimated

on clinical examination. VM appear as hyperintense on T2-weighted images and hypointense on T1-weighted images (**Fig. 5**). With hemorrhage or thrombosis, the VM may demonstrate increased heterogeneous signal on T1-weighted images.[34,36] Fluid-fluid levels can be seen in regions of low or no flow. These malformations commonly extend from the subcutaneous fat to involve muscle and fascia, sometimes involving the bone, tendons, and joints. In the extremities, they tend to be oriented along the long axis, parallel to fascial planes.[31] The characteristic phleboliths of VM and potential blood products/hemosiderin are best seen on GRE sequences.

Postcontrast, there is often marked but heterogeneous enhancement.[34,36] On SE sequences, there are no flow voids, as can be seen with high-flow vascular anomalies.[36] No prominent feeding artery or draining vein is seen.[31] Although two-dimensional time-of-flight venography may demonstrate dysplastic veins, it is rarely required to either establish a diagnosis or guide further management.

Initial assessment of VM should include a wide field of view, to assess the full extent of the lesion. This is important because incomplete resection of a VM can cause flare in size and symptoms of the residual malformation.[31]

MRI may also demonstrate soft tissue changes related to the VM, such as fatty replacement,

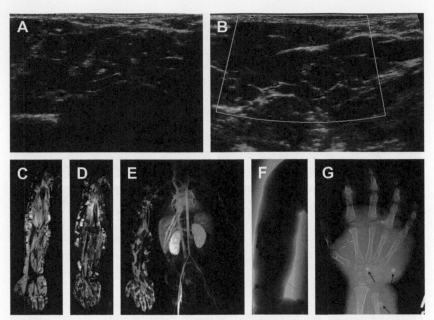

**Fig. 5.** Young girl with extensive venous malformation of the right arm. US images obtained at 3 years of age demonstrate a hypoechoic, spongiform malformation (*A*) with little flow seen on color Doppler (*B*). MRI also obtained at 3 years of age. Fluid-weighted (*C*) and postcontrast (*D*) sequences demonstrate hyperintense tubular and lobulated structures involving all the soft tissue layers with heterogeneous enhancement after contrast. Postcontrast MRI (*E*) and conventional venography (*F*) clearly demonstrate the associated abnormal ectatic veins. (*G*) Radiograph of the right hand shows multiple phleboliths (*arrows*).

atrophy of the adjacent musculature, or hypertrophy of the subcutaneous fat compared with the contralateral side.[31]

**Angiography** Angiographic evaluation of VM is best performed with direct intralesional injection of contrast. With arterial injection, normal arteries are seen with no evidence of AV shunting. There is also limited assessment of the VM, because of poor opacification of proximal veins caused by slow flow.[35,36] Therefore, there is no role for arteriography in the diagnosis or management of VM.

Direct venography and intralesional injection are sometimes better in characterizing the VM, but visualization is limited to the cannulated vessels and associated draining vein (**Fig. 5**F).[36] Using US guidance, a needle is advanced into the VM and a small volume of low osmolarity iodinated contrast is injected. Based on the venographic findings, some have characterized the VM as one of four types: (1) isolated VM with no visible draining veins, (2) drainage into normal veins, (3) dysplastic draining veins, and (4) venous ectasia. Type 3 or 4 lesions are higher risk for sclerotherapy because of the potential for distal embolization.[32,37]

**Radiographs and CT** Radiographs may reveal the presence of a soft tissue mass or phleboliths, which are highly suggestive of VM (**Fig. 5**G).

However, the main use of radiographs and CT is in assessing skeletal manifestation of VM, such as direct osseous involvement or associated bony overgrowth. The malformations appear as hypodense or heterogeneous in density, with slow, peripheral enhancement. CT is not as helpful as MRI in characterizing the type or extent of the lesion.[34] Extension of the malformation into the deep musculature and bone is best appreciated on MRI. Therefore, there is no role for routine use of CT in the assessment of VM.

*Treatment and complications*
VM are referred for treatment because of pain, cosmetic issues, or loss of function caused by location. They can cause localized intravascular coagulopathy, which is a separate entity from KMP.[3] Sclerotherapy is the primary treatment in most cases, with agents including Ethibloc (Ethnor Laboratories/Ethicon, Norderstedt, Germany), sodium tetradecyl sulfate, and absolute alcohol.[37] Direct injection and venography are performed before sclerotherapy to assess the VM and the deep venous anatomy. Local complications of sclerotherapy include skin necrosis, ulceration, and peripheral nerve damage. Rare systemic complications can occur if ethanol passes into the systemic circulation, causing hemolysis, renal toxicity, and cardiac arrest.[34]

Multiple treatments are often necessary. Interim MRI can be performed to assess response to treatment but there should be a delay between sclerotherapy and repeat imaging of several months to allow posttreatment inflammation to resolve. After treatment, the VM usually demonstrates increased heterogeneity on T1- and T2-weighted images and decrease in size. Postcontrast imaging can show potential areas of residual perfusion.[34] However, because the diagnosis is already established, the use of contrast is rarely necessary. Surgical resection may be performed if sclerotherapy does not provide adequate results.

## Lymphatic Malformation

### Background and clinical presentation
LM result from disordered development of the lymphatic system. Dilated lymphatic channels lack normal communication to the lymphatic system.[38] Depending on the size of these spaces, they can be characterized as microcystic, macrocystic, or mixed. There is considerable variability in the criteria used to designate a malformation as microcystic or macrocystic. At our institution, only lesions or parts of lesions containing cysts that are too small to be accessed and aspirated with a hypodermic needle are designated as microcystic.

Although congenital, only 50% of LM are seen at birth, with 90% diagnosed by the age of 2.[39] A total of 70% to 80% involve the head-neck region.[40] They usually present as asymptomatic masses, which enlarge because of hemorrhage or infection. The overlying skin usually appears normal, but may have capillary staining or cutaneous blebs or vesicles, which are pathognomonic for LM.[3] A small minority have been reported to spontaneously regress.[41]

### Radiologic imaging
**Ultrasound** Macrocystic LM appear as cysts, sometimes containing echogenic debris. No blood flow is identified within the cavities themselves, although small arteries and veins may be seen within the cyst walls or intervening stroma (**Fig. 6**A).[7] In microcystic LM, the individual cysts are too small to discern. They appear as echogenic regions with soft tissue thickening (**Fig. 7**A).

**Magnetic resonance imaging** Macrocystic LM are isointense to hypointense on T1-weighted and hyperintense on fluid sensitive/T2-weighted images (see **Fig. 6**). Fluid-fluid levels are common, especially when there is associated hemorrhage. They demonstrate no or minimal peripheral enhancement involving the cyst walls. The venous channels are usually normal, although occasionally large or anomalous veins can be seen.[8,42]

As on US, the individual cysts of microcystic LM cannot be discerned. They appear as a region of diffuse hypointense signal on T1-weighted images and hyperintense on T2-weighted images. Microcystic LM can on occasion show mild diffuse enhancement, which can lead to confusion with a solid mass (see **Fig. 7**).[8]

### Complications and treatment
In the extremity, LM can cause local gigantisim, with bony and soft tissue overgrowth. Diffuse LM of the chest can cause chronic chylous effusion, and in the gastrointestinal tract a protein-losing enteropathy. In Gorham-Stout disease, LM of the bone and surrounding soft tissue causes osteolysis.[3]

The two most common complications are bleeding and hemorrhage.[3] LM can cause significant morbidity depending on the area of involvement (eg, causing mass effect on the trachea in neck and mediastinal involvement, or speech difficulties if the tongue is involved). Treatment options include sclerotherapy and surgical resection. Sclerotherapy is primarily effective for macrocystic LM, or the macrocystic component of a mixed lesion, with agents including bleomycin, Ethibloc, ethanol, OK-432 (Chugai Pharmaceutical Co, Ltd, Tokyo, Japan), doxycycline, and sodium tetradecyl sulfate.[39,41,43] Microcystic LM has a much less favorable response to sclerotherapy, although there have been encouraging reports with the use of intralesional bleomycin.[44,45] Complete resection is more easily accomplished with macrocystic LM than the more infiltrative and diffuse microcystic LM.[39] When possible, microcystic LM are managed conservatively.

## FAST-FLOW LESIONS: AVM AND AVF
### Background and Clinical Presentation

AVM are rare, resulting from an error in vascular development. They are composed of a nidus of anomalous connections between arteries and veins without intervening capillary bed. Like all vascular malformations, they are present at birth, although they may not be clinically apparent until later. On examination, AVM may present as a pulsatile mass with thrill, warmth, and redness.[8] Clinically, they can be categorized according to the Schobinger classification: stage 1, quiescence; stage 2, expansion (with enlargement of the AVM); stage 3, destruction (skin ulceration and bleeding); and stage 4, decompensation (cardiac failure).[46,47]

AVM expand over time, not because of cellular proliferation, but related to increased blood flow and the recruitment of adjacent normal vessels by shunts across the low-resistance arteriovenous

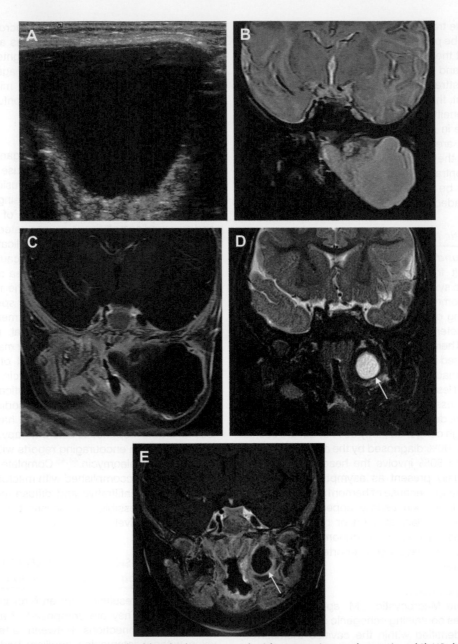

**Fig. 6.** Macrocystic LM in a 2-month-old girl who presented with upper airway obstruction. (*A*) US shows large anechoic cyst. (*B*) Coronal fluid-sensitive sequence demonstrates a hyperintense macrocystic lesion, with more complex lower-intensity component medially, reflecting hemorrhage. (*C*) Postcontrast coronal T1 FS image shows only peripheral enhancement. Patient underwent three sclerotherapy treatments with doxycycline, with significant decrease in size of the LM as seen on coronal FSEIR (*D*) and T1 FS postcontrast (*E*) images (*arrow*).

connections. Like VM, puberty and pregnancy can cause progression of the lesion.[47] AVM can also enlarge because of trauma, including the iatrogenic trauma of biopsy, ligation, or partial excision.[8,47]

AVF may be congenital or posttraumatic. Unlike AVM, there is usually a single arteriovenous communication present. However, if long-standing, AVF can also recruit additional vessels, simulating AVM.[48]

## Radiologic Imaging

US imaging shows no soft tissue mass. Multiple, enlarged subcutaneous arteries and veins are present, with high-flow, low-resistance wave forms in the arteries and arterialized wave forms in the draining veins.[7,8]

Similarly on MRI, the dominant feature of AVM and AVF are the dilated, often tortuous feeding

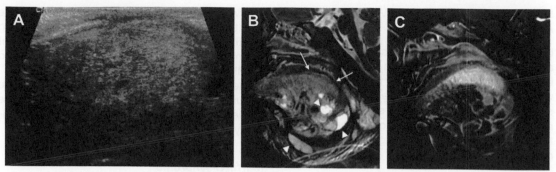

**Fig. 7.** A 2-year-old girl with microcystic LM of the tongue. (*A*) Ultrasound of the tongue shows heterogenous echotexture with innumberable hyperehcoic foci corresponding to the walls of the microcysts. Sagittal T2 FS image (*B*) shows soft tissue thickening and increased T2 signal within the tongue (*arrow*) with enhancement post-contrast (*C*). There is also a macrocystic component in the submandibular region that is bright on fluid-sensitive sequence (*B, arrowheads*), with only peripheral/septal enhancement after contrast (*C*).

arteries and draining veins with the absence of a mass (**Fig. 8**). These can be seen on SE sequences as flow-related signal void or as bright signal on GRE.[8,31] There may be edema and enhancement in the surrounding tissues, although no focal mass is present.[8] Similar to VM, associated soft tissue changes may be present, including fatty infiltration of the adjacent musculature, and prominence of subcutaneous fat compared with the contralateral side.[30] The enlarged feeding arteries, draining veins and nidus with shunt can be confirmed with angiography.[8]

## Complications and Treatment

AVM and AVF cause pain and ulceration secondary to ischemia from steal phenomenon. The shunting causes increased cardiac output.[3]

Treatment of AVM is complex. Options include surgery, embolization, or a combination of the two, although complete cure is often not achieved.

The treatment is primarily aimed at symptom relief and decreasing deformity. Embolization can be used preoperatively to reduce blood loss, or as primary therapy for lesions not amenable to surgery. Embolization agents include n-butyl cyanoacrylate, Onyx (ev3, Irvine, CA, USA), and ethanol. Surgery offers the best long-term outcome, but recurrence rates are still high, particularly if the AVM is not small and localized. Incomplete excision can lead to worsening of the malformation. The target of treatment should be the nidus of the AVM. It is important that proximal feeding arteries not be ligated with surgery or occluded with embolization because subsequent recanalization and vasculogenesis stimulate enlargement, and access to the nidus would be blocked for future embolization.[46,49]

AVF can be treated by obliterating the anomalous arteriovenous connection, most commonly with coils. As with AVM, occluding the proximal feeding artery leads to poor response.[50]

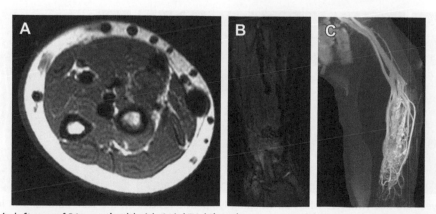

**Fig. 8.** AVM in left arm of 21-month-old girl. Axial T1 (*A*) and coronal STIR (*B*) images show large flow voids in the subcutaneous tissues and muscles corresponding to dilated arteries and veins. By 8 years of age, the AVM has progressed with markedly dilated, tortuous arteries and veins seen on postcontrast MR angiogram (*C*).

# SYNDROMES ASSOCIATED WITH VASCULAR ANOMALIES

Like IH, vascular malformations are also seen in a variety of syndromes, which can be grouped into those containing slow-flow lesions and those with fast-flow lesions. The role of imaging is to delineate the individual fast- or slow-flow components because each entity requires specifically tailored treatment, and to diagnose associated complications.

## Slow-Flow Combined Vascular Anomaly Syndromes

### Klippel-Trénaunay syndrome

Klippel-Trénaunay syndrome (KTS) affects one lower extremity in 95% of patients and is defined by at least two of the following abnormalities: cutaneous capillary malformations (port-wine stain) of the affected limb; VM or varicose veins; or soft tissue or bony overgrowth of the affected limb.[51,52] The port-wine stain is the most common feature, seen in 98% of patients.[52] KTS is frequently associated with persistent embryologic veins including the lateral vein of the thigh (also known as the marginal vein or the vein of Servelle), and persistent sciatic veins. There may be aplasia or hypoplasia of the lymphatic trunks, with associated lymphedema and cutaneous lymphatic vesicles; anomalies of the deep venous system, including aneurysmal dilatation, duplication, aplasia, and hypoplasia.[51,53–55]

At the orthopedic level, imaging is useful in assessing bony overgrowth, with the affected limb demonstrating increased size longitudinally and circumferentially. The limb overgrowth continues until physeal closure. It is best assessed with radiographs. In the case of lower-extremity involvement, frontal view of the legs from the hips to the ankles can be obtained to assess leg length discrepancy, and aid in possible treatment planning. Soft tissue overgrowth can be assessed by MRI.[56]

The LM and venous anomalies of KTS can be evaluated by the same techniques used for these entities in isolation, namely US, MRI, and venography (**Fig. 9**).

### Maffucci syndrome

Maffucci syndrome (MS) is the combination of enchondromas and VM, with bony and vascular lesions usually appearing in childhood. The enchondromas are most common in the hands and feet. There is a significant risk of malignant degeneration to chondrosarcoma with a wide range of reported incidence from 15% to 40%.[56–58] Patient's with MS also have an increased risk of noncartilaginous tumors, which is why the syndrome has been thought of as a generalized mesodermal dysplasia. The overall malignancy risk has been reported from 23% to 100%.[57] Reported neoplastic associations include spindle cell hemangioedotheliomas, ovarian tumors, and fibrosarcoma.[57,59]

In assessing the bony changes of MS, radiographs are particularly helpful to visualize the enchondromas, which appear as lucent expansile bony lesions, demonstrating the ring and arc appearance of cartilaginous matrix (**Fig. 10**A). Rapidly expanding lesions should be followed to assess for evidence of soft tissue mass and cortical destruction, which may indicate malignant degeneration. This can be further assessed by MRI, although biopsy is typically needed for confirmation.

The soft tissue abnormalities of MS are best evaluated by MRI (**Fig. 10**B), although radiographs

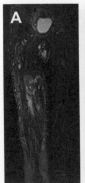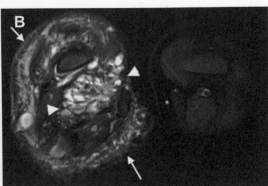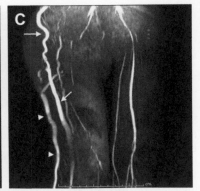

**Fig. 9.** A 3-year-old boy with KTS who had weeping lymphatic vesicles on the skin. Coronal STIR image of the right lower extremity (*A*) and axial T2 FS image through the distal femur (*B*) demonstrating subcutaneous microcystic LM (*arrows*) and intramuscular VM (*arrowheads*). (*C*) Two-dimensional time-of-flight MR venography shows persistent sciatic vein (*arrows*) and large marginal vein (*arrowheads*).

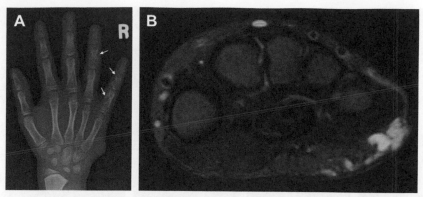

**Fig. 10.** Maffucci syndrome in a 9-year-old boy. (*A*) Frontal radiograph of the right hand shows lucent bone lesions consistent with enchondromas (*arrows*), and soft tissue mass adjacent to the fifth metacarpal. (*B*) Axial fluid-sensitive sequence demonstrates the mass represents a venous malformation.

may demonstrate phleboliths in the soft tissues related to the VM.

### Blue rubber bleb nevus syndrome

This syndrome is characterized by VM that involve the skin and viscera, predominately the gastrointestinal tract.[60] The name comes from the appearance of the skin lesions, which are small (millimeters to 4 cm) bluish protuberances that feel rubbery.[61,62]

The superficial VM can be imaged using US with Doppler, demonstrating the low flow in the lesions; MRI is needed to assess deeper lesions, with potential bone and joint involvement and solid organ involvement (**Fig. 11**).[52] Percutaneous contrast injection of the VM under fluoroscopy is used as a precursor to sclerotherapy in skin lesions.[61] The gastrointestinal tract lesions can be assessed with a variety of modalities, including barium studies, CT, MRI, endoscopy, or video capsule endoscopy. Patients with gastrointestinal VM may have anemia secondary to persistent bleeding and can be treated surgically.[63]

There can be associated skeletal deformity, with pressure effects on the bone from the VM or bony hypertrophy. Joint involvement can cause pain or decreased range of motion.[62]

### Fast-Flow Combined Vascular Anomaly Syndromes

#### Parkes Weber syndrome

Parkes Weber syndrome (PWS) must be distinguished from KTS. It is also characterized by cutaneous capillary malformation, with hypertrophy of the affected limb. However, it features AVF, making it a high-flow vascular syndrome lacking the low-flow venous and LM of KTS. The marginal vein of Servelle is not associated with PWS and there tends to be less musculoskeletal involvement.[64]

The AVF of PWS may be imaged using US with Doppler, although it may be challenging to demonstrate the full extent of the lesion. Alternatively, dynamic MRA or digital subtraction angiography can be performed, demonstrating enlarged feeding arteries and early draining veins (**Fig. 12**).[55] Because of the AVF, patients with PWS can have skin ulcerations and high-output cardiac failure, which can be treated with transarterial embolization of the fistula.[55]

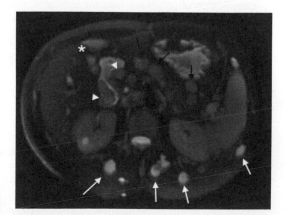

**Fig. 11.** A 41-year-old woman with blue rubber bleb nevus syndrome. Axial T2 FS image shows lobulated T2 hyperintense lesions in the soft tissues of the back consistent with venous malformations (*white arrows*). There are also gastrointestinal tract VM involving the duodenum (*arrowheads*), visceral malformations of the liver (*asterisk*), and in the peripancreatic region (*black arrows*).

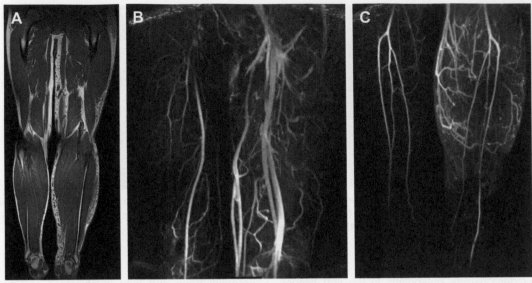

**Fig. 12.** A 17-year-old boy with Parkes Weber syndrome. (*A*) Coronal T1 image of the legs shows overgrowth of the left leg, affecting soft tissues and bone, with 2 cm measured leg length discrepancy. MR angiogram of the upper (*B*) and lower (*C*) leg show increased size of the arteries of the left thigh compared with the right, and increased size and number of draining veins, which opacify early.

## SUMMARY

US and MRI are the most useful imaging modalities in the evaluation of vascular anomalies. The lesions can be accurately characterized by imaging as hemangiomas or malformations, which can be further subdivided into fast flow or slow flow. Key imaging criteria in differentiating the various vascular anomalies include the presence or absence of a soft tissue mass, the flow characteristics of the lesion, and the pattern of enhancement with contrast.

## REFERENCES

1. Mulliken JB, Glowacki J. Hemangiomas and vascular malformations in infants and children: a classification based on endothelial characteristics. Plast Reconstr Surg 1982;69:412–22.
2. Dubois J, Alison M. Vascular anomalies: what a radiologist needs to know. Pediatr Radiol 2010;40:895–905.
3. Mulliken JB, Fishman SJ, Burrows PE. Vascular anomalies. Curr Probl Surg 2000;37:517–84.
4. Breugem CC, Maas M, Breugem SJ, et al. Vascular malformations of the lower limb with osseous involvement. J Bone Joint Surg Br 2003;85:399–405.
5. Haggstrom AN, Drolet BA, Baselga E, et al. Prospective study of infantile hemangiomas: demographic, prenatal, and perinatal characteristics. J Pediatr 2007;150:291–4.
6. Dubois J, Patriquin HB, Garel L, et al. Soft-tissue hemangiomas in infants and children: diagnosis using Doppler sonography. AJR Am J Roentgenol 1998;171:247–52.
7. Paltiel HJ, Burrows PE, Kozakewich HP, et al. Soft-tissue vascular anomalies: utility of US for diagnosis. Radiology 2000;214:747–54.
8. Konez O, Burrows PE. Magnetic resonance of vascular anomalies. Magn Reson Imaging Clin N Am 2002;10:363–88, vii.
9. Meyer JS, Hoffer FA, Barnes PD, et al. Biological classification of soft-tissue vascular anomalies: MR correlation. AJR Am J Roentgenol 1991;157:559–64.
10. Burrows PE, Mulliken JB, Fellows KE, et al. Childhood hemangiomas and vascular malformations: angiographic differentiation. AJR Am J Roentgenol 1983;141:483–8.
11. Koplewitz BZ, Springer C, Slasky BS, et al. CT of hemangiomas of the upper airways in children. AJR Am J Roentgenol 2005;184:663–70.
12. Rossler L, Rothoeft T, Teig N, et al. Ultrasound and colour Doppler in infantile subglottic haemangioma. Pediatr Radiol 2011;41:1421–8.
13. Haggstrom AN, Skillman S, Garzon MC, et al. Clinical spectrum and risk of PHACE syndrome in cutaneous and airway hemangiomas. Arch Otolaryngol Head Neck Surg 2011;137:680–7.
14. Frieden IJ, Reese V, Cohen D. PHACE syndrome. The association of posterior fossa brain malformations, hemangiomas, arterial anomalies, coarctation of the aorta and cardiac defects, and eye abnormalities. Arch Dermatol 1996;132:307–11.
15. Iacobas I, Burrows PE, Frieden IJ, et al. LUMBAR: association between cutaneous infantile hemangiomas of

the lower body and regional congenital anomalies. J Pediatr 2010;157:795–801.e1–7.

16. Schumacher WE, Drolet BA, Maheshwari M, et al. Spinal dysraphism associated with the cutaneous lumbosacral infantile hemangioma: a neuroradiological review. Pediatr Radiol 2012;42:315–20.

17. Stockman A, Boralevi F, Taieb A, et al. SACRAL syndrome: spinal dysraphism, anogenital, cutaneous, renal and urologic anomalies, associated with an angioma of lumbosacral localization. Dermatology 2007;214:40–5.

18. Huang SA, Tu HM, Harney JW, et al. Severe hypothyroidism caused by type 3 iodothyronine deiodinase in infantile hemangiomas. N Engl J Med 2000;343:185–9.

19. Mulliken JB, Enjolras O. Congenital hemangiomas and infantile hemangioma: missing links. J Am Acad Dermatol 2004;50:875–82.

20. Enjolras O, Mulliken JB, Boon LM, et al. Noninvoluting congenital hemangioma: a rare cutaneous vascular anomaly. Plast Reconstr Surg 2001;107:1647–54.

21. Gorincour G, Kokta V, Rypens F, et al. Imaging characteristics of two subtypes of congenital hemangiomas: rapidly involuting congenital hemangiomas and non-involuting congenital hemangiomas. Pediatr Radiol 2005;35:1178–85.

22. Krol A, MacArthur CJ. Congenital hemangiomas: rapidly involuting and noninvoluting congenital hemangiomas. Arch Facial Plast Surg 2005;7:307–11.

23. Rogers M, Lam A, Fischer G. Sonographic findings in a series of rapidly involuting congenital hemangiomas (RICH). Pediatr Dermatol 2002;19:5–11.

24. Konez O, Burrows PE, Mulliken JB, et al. Angiographic features of rapidly involuting congenital hemangioma (RICH). Pediatr Radiol 2003;33:15–9.

25. Sarkar M, Mulliken JB, Kozakewich HP, et al. Thrombocytopenic coagulopathy (Kasabach-Merritt phenomenon) is associated with Kaposiform hemangioendothelioma and not with common infantile hemangioma. Plast Reconstr Surg 1997;100:1377–86.

26. Lyons LL, North PE, Mac-Moune Lai F, et al. Kaposiform hemangioendothelioma: a study of 33 cases emphasizing its pathologic, immunophenotypic, and biologic uniqueness from juvenile hemangioma. Am J Surg Pathol 2004;28:559–68.

27. Hermans DJ, van Beynum IM, van der Vijver RJ, et al. Kaposiform hemangioendothelioma with Kasabach-Merritt syndrome: a new indication for propranolol treatment. J Pediatr Hematol Oncol 2011;33:e171–3.

28. Dubois J, Garel L, David M, et al. Vascular soft-tissue tumors in infancy: distinguishing features on Doppler sonography. AJR Am J Roentgenol 2002; 178:1541–5.

29. Chen YJ, Wang CK, Tien YC, et al. MRI of multifocal kaposiform haemangioendothelioma without Kasabach-Merritt phenomenon. Br J Radiol 2009; 82:e51–4.

30. Lopez V, Marti N, Pereda C, et al. Successful management of Kaposiform hemangioendothelioma with Kasabach-Merritt phenomenon using vincristine and ticlopidine. Pediatr Dermatol 2009;26:365–6.

31. Rak KM, Yakes WF, Ray RL, et al. MR imaging of symptomatic peripheral vascular malformations. AJR Am J Roentgenol 1992;159:107–12.

32. Dubois JM, Sebag GH, De Prost Y, et al. Soft-tissue venous malformations in children: percutaneous sclerotherapy with Ethibloc. Radiology 1991;180: 195–8.

33. Trop I, Dubois J, Guibaud L, et al. Soft-tissue venous malformations in pediatric and young adult patients: diagnosis with Doppler US. Radiology 1999;212: 841–5.

34. Dubois J, Soulez G, Oliva VL, et al. Soft-tissue venous malformations in adult patients: imaging and therapeutic issues. Radiographics 2001;21: 1519–31.

35. Laor T, Burrows PE, Hoffer FA. Magnetic resonance venography of congenital vascular malformations of the extremities. Pediatr Radiol 1996;26:371–80.

36. Claudon M, Upton J, Burrows PE. Diffuse venous malformations of the upper limb: morphologic characterization by MRI and venography. Pediatr Radiol 2001;31:507–14.

37. Puig S, Aref H, Chigot V, et al. Classification of venous malformations in children and implications for sclerotherapy. Pediatr Radiol 2003;33:99–103.

38. Cahill AM, Nijs EL. Pediatric vascular malformations: pathophysiology, diagnosis, and the role of interventional radiology. Cardiovasc Intervent Radiol 2011; 34:691–704.

39. Boardman SJ, Cochrane LA, Roebuck D, et al. Multimodality treatment of pediatric lymphatic malformations of the head and neck using surgery and sclerotherapy. Arch Otolaryngol Head Neck Surg 2010;136:270–6.

40. Puig S, Casati B, Staudenherz A, et al. Vascular low-flow malformations in children: current concepts for classification, diagnosis and therapy. Eur J Radiol 2005;53:35–45.

41. Nehra D, Jacobson L, Barnes P, et al. Doxycycline sclerotherapy as primary treatment of head and neck lymphatic malformations in children. J Pediatr Surg 2008;43:451–60.

42. Kern S, Niemeyer C, Darge K, et al. Differentiation of vascular birthmarks by MR imaging. An investigation of hemangiomas, venous and lymphatic malformations. Acta Radiol 2000;41:453–7.

43. Shiels WE II, Kenney BD, Caniano DA, et al. Definitive percutaneous treatment of lymphatic malformations of the trunk and extremities. J Pediatr Surg 2008;43:136–9 [discussion: 40].

44. Yang Y, Sun M, Ma Q, et al. Bleomycin A5 sclerotherapy for cervicofacial lymphatic malformations. J Vasc Surg 2011;53:150–5.

45. Bai Y, Jia J, Huang XX, et al. Sclerotherapy of microcystic lymphatic malformations in oral and facial regions. J Oral Maxillofac Surg 2009;67:251–6.

46. Greene AK, Orbach DB. Management of arteriovenous malformations. Clin Plast Surg 2011;38:95–106.

47. Kohout MP, Hansen M, Pribaz JJ, et al. Arteriovenous malformations of the head and neck: natural history and management. Plast Reconstr Surg 1998;102:643–54.

48. Lawdahl RB, Routh WD, Vitek JJ, et al. Chronic arteriovenous fistulas masquerading as arteriovenous malformations: diagnostic considerations and therapeutic implications. Radiology 1989;170:1011–5.

49. Do YS, Yakes WF, Shin SW, et al. Ethanol embolization of arteriovenous malformations: interim results. Radiology 2005;235:674–82.

50. Holt PD, Burrows PE. Interventional radiology in the treatment of vascular lesions. Facial Plast Surg Clin North Am 2001;9:585–99.

51. Jacob AG, Driscoll DJ, Shaughnessy WJ, et al. Klippel-Trenaunay syndrome: spectrum and management. Mayo Clin Proc 1998;73:28–36.

52. Elsayes KM, Menias CO, Dillman JR, et al. Vascular malformation and hemangiomatosis syndromes: spectrum of imaging manifestations. AJR Am J Roentgenol 2008;190:1291–9.

53. Bastarrika G, Redondo P, Sierra A, et al. New techniques for the evaluation and therapeutic planning of patients with Klippel-Trenaunay syndrome. J Am Acad Dermatol 2007;56:242–9.

54. Servelle M. Klippel and Trenaunay's syndrome. 768 operated cases. Ann Surg 1985;201:365–73.

55. Ziyeh S, Spreer J, Rossler J, et al. Parkes Weber or Klippel-Trenaunay syndrome? Non-invasive diagnosis with MR projection angiography. Eur Radiol 2004;14:2025–9.

56. Garzon MC, Huang JT, Enjolras O, et al. Vascular malformations. Part II: associated syndromes. J Am Acad Dermatol 2007;56:541–64.

57. Albregts AE, Rapini RP. Malignancy in Maffucci's syndrome. Dermatol Clin 1995;13:73–8.

58. Kessler HB, Recht MP, Dalinka MK. Vascular anomalies in association with osteodystrophies: a spectrum. Skeletal Radiol 1983;10:95–101.

59. Fanburg JC, Meis-Kindblom JM, Rosenberg AE. Multiple enchondromas associated with spindle-cell hemangioendotheliomas. An overlooked variant of Maffucci's syndrome. Am J Surg Pathol 1995;19:1029–38.

60. Moodley M, Ramdial P. Blue rubber bleb nevus syndrome: case report and review of the literature. Pediatrics 1993;92:160–2.

61. Kassarjian A, Fishman SJ, Fox VL, et al. Imaging characteristics of blue rubber bleb nevus syndrome. AJR Am J Roentgenol 2003;181:1041–8.

62. McCarthy JC, Goldberg MJ, Zimbler S. Orthopaedic dysfunction in the blue rubber-bleb nevus syndrome. J Bone Joint Surg Am 1982;64:280–3.

63. Barlas A, Avsar E, Bozbas A, et al. Role of capsule endoscopy in blue rubber bleb nevus syndrome. Can J Surg 2008;51:E119–20.

64. Redondo P, Aguado L, Martinez-Cuesta A. Diagnosis and management of extensive vascular malformations of the lower limb: part I. Clinical diagnosis. J Am Acad Dermatol 2011;65:893–906 [quiz: 907–8].

# Systemic Treatments for Severe Pediatric Psoriasis
## A Practical Approach

Ann L. Marqueling, MD[a], Kelly M. Cordoro, MD[b,*]

## KEYWORDS

- Pediatric • Psoriasis • Systemic • Phototherapy • Acitretin • Cyclosporine • Methotrexate
- Biologics

## KEY POINTS

- Systemic treatment is reserved for severe, recalcitrant psoriasis in children. All systemic treatments have potential adverse effects that require baseline and follow-up clinical and/or laboratory monitoring.
- Narrow-band ultraviolet B (NB-UVB) as monotherapy works best for guttate and thin-plaque psoriasis, but its use may be limited by the practicality of attending multiple weekly treatments. NB-UVB used in combination with acitretin is synergistic.
- Acitretin is a nonimmunosuppressive treatment and is a first-line choice for generalized pustular, diffuse guttate, and thin-plaque psoriasis.
- Methotrexate and cyclosporine are rescue drugs, ideally used to control the acute phase and flares of severe recalcitrant plaque, pustular, and erythrodermic psoriasis, with the goal of obtaining control and then tapering to other agents.
- All of the inhibitors of tumor necrosis factor α have demonstrated positive effects on refractory plaque and generalized pustular psoriasis. Of these agents, etanercept has the most longitudinal data to support its efficacy and safety in the pediatric population.

## INTRODUCTION

A subset of children with psoriasis will experience severe, debilitating, life-altering disease at some point. As with any severe disease, the exact approach will vary by the individual. The risks and benefits of potential treatments should be weighed against the risks of undertreated disease. In the case of children, this task can be daunting. Limited by lack of data, standardized approaches, and approved therapies, clinicians must combine experience with the best available evidence to create a safe and effective therapeutic plan for that moment in time. Many children will endure a lifetime of disease and the treatments required to manage it. With this in mind, optimal management calls for plans that use the time-honored strategies of sequential, combination, and rotational therapy to maximize the benefits and minimize cumulative toxicities of the treatments. The choice of treatment in patients with severe disease is determined by the primary morphology, speed of progression, patient's age, presence of comorbidities such as psoriatic arthropathy, impact on quality of life, and level of disability. Severity need not always be defined by objective criteria, such as extent. A patient with 5% body surface area (BSA) involvement may be deemed severe based on the distribution of lesions, whereas a patient with greater

[a] Departments of Dermatology and Pediatrics, School of Medicine, Stanford University, 700 Welch Road, Suite 301, Stanford, CA 94304, USA; [b] Department of Dermatology, University of California, San Francisco, 1701 Divisadero Street, third floor, San Francisco, CA 94143, USA
* Corresponding author.
*E-mail address:* cordorok@derm.ucsf.edu

Dermatol Clin 31 (2013) 267–288
http://dx.doi.org/10.1016/j.det.2012.12.005
0733-8635/13/$ – see front matter © 2013 Elsevier Inc. All rights reserved

than 30% BSA may perceive no effects on quality of life whatsoever. Discussion with the patient (if age appropriate) and family will assist with this determination. Finally, not all cases determined to be severe initially require immediate treatment with systemic therapy or phototherapy. In younger children in particular, it is reasonable to allow the disease to evolve for a period of time before starting a systemic agent (Case 1).

The current era of psoriasis research in adults has enjoyed an informational explosion with regard to risk factors for disease and associations with cardiovascular disease, metabolic syndrome, and depression.[1] Comorbidity in pediatric patients with psoriasis remains insufficiently investigated. To date, psoriasis has not been definitively determined to be an independent risk factor for any chronic disease in childhood; however, obesity has been discovered to be associated with pediatric psoriasis, but the direction of the association remains to be determined.[2,3] Of particular relevance in children is determining the influence that psoriasis severity may have on development of metabolic syndrome, cardiovascular disease, and other comorbidities. Whether controlling severe disease in childhood can affect future health is unclear. Until we learn more, a reasonable approach to children with severe psoriasis is heightened awareness of potential associations and regular follow-up. Laboratory and other evaluations beyond that required to monitor systemic medications should be directed by the history, review of systems, and physical examination.

This review focuses on treating patients with decidedly severe disease. First, individual medications are reviewed, followed by a series of illustrative cases featuring approaches to various presentations of severe plaque, palmoplantar, and generalized pustular psoriasis. A comprehensive review of all aspects of the management of pediatric psoriasis is available for reference, and may be used as a supplement to this article.[4]

## PHOTOTHERAPY

Ultraviolet (UV) light has been used as a treatment for psoriasis even before Goeckerman popularized UVB phototherapy in 1925.[5] Indications for phototherapy in children include diffuse involvement, disease refractory to combination topical therapy, contraindications to systemic therapy, and debilitating palmoplantar psoriasis. Three types of UV light are used for phototherapy: narrow-band UVB (NB-UVB, 311–313 nm), broadband UVB (BB-UVB, 290–320 nm) and UVA (320–400 nm). Although all 3 modalities may be used for children, including the original Goeckerman therapy, NB-UVB has

emerged as the treatment of choice because of its safety and ease of administration.[6] In children, starting and incremental dosing is usually based on Fitzpatrick skin type per established protocols.[7,8] Starting dose may also be calculated based on a percentage (50%–80%) of the predetermined minimal erythema dose established by phototesting; however, in most children this is cumbersome and impractical. The two phases of phototherapy are clearing and maintenance. In the clearing phase, the dose is increased based on clinical response and the absence of adverse effects (erythema, burn, or pruritus) or missed treatments. Once clear, the dose from the clearing phase is maintained and the frequency of treatments is decreased.[9] Note that dosing protocols are not interchangeable for BB-UVB and NB-UVB sources and between equipment from different manufacturers. To minimize the risk of adverse events, children should receive phototherapy at centers staffed by personnel with experience in treating pediatric patients. Phototherapy is not a practical option for every patient, as the time commitment is extensive and an optimal effect requires adherence to the routine.

### NB-UVB

NB-UVB encompasses the most biologically active radiation in sunlight, and is an ideal choice for both efficacy and safety.[7,10–12] Treatment with NB-UVB rapidly depletes infiltrating T cells from psoriatic plaques and leads to faster clearance, less erythema, and longer remission than BB-UVB.[7] NB-UVB has been proved to be effective for moderate to severe psoriasis in children across all skin types.[7,8,13,14] Guttate psoriasis responds best, but thin plaques will also respond. Clearance or near clearance is achieved in 50% to 88% of patients after 15 to 20 treatments, including those with skin type V.[13,15] Two to 3 treatments per week are recommended for children.[16,17] Patient age, duration, and extent of disease have little to no relationship to cumulative clearance dose, number of sittings, or duration of therapy.[13] Furthermore, verbal reports from patients regarding whether their psoriasis improves or not in response to natural sunlight do not correlate with their actual response to UVB phototherapy.[18]

Acute adverse effects of NB-UVB therapy are dose dependent and may include erythema, burning, pigmentation, and transient lesional blistering.[19] Suberythemogenic regimens should be used to minimize these risks. Short-term side effects are usually mild and consist of xerosis, erythema, pruritus, and photoactivation of herpes simplex virus. Long-term effects may include premature photoaging and cutaneous carcinogenesis,[14] although the precise long-term risks in children are unavailable.[20] As with all treatments in children, the potential benefits must be weighed against the risks of other systemic therapies and the severity of the disease in the individual patient.

Combination therapy with NB-UVB and topical agents, such as calcipotriene,[21] tazarotene,[22] and anthralin,[23] enhances the efficacy of both therapies and decreases overall exposure to UV radiation. Calcipotriene may be degraded by NB-UVB light and ideally should be applied after phototherapy.[24] Systemic acitretin combined with NB-UVB (RE-NB-UVB) may decrease the time to clearance and the overall exposure to both agents.[25,26] RE-NB-UVB is effective and well tolerated in severe generalized pustular psoriasis in children, and may be used within the context of a sequential regimen as transitional and maintenance therapy after the acute toxic stage is controlled with cyclosporine (CSA) (Cases 7 and 9).[27]

## UVA

Photochemotherapy with psoralen and UVA light (PUVA) remains a viable treatment option for children with severe psoriasis. Oral psoralen should be restricted to children who are at least 12 years old or weigh at least 100 lb (45.4 kg). It is taken 90 minutes before therapeutic UVA exposure. PUVA is slightly more effective than NB-UVB[28]; however, NB-UVB is logistically more feasible and may be safer.[29] Short-term effects of oral PUVA include nausea, vomiting, headache, keratitis, hepatotoxicity, and generalized photosensitization requiring 24 hours of photoprotection.[30,31] A helpful approach to minimize additional outdoor UV exposure after treatment is to schedule the child in the last appointment of the day.[9] Long-term risks of oral psoralen include premature photoaging, cutaneous malignancy, and cataracts.[31] Topical PUVA is often considered safer than oral PUVA, but lacks long-term carcinogenicity data in children.[32] Topical PUVA is a good choice for recalcitrant palmoplantar psoriasis (Case 6).[33]

## ACITRETIN (SORIATANE)

Retinoids are nonimmunosuppressive vitamin A analogues that bind to nuclear receptors and affect cellular metabolism, epidermal differentiation, and apoptosis.[34] Acitretin, a metabolite of etretinate, replaced etretinate in 1998. Long-term experience treating children with disorders of cornification with oral retinoids supports their safety in children, although laboratory monitoring is necessary (**Table 1**).[35] Acitretin works best for guttate and pustular psoriasis and has been used

in children as young as 6 months old. Time to response may be as little as 3 weeks.[36–38] Acitretin also is a good choice for palmoplantar psoriasis (Case 6) and is a first-line agent for initial control of, and intermittent rescue therapy for, generalized pustular psoriasis (Case 7). It also can be used as maintenance treatment for pustular, erythrodermic, severe guttate, or plaque psoriasis, alone or in combination with other treatments. Retinoids and NB-UVB phototherapy (RE-NB-UVB) are synergistic (Cases 7, 8, and 9).[36,39]

Acitretin doses should be kept at or below 0.5 to 1 mg/kg per day to limit short-term and long-term toxicities. Parents should be advised to avoid concomitant vitamin supplements containing greater than 5000 IU of vitamin A. Short-term mucocutanenous adverse effects are dose dependent and common at doses closer to 1 mg/kg per day or higher. Although these effects can be dose limiting, they are all reversible.[40] If cheilitis, xerosis, skin fragility, palmoplantar desquamation, epistaxis, hair thinning, brittle nails, or blepharoconjunctivitis arise, the dose should be decreased until the symptoms are tolerable and manageable. Unfortunately, acitretin may need to be discontinued because of inadequate efficacy at the low doses required to keep mucocutaneous side effects under control. Serious ocular toxicity, including corneal opacities, papilledema, cataracts, and abnormal retinal function, are very rare in children and typically reversible.[41] Back pain, myalgias, arthralgias, and (rarely) elevated creatine phosphokinase may be associated with early retinoid therapy, and occur more frequently in physically active patients. The mechanism is unknown, but the process is benign and transient in almost all cases and does not require cessation of therapy.[40]

Blood monitoring is necessary to detect alterations in lipids and liver enzymes during retinoid therapy (see **Table 1**). Transient hyperlipidemia, particularly hypertriglyceridemia, may occur in up to one-quarter of patients, but is dose dependent and reversible with dose reduction or discontinuation.[35] Triglyceride levels above 1000 mg/dL, though rare, increase the risk of eruptive xanthomas and pancreatitis. Mild transaminitis may be seen in up to 15% of patients and generally resolves without discontinuation of treatment. Hepatotoxicity from chronic use in children has not been reported.[40] Teratogenicity is a well-known and serious toxicity of retinoids. Acitretin is converted to etretinate in the presence of ethanol and remains in the system for 3 years; therefore, pregnancy must be avoided during and for 3 years following completion of acitretin treatment.[25] Isotretinoin, though not as effective

**Table 1**
Drug monitoring

| Drug | Mechanism of Action | Dosing | Baseline | Follow-up | Miscellaneous |
|---|---|---|---|---|---|
| Methotrexate (MTX)[25,46,47,52,54,59] | Folic acid analogue, inhibits DHFR and interferes with DNA synthesis and effects on T cells | 0.2–0.7 mg/kg/wk Start with test dose 1.25–5 mg; then increase by 1.25–5 mg per wk until therapeutic effect obtained | CBC/platelets Liver function Renal function Hepatitis A/B/C HIV if at risk | CBC, platelets, liver function 7 d after test dose, then: weekly for 2–4 wk and after each dose, then every 2 wk for 1 mo and every 2–3 mo while on stable doses Renal function every 6–12 mo | Liver enzymes transiently increase after MTX dosing; obtain labs 5–7 d after the last dose Liver biopsy: no standard recommendations; see text CXR if respiratory symptoms arise |
| Retinoids[34,35,40,40,54] | Vitamin A analogue, binds to nuclear receptors and affects cellular metabolism, epidermal differentiation, and apoptosis | 0.5–1 mg/kg/d | CBC/platelets Liver function Renal function Fasting lipid profile Pregnancy testing per FDA prevention program guidelines | Liver function and lipid profile after 1 mo of treatment and with dose increases, then every 3 mo Monthly pregnancy test | Baseline skeletal survey if long-term treatment anticipated: radiographs of all 4 limbs and spine, repeated yearly or as symptoms arise Ophthalmologic examination if symptoms arise |
| Cyclosporine (CSA)[25,54,115,116] | Calcineurin inhibitor, specifically and reversibly inhibits immunocompetent T cells and suppresses proinflammatory cytokines IL-2 and IFN-γ | 3–5+ mg/kg/d See text for details (4 mg/kg/d is recommended maximum for adults) | Blood pressure × 2 Renal function Urinalysis with micro Fasting lipid profile CBC/platelets Liver function Magnesium Potassium Uric acid HIV if at risk | Blood pressure every visit Every 2 wk for 1–2 mo, then monthly: renal function, liver function, lipids, CBC, Mg+, K+, uric acid | Whole-blood CSA trough level if inadequate clinical response or concomitant use of potentially interacting medications (see text) If Cr increases >25% above baseline, reduce dose by 1 mg/kg/d for 2–4 wk and recheck. Stop CSA if Cr remains >25% above baseline; hold lower dose if level is within 25% of baseline |

**Biologics**

| | Description | Dosing | Baseline evaluation | Monitoring | Vaccinations |
|---|---|---|---|---|---|
| TNF-α inhibitors Etanercept Infliximab Adalimumab[107,109,117,118] | Etanercept: Fully human fusion protein of TNF-α receptor II bound to the Fc component of human IgG1 Infliximab/adalimumab: Monoclonal antibodies that bind TNF-α | Etanercept: 0.8 mg/kg SC weekly Infliximab: 3.3–5 mg/kg IV at weeks 0, 2, 6, then every 7–8 wk Adalimumab: 24 mg/m² SC (maximum 40 mg) every 2 wk[a] | PPD Electrolytes Liver function CBC with differential Hepatitis A/B/C if at risk HIV if at risk Update vaccinations | CBC, liver function every 4–6 mo. Liver function more frequently with infliximab PPD annually Other labs/serologies Per signs and symptoms | Avoid live and live-attenuated vaccines (eg, varicella; MMR; oral typhoid; yellow fever; intranasal influenza; herpes zoster; BCG) Vaccinate household contacts before treatment initiation |
| Ustekinumab[112,113,118,119] | Human monoclonal antibody that binds the p40 subunit of IL-12 and IL-23 | Not specified; single case report of 45 mg at weeks 0, 4, then every 12 wk[b] | PPD Update vaccinations Not specific, likely similar to other biological agents | PPD annually Not specific, likely similar to other biological agents | Avoid live and live-attenuated vaccines (eg, varicella; MMR; oral typhoid; yellow fever; intranasal influenza; herpes zoster; BCG) Vaccinate household contacts before treatment initiation Ustekinumab has not been studied in HIV patients |

*Abbreviations:* BCG, bacillus Calmette-Guerin; CBC, complete blood count; Cr, creatinine; CSA, cyclosporine; CXR, chest radiograph; DHFR, dihydrofolate reductase; FDA, Food and Drug Administration; HIV, human immunodeficiency virus; IFN, interferon; IgG, immunoglobulin G; IL, interleukin; IV, intravenous; MMR, measles-mumps-rubella vaccine; MTX, methotrexate; PPD, purified protein derivative; SC, subcutaneous; TNF, tumor necrosis factor.

[a] Dosing from published experience in patients with juvenile idiopathic arthritis, in 2 case reports in pediatric psoriasis, dosing was 40 mg every 2 weeks in 2 adolescent patients.

[b] Dosing from single case report; adult dosing is either 45 mg or 90 mg at weeks 0, 4 and then every 12 weeks depending on weight.

*Adapted from* Refs.[4,25,34,35,40,46,47,52,54,59,107,109,112,113,115–119]

for psoriasis, clears from the system in 1 month,[34] and may be used in severe cases of pustular psoriasis in adolescent females provided appropriate contraceptive counseling and control measures are in place.[42]

Long-term, high-dose (>1 mg/kg/d) retinoid toxicity may include premature epiphyseal closure, hyperostosis resembling diffuse idiopathic skeletal hyperostosis (DISH), calcification of anterior spinal ligaments, formation of periosteal bone, and decreased bone mineral density.[43] Although these are rare in children on low-dose regimens (1 mg/kg/d or less) such as those used in psoriasis, they have been reported in patients on long-term, high-dose therapy such as those used for severe ichthyoses and related diseases.[34,35,43,44] Evidence linking long-term, low-dose acitretin with radiologic skeletal abnormalities is conflicting.[45] It is difficult to advise on the best course of action regarding bone monitoring because the evidence is mixed. In practice, a conservative approach is to obtain annual and symptom-driven radiographs of the long bones and spine, and closely monitor growth parameters in children on long-term retinoid therapy. If possible, long-term (>1 year) uninterrupted therapy is to be avoided in prepubertal children.[4]

## METHOTREXATE (RHEUMATREX, TREXALL)

Methotrexate (MTX) has been used to treat psoriasis since the 1950s and remains the most widely prescribed drug for severe psoriasis worldwide.[46] It is a folic acid analogue that reversibly inhibits dihydrofolate reductase, resulting in interference with DNA synthesis and effects on T cells.[46,47] De Jager and colleagues[48] recently deemed MTX the systemic treatment of choice for children with moderate to severe psoriasis based on a systematic literature review of published data from 1980 to 2008. The investigators noted that most of the available data are in reference to plaque psoriasis, and concluded that short-term side effects are usually mild and easily managed. MTX has been used safely and successfully in children from 2 to 16 years of age with erythrodermic, plaque, and pustular psoriasis, and psoriatic arthritis.[49–51]

In practice, MTX is typically reserved for patients with severe, recalcitrant plaque, erythrodermic or pustular psoriasis, or psoriatic arthritis (Cases 2 and 5). MTX is ideally suited as a rescue drug in sequential regimens whereby MTX is used to gain control during the acute phase or during flares, followed by tapering and transition to any combination of topicals, other systemic therapies, and/or phototherapy for maintenance. Using MTX in this way decreases the cumulative dose, thereby minimizing the risk of adverse effects. MTX can be used in other combinations and rotations, or as monotherapy. In all cases, laboratory monitoring is required (see **Table 1**).

The recommended therapeutic dose range for children is 0.2 to 0.7 mg/kg per week.[52] A test dose of 1.25 mg (half of a 2.5-mg tablet) to 5 mg is given initially, followed by a complete blood count 1 week later to detect early bone marrow toxicity. If laboratory tests are normal, weekly dosing begins with conservative dose escalations of 1.25 to 5 mg per week until a therapeutic effect is obtained. Slow taper to the lowest effective maintenance dose should be attempted after 2 or 3 months of remission or disease stability. Methotrexate can be given via oral or parenteral routes (intravenously or intramuscularly). Parenteral administration is recommended if adequate oral dosing is ineffective or intolerable because of nausea or vomiting.[53] The liquid formulation for injection can be given orally to children who cannot swallow pills.

When children taking MTX for psoriasis are appropriately counseled, dosed, and monitored, serious side effects are rare (see **Table 1**).[52,54,55] MTX interacts with numerous drugs; the most relevant in children are nonsteroidal anti-inflammatory drugs (NSAIDs)[56,57] and trimethoprim-sulfamethoxazole (TMP-SMX).[58] The most common side effects of MTX are nausea and appetite suppression. Vomiting and diarrhea are less frequent but may necessitate dose reduction or cessation of therapy. If nausea is severe, on should try dividing the total weekly dose into 3 administrations given 12 hours apart. Another alternative is changing the route to intramuscular to thus bypass the gut.

The most worrisome side effects of MTX are pulmonary toxicity, bone marrow toxicity, and hepatotoxicity. Pulmonary toxicity is extremely rare in children[55] but can present early in treatment as acute, idiosyncratic pneumonitis or later as pulmonary fibrosis.[25,59] Bone marrow toxicity is a potentially life-threatening short-term side effect and can occur early (first 4–6 weeks) in the treatment course.[59,60] Risk is increased in children with renal disease, concurrent major illness, and concomitant use of certain medications, including TMP-SMX and NSAIDs. Hepatotoxicity is much rarer in children than in adults taking MTX. Lower cumulative doses and absence of preexisting risk factors in children such as diabetes, obesity, and alcoholism may partly explain this observation. There is no reliable, specific, noninvasive screening test for the presence and severity of hepatic fibrosis. In adults, liver biopsy remains the gold standard for diagnosis of fibrosis and cirrhosis, although debate persists over the timing of liver biopsy.[61] There are no specific monitoring guidelines for liver biopsy in pediatric patients, although general consensus and expert opinion suggest it is not required unless there is clinical or laboratory evidence of abnormality or cumulative doses exceed 1.5 g.[52,54] In practice, it is best to avoid MTX if possible in children with baseline risk factors. Patients supplemented with folic acid have less risk of nausea, macrocytic anemia, pancytopenia, and liver-enzyme elevations without significant alteration of efficacy.[62–67]

## CYCLOSPORINE (GENGRAF, NEORAL)

CSA is an immunosuppressive agent that is used for the prevention and treatment of transplant rejection in children older than 6 months. There is substantial clinical experience with off-label use for refractory pediatric atopic dermatitis and psoriasis.[68–73] CSA is a good choice for rapidly evolving or recalcitrant plaque or pustular psoriasis (Case 3). Its use has been deemed effective and well tolerated in children as young as 11 months old at doses ranging from 1.5 to 5 mg/kg/d for 6 weeks to 2 years,[72–76] often in combination with topical agents and less commonly with acitretin.[72]

CSA acts rapidly. Clinical improvement may be observed as early as 2 weeks, but often takes 4 to 8 weeks or more for full response. Once psoriasis has been stable for 2 to 3 months, a gradual taper should be started and adjusted according to clinical response. Rebounds during or after tapering of CSA are not uncommon. Combination and sequential therapy with topical or systemic agents or phototherapy may be required to maintain disease control. Combination therapy with acitretin often results in decreased total dose and duration of both agents.[77] Although combining CSA and phototherapy is not routinely recommended because of the risk of squamous cell carcinoma, in severe psoriasis NB-UVB can be initiated as a transitional and maintenance modality once CSA controls the disease and is being tapered off (Cases 8 and 9).

The suggested maximum dose of CSA for adults with psoriasis is 4 mg/kg/d in the United States and 5 mg/kg/d internationally, to limit the risk of hypertension and immunosuppression. Continuous use for more than 1 to 2 years should be avoided owing to the risks of nephrotoxicity.[25,71,73] Because children have higher BSA to weight ratios and age-dependent differences in pharmacokinetics, they often require higher doses than those recommended for adults.[73] In children with severe or rapidly evolving disease, starting at 5 mg/kg/d is reasonable, followed by slow taper after control is

achieved. Dosage adjustments are based on clinical response, serum creatinine levels, and blood pressure. Although no clear guidelines exist for monitoring CSA trough levels during treatment of psoriasis in adults,[78,79] given the differences in metabolism of the drug in children, it is reasonable to check a trough if the disease is not responding as expected. This aspect is particularly important when concomitant medications are being used that may affect CSA metabolism.

The most important adverse effects of CSA are nephrotoxicity and hypertension. Close laboratory (see **Table 1**) and blood-pressure monitoring is necessary to detect dose-related side effects that typically can be controlled and reversed by appropriate dose modification. Additional side effects include nausea, diarrhea, myalgias, arthralgias, headache, paresthesias, gingival hyperplasia, and hypertrichosis, although these are rare in doses used for psoriasis in contrast to the high doses used in transplant patients.[72] Long-term risks of malignancy, skin cancer, and lymphoproliferative disorders are a concern in children; however, evidence suggests that risk is minimal if using 5 mg/kg/d or less in patients who are not on concomitant immunosuppressive medications.[80] Vaccination may be less effective, and live-attenuated vaccines must be avoided during treatment. CSA is metabolized by the hepatic cytochrome P450 system. Drug levels may be influenced by numerous medications that induce and inhibit these enzymes. A current list of all medications taken by the patient should be kept, and potential drug interactions checked for frequently.

## BIOLOGICS

Biological medications target and interrupt specific components of the inflammatory cascade involved in psoriasis pathogenesis. The details of mechanism of action, adverse effects, and contraindications of each agent have recently been reviewed.[81] Biological therapies are an attractive choice for treating psoriasis in children, but their proper role in the management of this disease remains to be defined. Biologics offer the convenience of less frequent dosing and far less laboratory monitoring than traditional systemic agents. Furthermore, targeted therapy lacks many of the potential end-organ toxicities of traditional agents. However, caution is advised. Biological therapies have not yet accumulated adequate long-term safety data in children with psoriasis to deem them completely safe. There has been only one randomized, double-blind trial in the United States[2]; all other reports in children are case series, case reports, and anecdotes. It is thus important that the decision to pursue biological therapy in a child with psoriasis must be individualized after a detailed discussion with the parents regarding the known and unknown benefits and risks.

Similar to the other systemic agents, none of the biologics are approved for psoriasis in patients younger than 18 years. Because of the lack of data, no formalized guidelines exist for dosing and laboratory monitoring in pediatric patients. As experience and evidence of safety expand, the biological agents may take a primary position in the treatment of children as they have done in adults. The advantages of less frequent dosing and monitoring, tolerance, and short-term safety must be fairly weighed against the exorbitant cost and unknown long-term toxicities in this specific patient population. In practice, because of long-term safety concerns and, more practically, insurance coverage issues, biologics often are used as second-line or third-line agents for refractory cases of plaque, erythrodermic, and pustular psoriasis in children. Before initiation of biological therapy, children should undergo tuberculosis screening, immunization updates, and baseline laboratory studies, followed by regularly scheduled clinical surveillance for adverse events, particularly infections, and follow-up laboratory monitoring (see **Table 1**).

### Etanercept (Enbrel)

Of all the biologics, etanercept has accumulated the most data in pediatric psoriasis.[2,82,83] Furthermore, etanercept is approved by the Food and Drug Administration (FDA) for use in children aged 2 years and older for inflammatory arthritides, and therefore has longer-term safety data to substantiate recommendations for its use in the pediatric population. Although comparing efficacy and safety of drugs in different disease populations is not ideal, the widespread and long-term use of tumor necrosis factor (TNF) inhibitors in other diseases affords a greater degree of comfort with these agents. Case reports have shown successful treatment of erythrodermic, plaque, generalized pustular, and palmoplantar psoriasis in patients from 22 months to 17 years old (Cases 4 and 5).[82–87] The best data supporting the efficacy and safety of etanercept in moderate to severe pediatric plaque psoriasis comes from a phase III double-blind randomized controlled trial comparing etanercept 0.8 mg/kg weekly to placebo in 211 patients ages 4 to 16 years over the course of 48 weeks.[2] No deaths, cancers, opportunistic infections, tuberculosis, or demyelination events were reported in the study. Data at the 96-week point of the ongoing 264-week open-label

extension of this study showed continued efficacy, tolerability, and safety of etanercept in 140 patients.[88] Etanercept is delivered via subcutaneous injection and dosed either weekly or biweekly. The dosages that have been used successfully in children are 0.8 mg/kg to a maximum of 50 mg once weekly[2] and 0.4 mg/kg twice weekly.[82–84] Intermittent use may be an effective and more convenient, cost-effective strategy for treating children.[89] Based on the efficacy and safety data reported thus far, in 2009 the European Commission approved the use of etanercept for treatment of children aged 8 years and older with chronic severe plaque psoriasis who are inadequately controlled by, or intolerant of, other systemic therapies or phototherapy.[90]

Much of the long-term safety data for TNF-$\alpha$ inhibitors in general is from their use in juvenile idiopathic arthritis (JIA) and Crohn disease. Etanercept has accumulated the most efficacy and safety data in pediatric psoriasis. Data from 96 weeks of follow-up of a planned 264-week study revealed the most common adverse events to be minor infections, such as upper respiratory tract infections (URI) and pharyngitis, injection-site reactions, and headaches.[2,88] Severe infections were rare, and their relationship to the drug is questionable (gastroenteritis-related dehydration, lobar pneumonia). Studies in JIA patients have reported neuropathy (nondemyelinating) and serious infections, including varicella with aseptic meningitis and sepsis.[91,92] One study in JIA patients with 8 years of follow-up data found a rate of serious adverse events of 0.12 per patient-year, which did not increase with length of exposure, and a rate of serious infections at 0.03 per patient-year.[92] There were no opportunistic infections, malignancies, demyelinating disorders, or deaths in the combined data from pediatric psoriasis and JIA populations.[88,91–93]

### Infliximab (Remicade)

Infliximab is FDA-approved for the treatment of Crohn disease in children 6 years and older.[94] Infliximab is a potent inhibitor of TNF-$\alpha$, although documented use in pediatric psoriasis is limited to case reports and anecdotal experience. Uniformly positive responses to infliximab for refractory plaque and generalized pustular psoriasis were observed at doses of 3.3 to 5 mg/kg administered at weeks 0, 2, 6, and every 7 or 8 weeks thereafter. Treatment duration varied from a single dose to 10 months or longer, and time to effect was as rapid as hours to days.[48,95–98] The authors have used infliximab as rescue therapy in refractory, rapidly progressive, debilitating pustular psoriasis (Case 10).

In comparison with etanercept, patients receiving infliximab for JIA were found to have more frequent and more serious adverse events.[99,100] In adult psoriasis patients, infliximab is reported to carry an increased risk of tuberculosis reactivation and congestive heart failure.[101] Sporadic use of infliximab is ideally avoided, as this may increase the induction of neutralizing antibodies against the murine portion of the molecule, resulting in waning efficacy and increased infusion reactions.[97] Adding an immunosuppressant agent to reduce formation of the antichimeric antibodies, however, may increase the risk of potentially fatal hepatosplenic T-cell lymphoma, which to date has been reported only in pediatric and young adult patients with Crohn disease on both infliximab and azathioprine or 6-mercaptopurine.[94,102] Close surveillance for infections or signs of malignancy is warranted in patients on infliximab.

### Adalimumab (Humira)

Adalimumab is FDA-approved for treatment of moderate to severe polyarticular JIA in children 4 years and older,[103,104] and is used off-label for the treatment of pediatric inflammatory bowel disease and uveitis.[81] There are 2 case reports using adalimumab to treat recalcitrant pustular psoriasis in adolescent girls, both of whom had failed multiple systemic and biological agents.[105,106] The authors have experience with adalimumab in refractory plaque and brittle pustular psoriasis; in all cases the children cleared and have had no adverse events (Case 10). Given its successful use in adult patients with psoriasis and psoriatic arthritis, convenience of every 2-week dosing, and emerging evidence of efficacy and safety in children, adalimumab is gaining popularity for individually selected cases. Long-term safety in children with psoriasis remains to be established.

Adalimumab use in pediatric patients with JIA and Crohn disease has shown an adverse-effect profile similar to that of other TNF-α inhibitors, with infections and injection-site reactions being most common.[107,108] The observation of serologic conversion to antinuclear antibody positivity in adults in the absence of other diagnostic criteria for autoimmune disease is of unknown clinical relevance.[109]

### Black-box warning for TNF-α inhibitors

The risk of lymphoma and other cancers in patients treated with TNF-α inhibitors is a matter of considerable controversy. At this time, TNF-α inhibitors carry a black-box warning for increased risk of malignancy in the pediatric population. The extent of this risk continues to be under investigation. There have been 48 reports of cancer, half of which were lymphomas, in patients starting TNF-α inhibitors before the age of 18 years.[110] In addition, there have been rare reports in adolescents and young adults of hepatosplenic T-cell lymphoma in patients taking infliximab in combination with azathioprine or 6-mercaptopurine, as already noted.[102,111] Although there have been no cases of malignancy reported in studies of pediatric psoriasis, this potential risk, and the black-box warning highlighting it, warrant discussion with patients and their families before treatment initiation.

### Ustekinumab (Stelara)

Ustekinumab has recently been FDA-approved for the treatment of moderate to severe plaque psoriasis in adults. It is administered via subcutaneous injection once monthly for 2 months, then every 12 weeks.[112] At the time of writing, there is one case report detailing the use of ustekinumab in a 14-year-old male with plaque psoriasis who failed sequential therapy with cyclosporine (4 mg/kg/d) and etanercept (0.8 mg/kg once weekly). Phototherapy was not a viable option because of distance from the center. Ustekinumab was initiated at a dose of 45 mg subcutaneously at weeks 0 and 4, and then every 12 weeks. All laboratory parameters remained normal, and near total clinical response was observed by week 16. The investigators reported maintenance of complete clearance at 1 year of follow-up without any adverse events.[113] Ustekinumab is attractive for use in children with rapidly progressive disease because of its rapid onset of action and convenient administration schedule. There are inadequate data to recommend its adoption for use in children at present; however, a phase III multicenter, randomized, double-blind, placebo-controlled study evaluating the efficacy and safety of ustekinumab in the treatment of adolescent subjects with moderate to severe plaque psoriasis (CADMUS trial) is under way outside the United States.[114]

## ILLUSTRATIVE CASES
### Severe Plaque Psoriasis

#### Case 1
A 3-year-old boy presents with a severe, explosive-onset psoriatic eruption on the trunk (Fig. 1A, B). It progresses rapidly over 4 days and then stabilizes. It is intensely pruritic. He presents to the office with a low-grade fever, mild cough, and nasal congestion. Assessment is severe plaque psoriasis and concomitant viral upper respiratory infection versus streptococcal pharyngitis. There is no evidence of arthritis. A throat culture is obtained. Treatment choices include the conventional

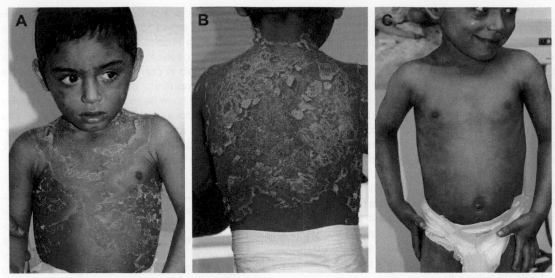

**Fig. 1.** (*A, B*) A 3-year-old boy with explosive-onset psoriasis during a viral upper respiratory infection. (*C*) Resolution 2 weeks after onset with topical therapy only.

systemic agents (CSA, MTX, retinoids), biological therapy, phototherapy, and empiric treatment for possible streptococcal pharyngitis. Because he has a symptomatic URI and is naïve to treatment, he is managed conservatively with oral antistreptococcal antibiotics and combination topical therapy with mid-potency topical corticosteroids (triamcinolone 0.1% ointment) twice daily and calcipotriene 0.005% ointment once daily. His throat culture is negative, and on follow-up visit 2 weeks later, his skin has cleared (**Fig. 1**C). This case illustrates explosive psoriasis in a genetically predisposed child (his father has psoriasis), likely triggered by a viral URI. Although the child in this case has severe psoriasis by all criteria (BSA, severe symptoms [pruritus], and effects on quality of life [inability to attend daycare; missed work days for parents]), systemic therapy is not necessarily the correct choice initially. Children with explosive-onset, or even slow-onset disease, with accompanying known triggers (infection, trauma, situational stress, triggering medication) can be observed for a few days to weeks to assess the evolution of the disease. In children without genetic susceptibility (ie, no known family history of psoriasis), the psoriasis may clear permanently on resolution of the triggering event or discontinuation of a triggering medication. In this case, the child remained clear for 8 months and returned to the clinic with a similar eruption, also triggered by infection and easily cleared. He remained clear for 6 months before flaring severely with full-body plaque psoriasis. MTX was initiated successfully as a rescue therapy; however, he is now undertreated, as his

parents fear the potential side effects of systemic agents and biologics, and phototherapy is not available in his area. Authorization for a home NB-UVB unit has been denied by his insurance. This case also illustrates several barriers to adequate care of children with severe disease including lack of approved medications, understandable parental fear of long-term side effects of systemic therapies, geographic isolation with high demand for specialty care, and insurance authorization and approval issues. In this case the authors are working with combination topical therapies to keep the patient's disease under control, and have appealed the denial for a phototherapy unit.

*Case 2*
The patient is a 15-year-old male with rashes on and off since 2 years of age. Prior biopsies of the trunk and palms have shown psoriasis. He has been treated with topical therapy only thus far because his physicians have told him that he "has to wait until he turns 18 because nothing is approved for use in children." On first visit to the office he is slightly overweight but otherwise healthy. Examination reveals diffuse confluent plaque psoriasis on the trunk and extremities, including the palms and soles (**Fig. 2**A, C, E). There is no evidence of psoriatic arthritis. He has been struggling in school in part because of severe pruritus, which is very distracting, and in part because of lack of self-esteem and willingness to participate. He has not participated in gym class for 3 years because of embarrassment over his skin disease and the bullying and teasing he has

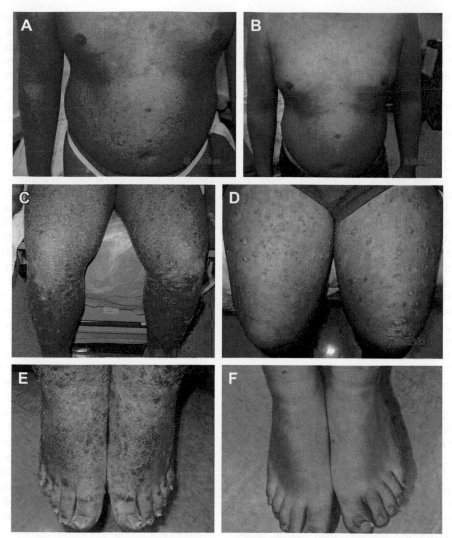

Fig. 2. (*A, C, E*) A 14-year-old boy with diffuse plaque psoriasis pretreatment. (*B, D, F*) Same patient status post 10 weeks of therapy with oral methotrexate (MTX).

suffered as a result of his appearance. There are no known triggering factors, and a baseline laboratory examination for metabolic syndrome and anticipation of the use of systemic therapy is within normal limits. The treatment choices in his case include the conventional systemic agents (CSA, MTX, retinoids), biological therapy, and phototherapy. Because of the chronicity and severity of his disease, he was started on MTX and combination topical therapy, and achieved near total clearance after 10 weeks of escalating doses to a maximum of 25 mg per week (**Fig.** 2B, D, F). He developed oral ulcerations, and the dose was decreased and maintained at 20 mg/wk, with folic acid 1 mg given daily except dose days, and topical mid-potency corticosteroids and calcipotriene ointment. He achieved complete clearance, and the oral ulcers resolved. On 3 months of remission,

the MTX was tapered by 1 2.5-mg tablet every 2 weeks. At 15 mg/wk, he flared and required dose escalation to 20 mg/wk. Folate was increased to 5 mg/d except on dose days that prevented recurrence of oral ulcerations, and he remains in remission. The next steps for him will be rotation to phototherapy, and if not successful a TNF-α inhibitor will be initiated. Many of the treatments mentioned will work effectively for severe, diffuse plaque psoriasis; in this case, the patient liked the idea of weekly therapy (more likely to be compliant) and he refused therapies requiring an injection.

## Case 3

A 5-year-old girl presents with rapidly progressive, inflammatory, secondarily infected plaque psoriasis. She has a personal history of early-onset psoriasis beginning in infancy. She is otherwise healthy, has no evidence of psoriatic arthritis, takes no medications, and has had no recent infections or other identifiable triggers for this acute flare. Examination reveals a mildly uncomfortable-appearing female with multiple edematous, inflamed, and fissured plaques, some with overlying serous and hemorrhagic crust, admixed with more typical guttate and plaque psoriasis on the scalp, face, periauricular areas, trunk, and extremities (**Fig. 3**A–C). There is no evidence of arthritis. Because of the rapidly progressive nature of her disease, a drug with a rapid onset of action is desirable. Baseline laboratory examination is normal, and streptococcal cultures from the throat and anus are negative. Cyclosporine at a dose of 5 mg/kg/d is initiated as well as oral antibiotics for the culture-proven methicillin-sensitive *Staphylococcus aureus* secondary skin infection. This case illustrates the need for rapid-acting medication in cases of severe and progressive psoriasis, particularly in children with a strong genetic predisposition in whom the psoriasis is likely to continue to worsen despite treatment for secondary infection and initiating trigger factors, if present. The goal for this patient's brittle disease is to establish control with CSA, followed by a taper and transition to maintenance therapy with another systemic agent, phototherapy, topical agents, or a combination thereof.

## Case 4

The patient is a 15-year-old male athlete with 3 years of severe, diffuse, large-plaque psoriasis without arthritis. He presents to the office with disease covering greater than 50% BSA (**Fig. 4**A). He is very healthy and has no family history of psoriasis, but his disease is taking its toll. He is depressed, socially withdrawn, and contemplating quitting the football team because of his appearance and the questions it provokes from others, including his coaches, who ask "What is it? Is it contagious?" His baseline laboratory work is normal. The patient lives 90 minutes

away in a group home. Given his social circumstances he is started on a nonimmunosuppressive drug, acitretin. The plaques thin modestly and after 6 months without much change, MTX is added. After 6 months of combined therapy with acitretin 25 mg/d, MTX 25 mg/wk, and topicals, he responds significantly but his disease persists (**Fig. 4**B), and he is deemed a treatment failure. Phototherapy is neither an optimal nor a feasible choice for him, given the distance from the nearest treatment center and his active schedule. He is therefore given etanercept subcutaneous injections, 50 mg twice weekly for 3 months followed by 25 mg twice weekly thereafter. The response is dramatic, with complete clearance after the first 3 months (**Fig. 4**C). However, when the dose is adjusted back to 25 mg twice weekly, plaques begin to develop on the shins, which are unresponsive to topical therapy. The authors are in the process of trying to increase his dose back to 50 mg twice weekly. This case reveals the difficulty in determining the precise role of biologics in therapy for children. On the one hand, the efficacy, ease of administration, convenient dosing schedule, and lack of monthly laboratory monitoring are attractive for the pediatric population. On the other hand, the lack of long-term data in pediatric patients with psoriasis specifically gives one pause. In this case, it could be argued that a TNF-α inhibitor should have been initiated earlier; thus the rationale for including cases like this one. Clinicians and researchers need to keep this discussion ongoing, and must continue to gather long-term data in children in an effort to better determine the precise place in management of these promising and effective medications.

## Case 5

A 9-year-old female has been followed in the authors' practice since the age of 3 years. She has had battled severe, diffuse, ostraceous, and rupioid psoriasis since 3 years of age. Her leg at the age of 4 years is shown in **Fig. 5**A; **Fig. 5**B and C show the same leg at age 9. She has

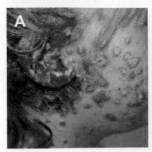
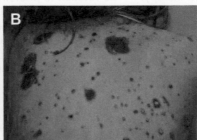
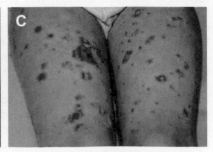

**Fig. 3.** (*A–C*) A 5-year-old girl with edematous, inflamed, fissured, superinfected plaque psoriasis.

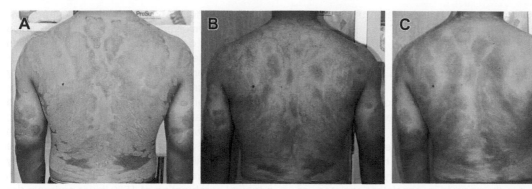

Fig. 4. (A) A 15-year-old male with diffuse, large-plaque psoriasis covering greater than 50% body surface area. (B) Persistent disease status post 6 months of combined therapy with acitretin, MTX, and topicals. (C) Complete clearance status post 3 months of etanercept therapy at 50 mg twice weekly.

been on various combinations through the years including combination topical therapy with ultra-potent corticosteroids, coal-tar formulations, calcipotriene, and various keratolytic agents. She has variably responded to and later failed various combinations of CSA, NB-UVB, and MTX. Most recently, she has been on 20 mg/wk of MTX and NB-UVB twice weekly, which held her disease reasonably well (almost clear) for more than 6 months, until she began to develop progressive ostraceous plaques again that rapidly became confluent (see **Fig. 5**B, C). After a long discussion of the options with her mother, etanercept was initiated at 25 mg weekly. Her psoriasis cleared within 3 months (**Fig. 5**D); however, she developed a swollen ankle joint on which she could not ambulate. This swelling was aspirated by

pediatric rheumatology and deemed to be consistent with psoriatic arthritis. In conjunction with rheumatology, MTX was restarted at 15 mg/wk, and her arthritis resolved. Now, after 6 months on combination etanercept and methotrexate, her psoriasis is returning on the extremities and trunk, but the arthritis has remained controlled. This case illustrates a complex and severe presentation, widely refractory to multiple agents. Of most interest is the appearance of psoriatic arthritis while on treatment with a TNF-α inhibitor, but not while on MTX. Her psoriatic arthritis has responded to MTX, but her cutaneous disease has proved too much for both MTX and etanercept, begging the question: where do we go next? Her dose of etanercept has been increased to 0.8 mg/kg/wk, and if this fails, the next steps

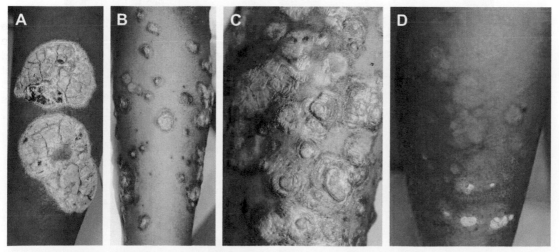

Fig. 5. (A) Leg of a patient at 4 years of age with ostraceous and rupioid psoriasis. (B, C) Same patient, same leg at age 9 years old, on MTX and narrow-band ultraviolet B (NB-UVB) therapy. (D) Same patient at age 9 years after 3 months of etanercept therapy at 25 mg weekly.

likely will be a transition to a different TNF-α inhibitor or a trial of ustekinumab.

## Palmoplantar Psoriasis

### Case 6

The patient is a 14-year-old boy with a 3 year history of severe palmoplantar psoriasis (**Fig. 6**A, B). He has been maintained at the current level with topical corticosteroids and emollients. At first presentation to the office, his hands are better managed than his feet primarily because of increased adherence to a consistent regimen, as he plays basketball and baseball and at one point was incapacitated by the severity of the palmar involvement. He recently has had to discontinue sports because the fingertips and feet have developed painful fissures that are not responding to topical therapy. He is otherwise healthy, and examination reveals patchy psoriatic plaques (less than 10% BSA) on his trunk and extremities, with diffuse involvement of the palms and soles with notable deep fissures. Treatment options for him include hand/foot topical PUVA, oral retinoids, MTX, or biologics. Because of the severity of the palms and soles, and no access to a phototherapy center, baseline labs were checked and acitretin initiated at 10 mg/d. He improved dramatically within 6 weeks, and at his 3-month follow-up he was nearly clear (**Fig. 6**B, D). He had mild cheilitis and xerosis but his laboratory parameters remained normal. Together with a topical combination of 15% liquor carbonis detergens compounded in triamcinolone 0.1% ointment applied nightly, he is maintained on acitretin 10 mg every other day. The goal is to taper the acitretin and maintain him with topical therapies only. Acitretin is an excellent choice for palmoplantar psoriasis, as are MTX and TNF-α inhibitors.

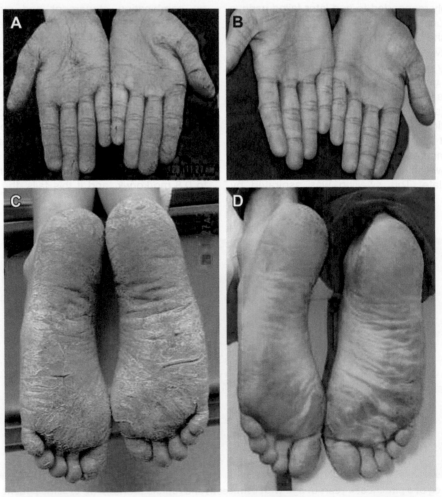

**Fig. 6.** (A, C) A 14-year-old boy with severe palmoplantar psoriasis on topical therapy. (B, D) Same patient status post acitretin 10 mg/d for 3 months.

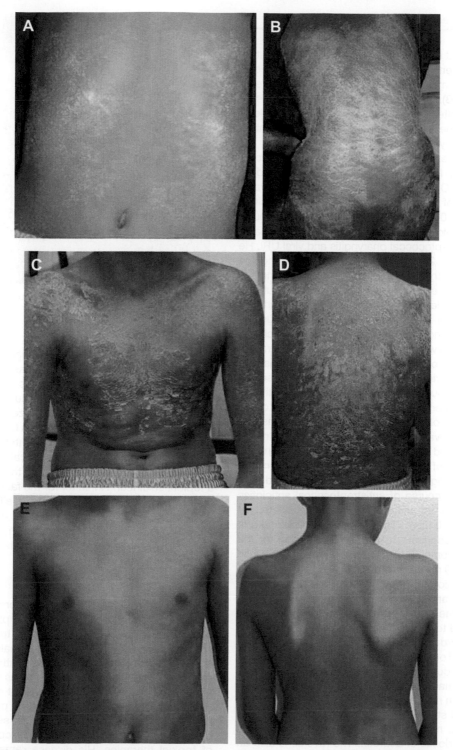

Fig. 7. (A, B) A 9-year-old boy with generalized pustular psoriasis. (C, D) Same patient with widespread exfoliation in areas of prior pustulation. (E, F) Same patient clear after a 3-month course of antistreptococcal antibiotics and acitretin, 10 mg/d.

## Generalized Pustular Psoriasis

### Case 7

The patient is a 9-year-old boy with a 5-year history of a recurrent, generalized pustular eruption accompanied by malaise, arthralgias, skin pain, and fever (**Fig. 7**A, B). He has been diagnosed for years as having acute generalized exanthematous pustulosis because the fever and malaise would prompt antibiotic therapy from his primary care physician, followed by eruption of pustules the following day, incorrectly interpreted as recurrent pustular drug eruption. On pustulation, the patient withdraws because of pain and remains in the fetal position for up to 10 days until the pustules spontaneously stop developing and heal. His triggers reliably include streptococcal pharyngitis and viral URI. He misses 1 to 2 weeks of school every few months because of the eruptions. On his initial visit, he has widespread exfoliation in areas of prior pustulation and no evidence of lymphadenopathy or arthritis (**Fig. 7**C, D). Assessment is generalized pustular psoriasis, and treatment options include acitretin and MTX as well as combination topical treatments at the time of pustulation. Because the episodes were occurring every few months, with severe disability, but spontaneously resolved within 2 weeks, an nonimmunosuppressive agent was opted for to control and maintain his disease. Baseline laboratory evaluation was normal except for a markedly elevated antistreptolysin O titer. Because of the possibility of a persistent streptococcal antigen effect driving his psoriasis, he was treated with a 3-month course of antistreptococcal antibiotics in addition to acitretin, which was initiated at a dose of 10 mg/d. Though less than 0.5 mg/kg/d, this was adequate to prevent pustulation for the next 18 months (**Fig. 7**E, F). His dose to was then tapered 10 mg 3 times a week, and this maintained his remission for another year, until he developed skin pain and a localized area of pustules on the arms in the context of a viral URI. His dose was increased to 20 mg/d during the flare then tapered to 10 mg/d after the flare was controlled, and he continued on this course over the next year. Eventually he required the addition of NB-UVB (RE-NB-UVB) to maintain his remission. Annual bone films have been normal and laboratory parameters have remained stable. The goal is to taper off the NB-UVB, and maintain his remission with the lowest possible doses of acitretin. The reverse is also an option (taper acitretin while maintaining NB-UVB) depending on the individual clinical situation.

### Case 8

This patient is a 3-year-old girl who presents with severe generalized pustular psoriasis (**Fig. 8**).

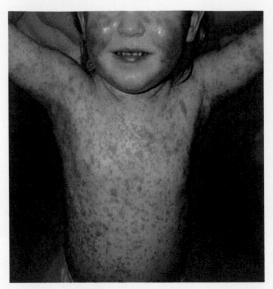

**Fig. 8.** A 3-year-old girl with severe generalized pustular psoriasis.

There are no identifiable disease triggers. Acitretin was initiated to gain control of her disease; despite doses of 1 mg/kg/d, her psoriasis progressed. Cyclosporine was added as a rescue therapy at 4 mg/kg/d and her disease stabilized. She was transitioned as follows. The CSA was tapered while the acitretin was continued for maintenance. She was adjunctively treated with topical corticosteroids and vitamin D analogues for the body and a topical calcineurin inhibitor for the face. She ultimately was able to be tapered off all systemic agents; however, at age 5 years her disease returned and required aggressive therapy (see Case 3). This case demonstrates the technique of combination and sequential therapy.

### Case 9

The patient is an 11-year-old boy who presents with his first episode of diffuse annular plaque and pustular psoriasis with no identifiable triggers and no comorbidities. Examination reveals a well-appearing child with diffuse plaques studded with pustules (**Fig. 9**A). He has no arthralgias or arthritis, and baseline laboratories and a throat culture are negative. The assessment is diffuse plaque and pustular psoriasis, and acitretin is selected to control his disease, together with a combination of topical therapies. His disease remains stable but does not improve over the ensuing 2 weeks, and during week 3 of therapy he endures a severe pustular flare with systemic toxicity (fevers, chills, arthralgias) and is admitted to the hospital. A 3-phase sequential therapy plan is initiated with CSA added to the acitretin as the rescue agent,

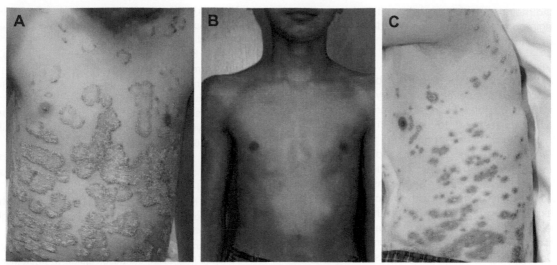

**Fig. 9.** (*A*) An 11-year-old boy with diffuse annular plaque psoriasis studded with pustules. (*B*) Same patient status post sequential therapy with cyclosporine and NB-UVB/acitretin. (*C*) Same patient at age 14 years with recurrence of severe generalized pustular psoriasis.

which results in stabilization of the disease. As he improves and is discharged from the hospital, the transition phase is entered and his CSA is tapered while starting NB-UVB at very conservative energies (as per skin type 1). Ultimately, the CSA is discontinued and remission is maintained with RE-NB-UVB (low-dose acitretin [10 mg every other day] and twice weekly NB-UVB), which is a synergistic combination (**Fig. 9**B). The acitretin is tapered off first, then the NB-UVB. He remains off all

medications and in remission for 2 years, followed by another episode of severe generalized pustular psoriasis for which a similar regimen is initiated (**Fig. 9**C). This case demonstrates a sequential 3-phase approach to therapy (clearing, transition, and maintenance), which limits undue exposure for long periods of time to any individual agent(s). The idea is to use synergistic combinations to gain control and clear the psoriasis, followed by transitioning to a less potentially toxic regimen

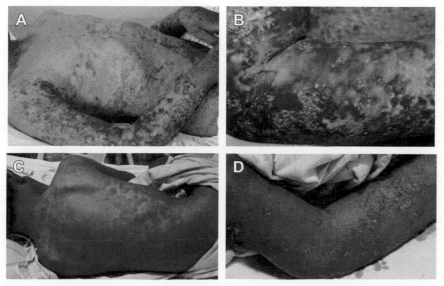

**Fig. 10.** (*A, B*) An 8-year-old boy with severe refractory generalized pustular psoriasis, covering 100% body surface area. (*C, D*) Same patient 48 hours status post rescue infusion with infliximab, 5 mg/kg.

and maintaining the remission with a conservative regimen or the lowest possible dose of the drug, phototherapy, or combination.[27,36,77]

### Case 10

This patient is an 8-year-old boy admitted to hospital with a severe flare of erythrodermic generalized pustular psoriasis covering 100% BSA, failing to respond to acitretin 1 mg/kg/d, CSA 5 mg/kg/d, and aggressive topical therapy (**Fig. 10**A, B). His disease is rapidly progressing and he has electrolyte dysregulation and systemic toxicity (fevers, chills, arthralgias, malaise, and skin pain). He is treated with a rescue infusion of infliximab 5 mg/kg. Within 48 hours there is a dramatic response with cessation of pustulation, and healing of existing pustules and erythroderma (**Fig. 10**C, D). On discharge he has a very unstable course, with multiple severe exacerbations requiring admission. He was unable to make clinic appointments for infusions with infliximab, and his disease is now maintained with adalimumab. TNF-α inhibitors for the treatment of severe generalized pustular psoriasis in children have been reported by others as well.[97,105]

### SUMMARY

Treating severe psoriasis in children is not an exact science. As we accumulate data and gain familiarity with new and emerging targeted therapies, we continue to build on the collective experience using conventional therapies. Children have a potential lifetime of treatment ahead of them. As such, we should consider not only today's known and unknown effects of various treatments but also tomorrow's. Although psoriasis is one of the most common diseases of childhood, several key issues remain in terms of standardizing care for children: FDA approval, standardized dosing and monitoring protocols, and long-term safety data for the newest group of therapies. Pooling our resources for data collection will bring us closer to more definitive therapeutic guidelines and protocols for the evaluation of potential comorbidities. Until more data on children are accumulated to advance the science, we will continue to rely more on the art of management.

### REFERENCES

1. Gelfand JM, Neimann AL, Shin DB, et al. Risk of myocardial infarction in patients with psoriasis. JAMA 2006;296:1735–41.
2. Paller AS, Siegfried EC, Langley RG, et al. Etanercept treatment for children and adolescents with plaque psoriasis. N Engl J Med 2008;358: 241–51.
3. Augustin M, Glaeske G, Radtke MA, et al. Epidemiology and comorbidity of psoriasis in children. Br J Dermatol 2010;162:633–6.
4. Cordoro KM. Management of childhood psoriasis. Adv Dermatol 2008;24:125–69.
5. Goeckerman WH. The treatment of psoriasis. Northwest Med 1925;24:229–31.
6. MacDonald A, Burden AD. Psoriasis: advances in pathophysiology and management. Postgrad Med J 2007;83:690–7.
7. Jain VK, Aggarwal K, Jain K, et al. Narrow-band UV-B phototherapy in childhood psoriasis. Int J Dermatol 2007;46:320–2.
8. Tay YK, Morelli JG, Weston WL. Experience with UVB phototherapy in children. Pediatr Dermatol 1996;13:406–9.
9. McClelland PB. Fundamentals of phototherapy. National Psoriasis Foundation guide to phototherapy. San Francisco (CA): National Psoriasis Foundation; 2008.
10. Parrish JA, Jaenicke KF. Action spectrum for phototherapy of psoriasis. J Invest Dermatol 1981;76: 359–62.
11. Walters IB, Burack LH, Coven TR, et al. Suberythemogenic narrow-band UVB is markedly more effective than conventional UVB in treatment of psoriasis vulgaris. J Am Acad Dermatol 1999; 40:893–900.
12. Dawe RS, Cameron H, Yule S, et al. A randomized controlled trial of narrowband ultraviolet B vs bathpsoralen plus ultraviolet A photochemotherapy for psoriasis. Br J Dermatol 2003;148:1194–204.
13. al-Fouzan AS, Nanda A. UVB phototherapy in childhood psoriasis. Pediatr Dermatol 1995;12:66.
14. Pasić A, Ceović R, Lipozencić J, et al. Phototherapy in pediatric patients. Pediatr Dermatol 2003; 20:71–7.
15. Ibbotson SH, Bilsland D, Cox NH, et al. An update and guidance on narrowband ultraviolet B phototherapy: a British Photodermatology Group Workshop Report. Br J Dermatol 2004;151:283–97.
16. Dawe RS, Wainwright NJ, Cameron H, et al. Narrow-band (TL-01) ultraviolet B phototherapy for chronic plaque psoriasis: three times or five times weekly treatment? Br J Dermatol 1998;138: 833–9.
17. Leenutaphong V, Nimkulrat P, Sudtim S. Comparison of phototherapy two times and four times a week with low doses of narrow-band ultraviolet B in Asian patients with psoriasis. Photodermatol Photoimmunol Photomed 2000;16:202–6.
18. Dawe RS, Ferguson J. History of psoriasis response to sunlight does not predict outcome of UVB phototherapy. Clin Exp Dermatol 2004;29:413–4.
19. Calzavara-Pinton PG, Zane C, Candiago E, et al. Blisters on psoriatic lesions treated with TL-01 lamps. Dermatology 2000;200:115–9.

20. Diffey BL, Farr PM. The challenge of follow-up in narrowband ultraviolet B phototherapy. Br J Dermatol 2007;157:344–9.
21. Woo WK, McKenna KE. Combination TL01 ultraviolet B phototherapy and topical calcipotriol for psoriasis: a prospective randomized placebo-controlled clinical trial. Br J Dermatol 2003;149: 146–50.
22. Behrens S, Grundmann-Kollmann M, Schiener R, et al. Combination phototherapy of psoriasis with narrow-band UVB irradiation and topical tazarotene gel. J Am Acad Dermatol 2000;42:493–5.
23. Carrozza P, Hausermann P, Nestle FO, et al. Clinical efficacy of narrow-band UVB (311 nm) combined with dithranol in psoriasis. An open pilot study. Dermatology 2000;200:35–9.
24. Lebwohl M, Hecker D, Martinez J, et al. Interactions between calcipotriene and ultraviolet light. J Am Acad Dermatol 1997;37:93–5.
25. Lebwohl M, Ali S. Treatment of psoriasis. Part 2. Systemic therapies. J Am Acad Dermatol 2001; 45:649–61.
26. Spuls PI, Rozenblit M, Lebwohl M. Retrospective study of the efficacy of narrowband UVB and acitretin. J Dermatolog Treat 2003;14(Suppl 2):17–20.
27. Kim HS, Kim GM, Kim SY. Two-stage therapy for childhood generalized pustular psoriasis: low-dose cyclosporin for induction and maintenance with acitretin/narrowband ultraviolet B phototherapy. Pediatr Dermatol 2006;23:306–8.
28. Tahir R, Mujtaba G. Comparative efficacy of psoralen-UVA photochemotherapy versus narrow band UVB phototherapy in the treatment of psoriasis. J Coll Physicians Surg Pak 2004;14:593–5.
29. van Weelden H, Baart de la Faille H, Young E, et al. Comparison of narrow-band UV-B phototherapy and PUVA photochemotherapy in the treatment of psoriasis. Acta Derm Venereol 1990;70:212–5.
30. Schiener R, Brockow T, Franke A, et al. Bath PUVA and saltwater baths followed by UV-B phototherapy as treatments for psoriasis: a randomized controlled trial. Arch Dermatol 2007;143:586–96.
31. Wolff K. Side-effects of psoralen photochemotherapy (PUVA). Br J Dermatol 1990;122(Suppl 36): 117–25.
32. Delrosso G, Bornacina C, Farinelli P, et al. Bath PUVA and psoriasis: is a milder treatment a worse treatment? Dermatology 2008;216:191–3.
33. Spuls PI, Hadi S, Rivera L, et al. Retrospective analysis of the treatment of psoriasis of the palms and soles. J Dermatolog Treat 2003;14(Suppl 2):21–5.
34. Patton TJ, Zirwas MJ, Wolverton SE. Systemic retinoids. In: Wolverton SE, editor. Comprehensive dermatologic drug therapy. 2nd edition. Philadelphia: Saunders (Elsevier); 2007. p. 275–300.
35. Lacour M, Mehta-Nikhar B, Atherton DJ, et al. An appraisal of acitretin therapy in children with inherited disorders of keratinization. Br J Dermatol 1996;134:1023–9.
36. Kopp T, Karlhofer F, Szepfalusi Z, et al. Successful use of acitretin in conjunction with narrowband ultraviolet B phototherapy in a child with severe pustular psoriasis, von Zumbusch type. Br J Dermatol 2004;151:912–6.
37. Rosinska D, Wolska H, Jablonska S, et al. Etretinate in severe psoriasis of children. Pediatr Dermatol 1988;5:266–72.
38. Shelnitz LS, Esterly NB, Honig PJ. Etretinate therapy for generalized pustular psoriasis in children. Arch Dermatol 1987;123:230–3.
39. Lee CS, Koo J. A review of acitretin, a systemic retinoid for the treatment of psoriasis. Expert Opin Pharmacother 2005;6:1725–34.
40. Brecher AR, Orlow SJ. Oral retinoid therapy for dermatologic conditions in children and adolescents. J Am Acad Dermatol 2003;49:171–82 [quiz: 183–6].
41. Gold JA, Shupack JL, Nemec MA. Ocular side effects of the retinoids. Int J Dermatol 1989;28: 218–25.
42. Al-Shobaili H, Al-Khenaizan S. Childhood generalized pustular psoriasis: successful treatment with isotretinoin. Pediatr Dermatol 2007;24:563–4.
43. Nesher G, Zuckner J. Rheumatologic complications of vitamin A and retinoids. Semin Arthritis Rheum 1995;24:291–6.
44. Ruiz-Maldonado R, Tamayo-Sanchez L, Orozco-Covarrubias ML. The use of retinoids in the pediatric patient. Dermatol Clin 1998;16:553–69.
45. Halverstam CP, Zeichner J, Lebwohl M. Lack of significant skeletal changes after long-term, low-dose retinoid therapy: case report and review of the literature. J Cutan Med Surg 2006;10:291–9.
46. MacDonald A, Burden AD. Noninvasive monitoring for methotrexate hepatotoxicity. Br J Dermatol 2005; 152:405–8.
47. Cronstein BN. The mechanism of action of methotrexate. Rheum Dis Clin North Am 1997;23:739–55.
48. de Jager ME, de Jong EM, van de Kerkhof PC, et al. Efficacy and safety of treatments for childhood psoriasis: a systematic literature review. J Am Acad Dermatol 2010;62:1013–30.
49. Kumar B, Dhar S, Handa S, et al. Methotrexate in childhood psoriasis. Pediatr Dermatol 1994;11:271–3.
50. Dogra S, Handa S, Kanwar AJ. Methotrexate in severe childhood psoriasis. Pediatr Dermatol 2004;21:283–4.
51. Kaur I, Dogra S, De D, et al. Systemic methotrexate treatment in childhood psoriasis: further experience in 24 children from India. Pediatr Dermatol 2008;25:184–8.
52. Paller AS. Dermatologic uses of methotrexate in children: indications and guidelines. Pediatr Dermatol 1985;2:238–43.

53. Hendel L, Hendel J, Johnsen A, et al. Intestinal function and methotrexate absorption in psoriatic patients. Clin Exp Dermatol 1982;7:491–7.

54. Swords S, Lauer SJ, Nopper AJ. Principles of treatment in pediatric dermatology: systemic treatment. In: Schachner LA, Hansen RC, Hodgson S, editors. Pediatric dermatology. 3rd edition. Philadelphia: Mosby (Elsevier); 2003. p. 133–43.

55. Graham LD, Myones BL, Rivas-Chacon RF, et al. Morbidity associated with long-term methotrexate therapy in juvenile rheumatoid arthritis. J Pediatr 1992;120:468–73.

56. Kremer JM, Hamilton RA. The effects of nonsteroidal antiinflammatory drugs on methotrexate (MTX) pharmacokinetics: impairment of renal clearance of MTX at weekly maintenance doses but not at 7.5 mg. J Rheumatol 1995;22:2072–7.

57. Wallace CA, Smith AL, Sherry DD. Pilot investigation of naproxen/methotrexate interaction in patients with juvenile rheumatoid arthritis. J Rheumatol 1993;20: 1764–8.

58. Thomas DR, Dover JS, Camp RD. Pancytopenia induced by the interaction between methotrexate and trimethoprim-sulfamethoxazole. J Am Acad Dermatol 1987;17:1055–6.

59. Callen JP, Kulp-Shorten CL, Wolverton SE. Methotrexate. In: Wolverton SE, editor. Comprehensive dermatologic drug therapy. 2nd edition. Philadelphia: Saunders (Elsevier); 2007. p. 163–81.

60. Gutierrez-Urena S, Molina JF, Garcia CO, et al. Pancytopenia secondary to methotrexate therapy in rheumatoid arthritis. Arthritis Rheum 1996;39: 272–6.

61. Kalb RE, Strober B, Weinstein G, et al. Methotrexate and psoriasis: 2009 National Psoriasis Foundation Consensus Conference. J Am Acad Dermatol 2009;60:824–37.

62. Gisondi P, Fantuzzi F, Malerba M, et al. Folic acid in general medicine and dermatology. J Dermatolog Treat 2007;18:138–46.

63. Morgan S, Alarcon GS, Krumdieck CL. Folic acid supplementation during methotrexate therapy: it makes sense. J Rheumatol 1993;20:929–30.

64. Morgan SL, Baggott JE, Lee JY, et al. Folic acid supplementation prevents deficient blood folate levels and hyperhomocysteinemia during longterm, low dose methotrexate therapy for rheumatoid arthritis: implications for cardiovascular disease prevention. J Rheumatol 1998;25:441–6.

65. Morgan SL, Baggott JE, Vaughn WH, et al. Supplementation with folic acid during methotrexate therapy for rheumatoid arthritis. A double-blind, placebo-controlled trial. Ann Intern Med 1994;121:833–41.

66. Morgan SL, Baggott JE, Vaughn WH, et al. The effect of folic acid supplementation on the toxicity of low-dose methotrexate in patients with rheumatoid arthritis. Arthritis Rheum 1990;33:9–18.

67. van Ede AE, Laan RF, Rood MJ, et al. Effect of folic or folinic acid supplementation on the toxicity and efficacy of methotrexate in rheumatoid arthritis: a forty-eight week, multicenter, randomized, double-blind, placebo-controlled study. Arthritis Rheum 2001;44: 1515–24.

68. Harper JI, Ahmed I, Barclay G, et al. Cyclosporin for severe childhood atopic dermatitis: short course versus continuous therapy. Br J Dermatol 2000;142:52–8.

69. Leonardi S, Marchese G, Rotolo N, et al. Cyclosporin is safe and effective in severe atopic dermatitis of childhood. Report of three cases. Minerva Pediatr 2004;56:231–7.

70. Zaki I, Emerson R, Allen BR. Treatment of severe atopic dermatitis in childhood with cyclosporin. Br J Dermatol 1996;135(Suppl 48):21–4.

71. Berth-Jones J, Voorhees JJ. Consensus conference on cyclosporin A microemulsion for psoriasis, June 1996. Br J Dermatol 1996;135:775–7.

72. Pereira TM, Vieira AP, Fernandes JC, et al. Cyclosporin A treatment in severe childhood psoriasis. J Eur Acad Dermatol Venereol 2006;20:651–6.

73. Perrett CM, Ilchyshyn A, Berth-Jones J. Cyclosporin in childhood psoriasis. J Dermatolog Treat 2003;14:113–8.

74. Alli N, Gungor E, Karakayali G, et al. The use of cyclosporin in a child with generalized pustular psoriasis. Br J Dermatol 1998;139:754–5.

75. Kilic SS, Hacimustafaoglu M, Celebi S, et al. Low dose cyclosporin A treatment in generalized pustular psoriasis. Pediatr Dermatol 2001;18: 246–8.

76. Mahe E, Bodemer C, Pruszkowski A, et al. Cyclosporine in childhood psoriasis. Arch Dermatol 2001;137:1532–3.

77. Koo J. Systemic sequential therapy of psoriasis: a new paradigm for improved therapeutic results. J Am Acad Dermatol 1999;41:S25–8.

78. Heydendael VM, Spuls PI, Berge Ten IJ, et al. Cyclosporin trough levels: is monitoring necessary during short-term treatment in psoriasis? A systematic review and clinical data on trough levels. Br J Dermatol 2002;147:122–9.

79. Mockli G, Kabra PM, Kurtz TW. Laboratory monitoring of cyclosporine levels: guidelines for the dermatologist. J Am Acad Dermatol 1990;23: 1275–8 [discussion: 1278–9].

80. Ellis CN. Safety issues with cyclosporine. Int J Dermatol 1997;36(Suppl 1):7–10.

81. Wright NA, Piggott CD, Eichenfield LF. The role of biologics and other systemic agents in the treatment of pediatric psoriasis. Semin Cutan Med Surg 2010;29:20–7.

82. Hawrot AC, Metry DW, Theos AJ, et al. Etanercept for psoriasis in the pediatric population: experience in nine patients. Pediatr Dermatol 2006;23:67–71.

83. Papoutsaki M, Costanzo A, Mazzotta A, et al. Etanercept for the treatment of severe childhood psoriasis. Br J Dermatol 2006;154:181–3.

84. Kress DW. Etanercept therapy improves symptoms and allows tapering of other medications in children and adolescents with moderate to severe psoriasis. J Am Acad Dermatol 2006;54: S126–8.

85. Fabrizi G, Guerriero C, Pagliarello C. Etanercept in infants: suberythrodermic, recalcitrant psoriasis in a 22 month-old child successfully treated with etanercept. Eur J Dermatol 2007;17:245.

86. Safa G, Loppin M, Bousser AM, et al. Etanercept in a 7-year-old boy with severe and recalcitrant psoriasis. J Am Acad Dermatol 2007;56: S19–20.

87. Floristan U, Feltes R, Ramírez P, et al. Recalcitrant palmoplantar pustular psoriasis treated with etanercept. Pediatr Dermatol 2011;28:349–50.

88. Paller AS, Siegfried EC, Eichenfield LF, et al. Long-term etanercept in pediatric patients with plaque psoriasis. J Am Acad Dermatol 2010;63: 762–8.

89. Siegfried EC, Eichenfield LF, Paller AS, et al. Intermittent etanercept therapy in pediatric patients with psoriasis. J Am Acad Dermatol 2010;63: 769–74.

90. European Medicines Agency. Human medicines—CHMP post-authorisation summary of positive opinion for Enbrel II-126. Available at: http://www.ema.europa.eu/ema/index.jsp?curl=pages/medicines/human/medicines/000262/smops/Positive/human_smop_000264.jsp&mid=WC0b01ac058001d127&murl=menus/medicines/medicines.jsp. Accessed February 20, 2012.

91. Prince FH, Twilt M, ten Cate R, et al. Long-term follow-up on effectiveness and safety of etanercept in juvenile idiopathic arthritis: the Dutch national register. Ann Rheum Dis 2009;68:635–41.

92. Lovell DJ, Reiff A, Ilowite NT, et al. Safety and efficacy of up to eight years of continuous etanercept therapy in patients with juvenile rheumatoid arthritis. Arthritis Rheum 2008;58:1496–504.

93. Giannini EH, Ilowite NT, Lovell DJ, et al. Long-term safety and effectiveness of etanercept in children with selected categories of juvenile idiopathic arthritis. Arthritis Rheum 2009;60:2794–804.

94. Janssen Biotech, Inc. REMICADE (infliximab) [full prescribing information]. Available at: http://www.remicade.com/hcp/remicade/assets/hcp_ppi.pdf. Accessed February 20, 2012.

95. Farnsworth NN, George SJ, Hsu S. Successful use of infliximab following a failed course of etanercept in a pediatric patient. Dermatol Online J 2005;11:11.

96. Menter MA, Cush JM. Successful treatment of pediatric psoriasis with infliximab. Pediatr Dermatol 2004;21:87–8.

97. Pereira TM, Vieira AP, Fernandes JC, et al. Anti-TNF-alpha therapy in childhood pustular psoriasis. Dermatology 2006;213:350–2.

98. Weishaupt C, Metze D, Luger TA, et al. Treatment of pustular psoriasis with infliximab. J Dtsch Dermatol Ges 2007;5:397–9.

99. Lahdenne P, Vähäsalo P, Honkanen V. Infliximab or etanercept in the treatment of children with refractory juvenile idiopathic arthritis: an open label study. Ann Rheum Dis 2003;62:245–7.

100. Pontikaki I, Gerloni V, Gattinara M, et al. Side effects of anti-TNFalpha therapy in juvenile idiopathic arthritis. Reumatismo 2006;58:31–8 [in Italian].

101. Papp KA. The long-term efficacy and safety of new biological therapies for psoriasis. Arch Dermatol Res 2006;298:7–15.

102. Mackey AC, Green L, Liang LC, et al. Hepatosplenic T cell lymphoma associated with infliximab use in young patients treated for inflammatory bowel disease. J Pediatr Gastroenterol Nutr 2007; 44:265–7.

103. Abbott-Laboratories. Humira (adalimumab) [full prescribing information]. Available at: http://www.rxabbott.com/pdf/humira.pdf. Accessed February 20, 2012.

104. Sukhatme SV, Gottlieb AB. Pediatric psoriasis: updates in biologic therapies. Dermatol Ther 2009; 22:34–9.

105. Callen JP, Jackson JH. Adalimumab effectively controlled recalcitrant generalized pustular psoriasis in an adolescent. J Dermatolog Treat 2005; 16:350–2.

106. Alvarez AC, Rodríguez-Nevado I, De Argila D, et al. Recalcitrant pustular psoriasis successfully treated with adalimumab. Pediatr Dermatol 2011; 28:195–7.

107. Lovell DJ, Ruperto N, Goodman S, et al. Adalimumab with or without methotrexate in juvenile rheumatoid arthritis. N Engl J Med 2008;359: 810–20.

108. Rosh JR, Lerer T, Markowitz J, et al. Retrospective Evaluation of the Safety and Effect of Adalimumab Therapy (RESEAT) in pediatric Crohn's disease. Am J Gastroenterol 2009;104:3042–9.

109. Menter A, Gottlieb A, Feldman SR, et al. Guidelines of care for the management of psoriasis and psoriatic arthritis: section 1. Overview of psoriasis and guidelines of care for the treatment of psoriasis with biologics. J Am Acad Dermatol 2008;58: 826–50.

110. Diak P, Siegel J, La Grenade L, et al. Tumor necrosis factor alpha blockers and malignancy in children: forty-eight cases reported to the Food and Drug Administration. Arthritis Rheum 2010; 62:2517–24.

111. Thayu M, Markowitz JE, Mamula P, et al. Hepatosplenic T-cell lymphoma in an adolescent patient

after immunomodulator and biologic therapy for Crohn disease. J Pediatr Gastroenterol Nutr 2005; 40:220–2.

112. Janssen Biotech, Inc: Stelara (ustekinumab) [full prescribing information]. Available at: http://www.stelarainfo.com/pdf/PrescribingInformation.pdf#zoom=100. Accessed February 20, 2012.

113. Fotiadou C, Lazaridou E, Giannopoulou C, et al. Ustekinumab for the treatment of an adolescent patient with recalcitrant plaque psoriasis. Eur J Dermatol 2011;21:117–8.

114. ClinicalTrials.gov. A Study of the Safety and Efficacy of Ustekinumab in Adolescent Patients With Psoriasis (CADMUS). Available at: http://clinicaltrialsgov/ct2/show/study/NCT01090427. Accessed February 20, 2012.

115. Lee CS, Koo JY. Cyclosporine. In: Wolverton SE, editor. Comprehensive dermatologic drug therapy.

2nd edition. Philadelphia: Saunders (Elsevier); 2007. p. 219–37.

116. Pereira GM, Miller JF, Shevach EM. Mechanism of action of cyclosporine A in vivo. II. T cell priming in vivo to alloantigen can be mediated by an IL-2-independent cyclosporine A-resistant pathway. J Immunol 1990;144:2109–16.

117. Lebwohl M, Bagel J, Gelfand JM, et al. From the Medical Board of the National Psoriasis Foundation: monitoring and vaccinations in patients treated with biologics for psoriasis. J Am Acad Dermatol 2008;58:94–105.

118. Hsu S, Papp KA, Lebwohl MG, et al. Consensus guidelines for the management of plaque psoriasis. Arch Dermatol 2012;148:95–102.

119. Croxtall JD. Ustekinumab: a review of its use in the management of moderate to severe plaque psoriasis. Drugs 2011;71:1733–53.

# Approach to the Patient with an Infantile Hemangioma

Kristen E. Holland, MD[a],*, Beth A. Drolet, MD[b]

## KEYWORDS

- Infantile hemangioma • Treatment • Complications

## KEY POINTS

- Infantile hemangioma is the most common soft tissue tumor of childhood.
- Although spontaneous resolution of these lesions occurs, they can be a significant source of functional impairment and present risk for permanent cosmetic disfigurement.
- Awareness of risk factors predictive of complications and the need for treatment are key to ensuring appropriate management and optimizing patient outcomes.
- Discovery of the efficacy of β-blockers for the treatment of IH and its perceived lower side effect profile than medications traditionally used have resulted in widespread use. As the widespread use in infants is relatively new, the nature and true frequency of adverse effects are still being determined, and recommendations for monitoring are expected to evolve.

Infantile hemangioma (IH), or hemangioma of infancy, is the most common soft tissue tumor of childhood. Despite their frequency, it has only been in the last decade that these lesions have been better characterized and have become the subject of significant clinical and translational research. Recognition of the importance of defining subtypes and risks of IH has begun to lay the groundwork to develop future studies to create evidence-based guidelines for management and to care for affected patients better. Although most IHs are uncomplicated and do not require intervention, they can be a significant source of parental distress, cosmetic disfigurement, and morbidity. The wide spectrum of disease both in the morphology of these lesions and, more importantly, in their behavior has made it difficult to predict the need for treatment and has made it challenging to establish a standardized approach to management.

## EPIDEMIOLOGY

The incidence of IHs has been difficult to ascertain because IHs may not appear until after the immediate newborn period; as such, they have not traditionally been included in birth defect registries or surveillance systems. Inconsistent nomenclature used in older studies evaluating the incidence of hemangioma, whereby terms included "strawberry mark," "cavernous hemangiomata," "hemangioma," "strawberry nevi," and "angiomas," has made the interpretation of the findings less reliable.[1] A recent prospective study of newborns followed for the first 9 months of life demonstrated an incidence of 4.5% overall, with close to 10% in preterm infants.[2] Demographic risk factors for the development of IH include Caucasian race, female gender (female-to-male ratio of 1.8–2.4:1), and prematurity.[3,4] Additional perinatal characteristics associated with a higher risk of IH include preeclampsia, multiple gestation, and low birth

Conflicts of Interest: None.
[a] Department of Dermatology, Medical College of Wisconsin, 9000 West Wisconsin Avenue, Suite B260, Milwaukee, WI 53226, USA; [b] Children's Hospital of Wisconsin, Department of Dermatology, Medical College of Wisconsin, 9000 West Wisconsin Avenue, Suite B260, Milwaukee, WI 53226, USA
* Corresponding author.
*E-mail address:* kholland@mcw.edu

Dermatol Clin 31 (2013) 289–301
http://dx.doi.org/10.1016/j.det.2012.12.006
0733-8635/13/$ – see front matter © 2013 Elsevier Inc. All rights reserved.

weight.[3] Although some of these observed risk factors are potentially confounding, low birth weight has been found to be the most significant risk factor through multivariate analysis.[5] IHs have previously been considered sporadic; however, clinicians have noted a familial tendency, often caring for multiple siblings with hemangiomas. A recent case-control study in a Chinese population observed that 37% of patients with IH had a history of an IH in a first-degree relative, consistent with an earlier report.[5,6] Walter and colleagues[7] studied 5 families (22 individuals) with hemangiomas and vascular malformations and found a linkage to a locus on chromosome 5q31–33, suggesting that genes are located on this part of the chromosome, which contributes to the development of hemangiomas. Although these data provide compelling evidence that genetic factors contribute significantly to the development of hemangiomas, to the authors' knowledge, none of these studies have yet led to identification of a specific gene.

## PATHOGENESIS

Despite the frequency of this tumor, understanding of the pathogenetic mechanisms of IH is still in its infancy. IH pathogenesis is generally believed to be a complex interaction of both genetic and environmental factors.[5] Although early research focused on angiogenesis as the mechanism by which IHs form, more recent efforts have identified postnatal vasculogenesis as a possible pathway for development of IH. Tissue ischemia resulting in neovascularization has been proposed as the stimulus leading to the development of IH. Clinically, in support of this, an area of pallor or decreased blood flow on the skin has been noted to precede the development of IH.[8]

Histologic and immunohistochemical studies have demonstrated that IH is *not* a neoplasm of normal cutaneous capillaries.[9] Histologically, IHs have markedly increased cellularity with clusters of plump cells that are positive for markers of immature endothelial cells. North and colleagues[10] were the first to note that the endothelial-like cells of the hemangioma expressed GLUT-1, the erythrocyte-type glucose transporter protein that has been shown to be upregulated in zones of hypoxia. GLUT-1 seems to be an exclusive marker for IH and is an invaluable tool used to distinguish hemangiomas from other vascular lesions. The immunohistochemical phenotype of endothelial cells in hemangiomas is identical to that of the chorionic villus cells of the placenta, expressing GLUT-1 at all stages of development, from precursor lesions to fully involuted hemangiomas.[10,11] Although some have speculated that

IH may represent embolization of placenta,[12] an alternative explanation is that the phenotypic similarities instead represent an early, immature progenitor cell, which via its immature fetal phenotype shares common attributes.

In further support of hypoxia's role in pathogenesis, proliferating hemangiomas have been shown to contain cell types known to preferentially home to hypoxic sites.[13] Hypoxia-induced factors produced by hypoxic endothelial cells play an important role in trafficking of progenitor cells to ischemic tissue. Kleinman and colleagues[14] have demonstrated these factors to be upregulated in the blood (vascular endothelial growth factor A [VEGF-A], matrix metallopeptidase-9) and hemangioma tissue (stromal cell-derived factor-1$\alpha$, matrix metallopeptidase-9, VEGF-A, and hypoxia-inducible growth factor-1$\alpha$) from children with proliferating hemangiomas. Recently, Khan and colleagues[15] have characterized multipotential stem cells derived from IH specimens (HemSCs) and have demonstrated their ability to recapitulate human IH in immunodeficient mice, creating the first in vivo model. These hemangioma stem cells and cord blood endothelial progenitor cells are similar to each other in several in vitro assays, suggesting that circulating progenitor cells may be recruited into proliferating IH lesions.[11] The concept that IHs originating from circulating multipotent progenitor cells could also help explain the shared features with placental blood vessels. However, the origin of these hemangioma stem cells remains unknown and remains an area of future study.

Molecular and cellular mediators implicated in the proliferative and involutive phases of hemangiomas include VEGF, basic fibroblast growth factor, insulin-like growth factor-2, tissue inhibitor of metalloproteinase type 1, type IV collagenase, urokinase, hypoxia-inducible growth factor, and mast cells.[9,10,13,16–18] The importance of the VEGF signaling pathway and its known role in angiogenesis has been identified as a key part of IH proliferation and may account, in part, for the response to corticosteroids and propranolol.[19,20] Significant investigation into IH pathogenesis is currently underway, which will continue to advance the understanding of the mechanisms involved in IH growth and involution and lead to new, targeted therapy.

## DIAGNOSIS

The diagnosis of an IH is typically made clinically based on its appearance and characteristic behavior. Although their appearance may be quite variable, ranging from small, red lesions to large and bulky tumors, it is their behavior that helps to distinguish them from other vascular lesions. Early on, they can appear as a telangiectatic patch or an area of pallor and are often unrecognized until a few weeks of age when they begin to proliferate. The natural history of IH is characterized by an initial proliferative or growth phase followed by a plateau phase, and finally, the involution phase. In the proliferative phase, IHs tend to be firm and noncompressible and become softer and more compressible as they begin to involute. A change in color from bright red to purple or gray can often signal transition to the involution phase. However, the transition from the growth phase to involution may be more dynamic than previously thought, reflecting a balance between local proliferative factors and factors involved in apoptosis.[21] Chang and colleagues[21] detailed the growth characteristics of 526 IHs in 433 children, noting that most hemangioma growth occurs in the first 5 months. However, some IHs exhibit minimal proliferation, remain flat, and may be reticular or networklike in appearance. On average, IHs typically reach their maximum size by 9 months, but deep hemangiomas may proliferate longer. Albeit rare, IHs with an extended growth phase (up to 2 years) have been reported; these tend to be larger lesions and more often segmental or indeterminate rather than localized.[22] A subset of 23 IHs from a large prospective study of 1530 IHs that demonstrated prolonged growth were all of the deep or combined subtype, and it was the deep component that was subjectively thought to have the continued growth in the majority of IHs.[22]

In the past, IHs have been classified by their depth of soft tissue involvement (superficial, deep, and mixed).[23–25] Superficial hemangiomas (**Fig. 1**) appear as bright red lesions, which may be plaquelike or more rounded papules or nodules. Deep hemangiomas (**Fig. 2**) involve the deep dermis and subcutis and present as bluish to skin-colored nodules. Mixed hemangiomas

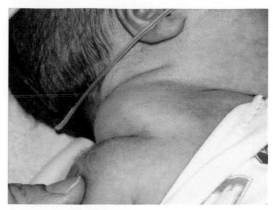

**Fig. 2.** Deep hemangioma.

(**Fig. 3**) clinically have features of both superficial and deep hemangiomas, often with a red plaque overlying a bluish nodule. However, another classification based on morphology has proven to have greater prognostic value and be more predictive of risk of complications or need for treatment. In this classification system, hemangiomas are defined as localized or segmental or indeterminate.[24,25] Localized hemangiomas are discrete, usually oval or round, and appear to grow from a single focal point. In contrast, the term "segmental" has been used to describe hemangiomas that demonstrate a geographic shape and involve a broad anatomic region or a recognized developmental unit (**Fig. 4**). The distinction between these morphologic subtypes is an important one, as segmental hemangiomas are at higher risk of complications and associated anomalies. Although the classification of an IH as segmental may be difficult at times to make with certainty, their larger size may assist with recognition of this subtype because they have been shown to

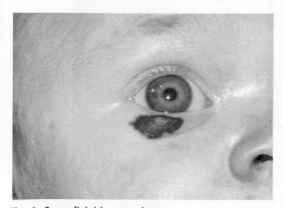

**Fig. 1.** Superficial hemangioma.

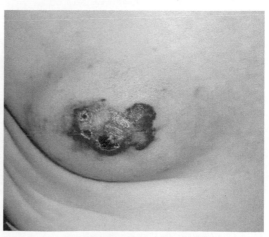

**Fig. 3.** Mixed hemangioma with focal secondary ulceration.

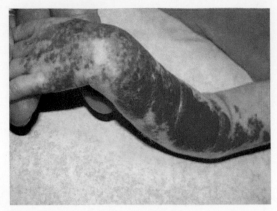

**Fig. 4.** Segmental hemangioma.

cover 4 times greater surface area than localized lesions.[24]

IHs may occur anywhere on the skin, but are most common on the head and neck. Reproducible patterns of segmental hemangiomas on the face have been demonstrated and mapped.[25,26] Although involvement of the lower face corresponds to known embryologic facial prominences (maxillary, mandibular, and frontonasal), involvement of the upper face (forehead) does not.

## COMPLICATIONS

Although most IHs are uncomplicated and do not require treatment, 24% of those referred to tertiary institutions had complications.[27] Providers should be aware of risk factors predictive of complications and the need for treatment to facilitate early referral to a physician with expertise in the management of IHs. Size, location, and subtype (localized vs segmental) are major factors to consider in evaluating an infant's risk.[27] Specifically, for every 10 cm² increase in size, a 5% increase in likelihood

of complications as well as a 4% increase in likelihood of treatment has been reported.[27] Although segmental hemangiomas tend to be larger lesions, this subtype has been shown to be an independent risk factor for the development of complications and/or need for treatment.[27] In a prospective IH study reported by Haggstrom and colleagues,[27] segmental IHs were 8 times more likely to receive treatment and 11 times more likely to develop complications compared with localized IHs after controlling for IH size. In this same study, the perceived risk of permanent disfigurement was the leading indication for treatment. The risk of disfigurement depends on the hemangioma subtype, location, and extent of proliferation. Minimally elevated IHs with a gentle slope noted at the edges are at risk for minimal residual telangiectasia or textural change, in contrast to more exophytic IHs with a steeper slope and more prominent superficial component, which are more likely to leave fibrofatty tissue and a resultant scar (**Fig. 5**).[28] Permanent distortion of anatomic landmarks can occur as the result of location (eg, nasal tip, involvement of ear cartilage) or secondary to ulceration (eg, lip).[28] Additional complications of IHs include ulceration, functional impairment (visual compromise, airway obstruction, auditory canal obstruction, feeding difficulty), and cardiac compromise. **Box 1** outlines locations at high risk for the development of hemangioma-specific complications or associated anomalies.

### Ulceration

Ulceration is the most common complication (reported in 16% of patients in a large prospective study)[29] and can result in pain, infection, bleeding, and permanent scarring. Associated pain can interfere with sleep as well as feeding. Locations

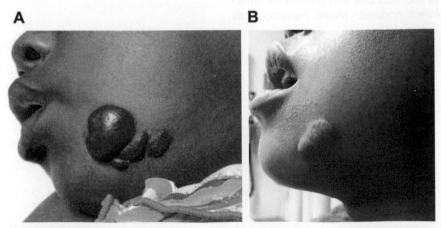

**Fig. 5.** (*A*) Patient with a protuberant superficial IH during the proliferative phase. (*B*) Same patient with resolved IH with residual fibrofatty tissue and scar.

**Box 1**
**High risk locations of IH**

| Location | Potential Complications or Associated Anomalies |
| --- | --- |
| Periocular | Functional compromise |
| Nasal tip | Cosmetic disfigurement |
| Lip or perioral | Ulceration |
| | Cosmetic disfigurement |
| | Functional compromise |
| Ear | Ulceration |
| | Cosmetic disfigurement |
| | Functional compromise |
| Other facial | Cosmetic disfigurement |
| | Risk for PHACE syndrome (with segmental morphology) |
| | Risk of airway hemangioma (with "beard" distribution) |
| Perineal, perianal | Ulceration |
| | Risk of LUMBAR syndrome (with segmental morphology) |
| Lumbosacral | Risk of spinal dysraphism, intraspinal IH, LUMBAR syndrome |
| Hepatic (large) | Congestive heart failure |

at high risk for ulceration and the associated frequency of this complication include anogenital (50%) (**Fig. 6**), lower lip (30%), and neck (25%).[29] IHs that are larger in size or of the segmental subtype are more likely to develop ulceration. Of the clinical subtypes (ie, superficial, mixed, and deep), the mixed subtype (having both superficial and deep components) has most frequently been associated with ulceration and is another independent risk factor.[29,30] The cause of ulceration is not well understood, but maceration and friction are likely contributing factors given the higher frequency in locations prone to this. Although

ulceration can be complicated by bleeding, clinically significant bleeding (ie, requiring hospitalization/transfusion) is rare.[29]

## Visual Compromise

Threat to vision is a common reason for treatment in the IH population.[27] Infants are at particular risk because stimulus deprivation for as little as 1 week can interrupt visual development and result in permanent visual impairment.[31] Periocular IH may cause ptosis, strabismus, and anisometropia, each of which may result in astigmatism, amblyopia, or blindness.[31] In addition, periocular IH can cause proptosis, exposure keratopathy, tear duct obstruction, and rarely, compressive optic neuropathy.[32] Amblyopia can develop in 3 ways, all of which are applicable to periocular IH: refractive-error differences, visual deprivation, and strabismus. Astigmatism, resulting from distortion of the cornea from pressure of the IH, is the most common cause of amblyobia.[31] If the IH affects growth of the eye, anisometropic (refractive error difference) amblyopia can occur. Strabismus may occur in rare cases from direct effects on extraocular muscles. Given the threat of permanent visual impairment, patients with periorbital hemangiomas should be referred early to a physician with an expertise in the treatment of IH and should be closely monitored by ophthalmology, including a retinal examination.[33]

## Visceral Involvement and Complications

Although solitary lesions are most common, multifocal cutaneous hemangiomas (**Fig. 7**) may occur in 30% of patients, although only 3% have greater than 6 lesions.[27] Historically, patients with numerous lesions have been placed into at least 2 categories: disseminated neonatal hemangiomatosis and benign neonatal hemangiomatosis, with

**Fig. 6.** Ulceration is a common complication of IH in the diaper area.

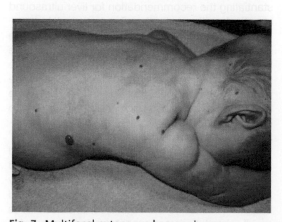

**Fig. 7.** Multifocal cutaneous hemangiomas.

the former considered to be more severe with multiple sites of potential extracutaneous disease and a rate of mortality as high as 60%.[34] However, in the past, all multifocal vascular lesions were considered to be hemangiomas, and with advances in histopathologic and radiologic diagnosis (ie, GLUT-1 stain), it is recognized that some of these severe cases represent other multifocal vascular anomalies (ie, multifocal lymphangioendotheliomatosis or cutaneovisceral angiomatosis) rather than true IHs.[35] Many of these other multifocal vascular lesions have a more aggressive course, often with coagulopathy and bleeding, and account for the high mortality historically reported with disseminated neonatal hemangiomatosis. In a critical review of 73 cases reported in the literature as diffuse neonatal hemangiomatosis, 43 were reclassified as IHs or probable IHs with death occurring in only 2 cases (5% of these patients). In contrast, 11 of the 17 (65%) patients were reclassified as multifocal lymphangioendotheliomatosis with thrombocytopenia (MLT)/probable MLT.[35] With greater recognition of other multifocal vascular tumors and improved diagnostics, overly aggressive intervention in infants with asymptomatic multifocal IH may be avoided in the future.

Patients with true multifocal cutaneous IH are recognized to have a higher risk of visceral hemangiomas, with liver and gastrointestinal involvement being most common. Ultrasound of the liver has been recommended in those patients with greater than 5 cutaneous hemangiomas.[36] A recent prospective study investigated the incidence of hepatic involvement in patients with more than 5 cutaneous IHs compared with those with 1 to 4 cutaneous lesions and demonstrated a significantly increased risk in patients with greater than 5 cutaneous lesions. In this study, 24 (16%) of the infants with 5 or more cutaneous IHs had hepatic hemangiomas, whereas none of the infants with less than 5 cutaneous IHs had hepatic hemangiomas (P<.003), substantiating the recommendation for liver ultrasound in patients with greater than 5 cutaneous IHs.[37]

Similar to cutaneous IH, the nomenclature surrounding liver involvement with IH (infantile hepatic hemangiomas) has been confusing; the term hemangioma has been used to describe venous malformations and IHs in the liver have been referred to as hemangioendothelioma, not to be confused with epithelioid hemangioendothelioma, a malignant tumor with metastatic potential.[38] Infantile hepatic hemangiomas have been subtyped into the 3 following subtypes: focal, multifocal, and diffuse. Focal involvement is typically a solitary lesion that undergoes spontaneous regression and has been likened to the equivalent of a cutaneous rapidly involuting congenital hemangioma; skin

involvement in this setting is unusual. Similar to congenital hemangioma and unlike true IH, these lesions are GLUT-1-negative. Multifocal involvement is the subtype typically seen in the setting of multiple cutaneous IHs. Although these are often asymptomatic, high-output cardiac failure may be seen secondary to arteriovenous or portovenous shunting. In a prospective study of infants with multiple cutaneous IHs reported by Horii and colleagues,[37] only 2 of the 24 infants (8%) found to have hepatic involvement required treatment of their hepatic hemangioma. Finally, diffuse involvement with near-total replacement of hepatic parenchyma may be seen. The resulting mass effect can result in abdominal compartment syndrome and multisystem organ failure. Overproduction of type 3 iodothyronine deiodinase by IH resulting in accelerated inactivation of thyroid hormone can result in acquired hypothyroidism in patients with multifocal or diffuse hepatic involvement.[39,40] These patients should be screened with a serum TSH to ensure that hypothyroidism is not missed, because mental retardation and cardiac failure can ensue if hypothyroidism not detected.

### Anomalies Associated with Anatomic Location of IH

The presence of IH in particular locations can be a marker for underlying or associated anomalies. The "beard" distribution (**Fig. 8**) of an IH, in which preauricular areas, chin, anterior neck, and lower lip is involved, has been associated with the presence of airway hemangiomas. In 2 retrospective studies, 29% to 63% of patients with large IHs on the lower lip, chin, neck, and preauricular region (beard) had airway involvement.[41,42] Airway hemangiomas typically present between 6 and 12 weeks of age with biphasic inspiratory and expiratory stridor and retractions.[41,43] Cough may be associated and may mimic croup. Infants with IH in the beard distribution should be monitored closely for

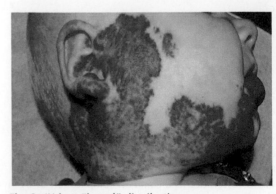

Fig. 8. IH in a "beard" distribution.

respiratory difficulties and referred to an ear, nose and throat specialist for evaluation. Serial evaluations may be required in young infants because the skin hemangioma may precede the development of symptomatic airway IH.

Cutaneous hemangiomas in the lumbosacral area have also been reported in association with underlying developmental anomalies. Because the skin overlying the lumbosacral region has an intimate developmental relationship with the neural tube, hemangiomas in this location have been recognized as one of the cutaneous markers associated with occult spinal dysraphism, including tethered cord, lipomyelomeningocele, intraspinal lipoma, and tight fila terminalia.[44,45] In a prospective cohort study evaluating the risk of spinal anomalies in patients with a midline lumbosacral IH, 51% of the patients evaluated by magnetic resonance imaging demonstrated spinal anomalies (intraspinal hemangioma or lipoma, structural malformation of the cord, or tethered cord).[46] Of these, 35% had an isolated IH without other signs of spinal dysraphism, which corresponded to a relative risk of spinal anomalies of 640 (children with IH plus another cutaneous sign of spinal dysraphism) and 438 (children with isolated IH). Given the low sensitivity of ultrasound (50%) demonstrated in the aforementioned study, magnetic resonance imaging should be performed in these patients to look for these anomalies to prompt early detection and prevention of neurologic impairment. Additional anomalies have been reported in association with lumbosacral IH, typically of the segmental morphologic subtype, resulting in the acronym LUMBAR being coined (Lower body IH and other skin defects, Urogenital anomalies, Myelopathy, Bony deformities, Anorectal malformations and Arterial anomalies, and Renal anomalies).[47] These malformations are typically evident at birth, prompting further evaluation to determine the extent of the associated anomalies; however, it has been suggested that systematic pelviperineal imaging should be performed even in the absence of obvious malformations because the potential for occult anomalies exists.[44] Recommendations for imaging based on region of involvement by IH have been outlined by Iacobas and colleagues.[47]

## PHACE Syndrome

Large facial hemangiomas have been described in association with posterior fossa brain malformations, arterial cerebrovascular anomalies, cardiovascular anomalies, eye anomalies, and ventral developmental defects, specifically, sternal defects and/or supraumbilical raphe.[48] PHACE (the neurocutaneous disorder characterized by posterior fossa abnormalities [P], large facial hemangiomas [H], arterial anomalies [A], cardiac defects [C], and eye anomalies [E]) syndrome refers to the constellation of findings in this neurocutaneous syndrome; recently, diagnostic criteria have been established to define this syndrome more precisely.[49] Little is known about the pathogenesis, natural history, or long-term outcome of PHACE syndrome. There is a strong female predominance, with nearly 90% of cases being girls.[50] Unlike isolated IH, patients with PHACE tend to be born full term, of normal birth weight, and born a singleton, suggesting a different pathogenesis.

Hemangiomas associated with PHACE syndrome tend to be large plaquelike, segmental facial hemangiomas (**Fig. 9**). In a recent prospective study systematically evaluating 108 patients with large facial hemangiomas at risk for PHACE syndrome, 33 (31%) met criteria for PHACE syndrome.[51] Structural cerebral and/or cerebrovascular anomalies are the most common extracutaneous findings associated with PHACE syndrome and have been described in 72% of PHACE patients in 1 study; however, this number may have underestimated the true incidence because not all at-risk patients were thoroughly evaluated for associated anomalies in this study.[50] Using standardized screening with magnetic resonance imaging/magnetic resonance angiography of the head and neck and echocardiogram, 94% had cerebrovascular anomalies, and 67% had cardiovascular anomalies.[51] The cerebrovascular anomalies in PHACE have been classified into the 5 following categories: narrowing (hypoplasia or stenosis), nonvisualization (aplasia or occlusion), dysgenesis (kinking, looping, tortuosity, dolichoectasia, or aneurysm), aberrant origin or course, and persistent embryonic arteries.[52] Neurologic sequelae, including seizures, developmental delay, focal motor impairments, headache, and stroke, have been reported.[50,53] Aortic arch anomalies are the most frequent cardiovascular finding; these anomalies include aortic coarctation, aortic

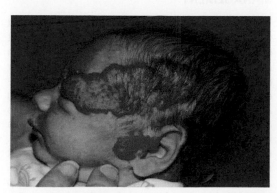

**Fig. 9.** Patient with segmental facial hemangioma associated with PHACE syndrome.

interruption, and tortuous aorta and are often associated with anomalous subclavian arteries. Ocular and ventral developmental anomalies occur less commonly, reported in 7% to 17% and 5% to 25%, respectively.[50,51] Rarely, endocrine abnormalities may be associated, including structural pituitary anomalies and endocrinopathies, including hypopituitarism, hypothyroidism, growth hormone deficiency, and diabetes insipidus.[50] All patients with large facial IHs at risk for PHACE syndrome should have a thorough investigation of the brain, heart, and eyes to evaluate for PHACE-associated anomalies. Although magnetic resonance imaging can demonstrate certain cerebrovascular anomalies, magnetic resonance angiography is necessary to characterize the cerebrovasculature fully.

A literature review of 22 PHACE patients with acute ischemic stroke examined clinical features of these patients to determine risk factors for stroke and found that severe underlying arteriopathy with narrowing or nonvisualization of a major cerebral artery (often ≥1) was noted more frequently (seen in 21 patients) than previously reported in a general PHACE cohort.[53] Furthermore, aortic anomalies were frequent (15 of 22 patients). None of these patients had arterial dysplasia as the sole class of arteriopathy. As imaging was often performed at the time of neurologic symptoms or stroke, the possibility that flow-related apparent narrowing occurred exists. Future prospective studies with standardized imaging protocols of patients with PHACE syndrome will better stratify the risk of stroke in patients with cerebrovascular anomalies.

Several similarities between PHACE and LUMBAR syndromes have been observed (segmental IH, female predisposition, arterial anomalies, and regional association with underlying anomalies), suggesting that these may be analogous syndromes occurring in different anatomic locations.[47]

## MANAGEMENT

The clinical heterogeneity and unpredictable and variable course of IHs complicate management decisions and have contributed to the lack of an evidenced-based standard of care. There are few prospective studies looking at the safety and efficacy of therapies for IH, and no Food and Drug Administration–approved agents for IH exist. As a result, the selection of therapeutic modalities is based on anecdote and small case series. Physicians caring for an infant with IH must first determine whether treatment is indicated. Although most hemangiomas are self-limited, up to 38% of hemangiomas referred to tertiary care specialists require systemic treatment because of

complications such as ulceration, bleeding, risk for permanent disfigurement, obstruction of vision, airway obstruction, or high-output cardiac failure.[27] Location, age of the patient, presence of or risk for complications, and growth rate are all factors that must be considered by physicians managing patients with IH.

### Ulceration

Initial therapy for most ulcerated hemangiomas, a common indication for treatment, is local wound care. Gentle debridement of the crust overlying the ulceration can be achieved with wet compresses with astringent solutions of aluminum acetate (ie, Domeboro solution; Bayer Healthcare, Morristown, NJ). In the diaper area, barrier creams containing zinc oxide or petrolatum play an important role in protecting the skin from maceration and irritation from urine and stool, which may inhibit healing. Nonadherent dressings such as petrolatum gauze or extrathin hydrocolloid dressings may act as an additional barrier to outside pathogens or irritants and promote healing. As secondary infection can develop in ulcerated IHs, cultures should be obtained in nonhealing lesions and topical antibiotics (ie, polymyxin-bacitracin, mupirocin, metronidazole) should be used. Oral antibiotics may be necessary in patients with evidence of infection nonresponsive to topical measures.

In ulcerations recalcitrant to the initial topical measures outlined above, topical application of becaplermin gel, a recombinant human platelet-derived growth factor, has been shown in a small case series to be effective at speeding healing.[54] More recently, a boxed warning was placed on this medication about the possible increased risk of mortality secondary to malignancy in some patients. As a result, its role is generally reserved as a second-line or third-line agent for patients who have failed other treatment modalities.[55]

Other modalities, including propranolol and pulse dye laser, have shown some benefit in the management of ulcerated IHs. These modalities are discussed in more detail later in the article.

### β-Blockers

The efficacy of propranolol for IH was first reported by Leaute-Labreze and colleagues[56] in 2008. After this initial report, the use of propranolol for IH quickly gained favor, because it has been perceived to have a lower side-effect profile than other systemic therapies used for treating IH. Its mechanism of action in the treatment of IH is unknown. Possible mechanisms of action purported include vasoconstriction, inhibition of angiogenesis, and induction of apoptosis.[20] Improvement in color, softening, growth arrest, and regression of IH have been observed with the administration of propranolol.[57–60] In contrast to corticosteroids, the former mainstay of therapy for complicated IH, the benefits of propranolol have been shown to extend beyond the proliferative phase. Successful treatment with more rapid resolution than expected for natural involution has been reported, when propranolol has been used in older patients.[58,59,61] A larger retrospective series of 42 patients initially treated over the age of 12 months or after documentation of growth arrest was examined to characterize the utility of propranolol better in this age group.[61] Doses of 1 to 3 mg/kg/d divided equally twice a day or three times a day have been reported to be effective for IH. In a case series of 55 infants treated with 2 mg/kg/d in 3 divided doses, 14.5% showed complete regression of the IH, 83.4% showed partial regression, and only 1 case (aged 18 months) did not show regression.[59] Most of these patients required treatment for several months; although 38.2% of these patients required dose-adjustment for weight over this time, more than half continued to show good response on the initial dose. Relapse or delayed growth of IH on discontinuation of the propranolol has been described.[59,62] Significant controversy still exists regarding recommended evaluation (ie, electrocardiogram, echocardiography, cardiology consultation) before initiation of therapy, monitoring with initiation (outpatient vs inpatient), dose escalation protocols, and toxicity monitoring. As such, considerable variation in clinical practice exists.

Although propranolol has been used for other indications in the pediatric population for decades, pharmacokinetics and safety in children have not been rigorously studied. In the IH literature, reported adverse effects of propranolol include hypotension, bronchospasm (particularly in patients with asthma or acute respiratory infection), hypoglycemia,[63,64] cold hands or feet,[58,59] sleep disturbance (insomnia, transient nightmares, sleepwalking), exanthema, fatigue/somnolence, gastroesophageal problems including diarrhea and constipation, and bronchospasm.[60] The most common serious side effects of propranolol include bradycardia and hypotension. Given the variation in monitoring practices described in the literature, the true incidence of hypotension or bradycardia in children on propranolol is not known. Hypoglycemia has most commonly been reported in the setting of concurrent illness with decreased oral intake or after fasting (ie, overnight).[63] This particular side effect has been unpredictable and does not seem to be dose-related.

Contraindications for the use of propranolol are outlined in **Box 2**. In addition, there are theoretical

---

**Box 2**
**Contraindications/precautions for treatment with propranolol**

Cardiogenic shock

Bradycardia

Hypotension

Second-degree or third-degree heart block

Sick sinus syndrome

Asthma/reactive airway disease

Hypersensitivity to propranolol

---

considerations specific to using oral propranolol for the treatment of IH.[63] Regarding hypoglycemia, most patients for whom propranolol will be prescribed for an IH will be less than 1 year of age, have limited glycogen stores and a relative inability to communicate, recognize, or treat symptoms. Furthermore, low birth weight, an important risk factor for the development of IH, also confers a greater risk of hypoglycemia. Oral corticosteroids are used frequently for the treatment of IHs; during treatment, there may be some protective effect as steroids inhibit insulin action. However, after prolonged steroid use there may be residual adrenal suppression and subsequent loss of the counterregulatory cortisol response, thus increasing the risk of hypoglycemia.[65] In patients with PHACE syndrome and cerebrovascular or aortic arch anomalies, lower blood pressure may decrease blood flow through stenotic or dysplastic vessels, resulting in hypoperfusion of the brain (when cerebrovascular vessels are involved) or the lower body (when aortic coarctation is present). Finally, in patients with high-output cardiac failure secondary to a large liver hemangioma, the use of propranolol could result in decompensation secondary to drug-induced suppression of heart rate/contractility. Until the safety of propranolol in these patients can be established and these theoretic concerns allayed, caution should be exercised when prescribing propranolol.

After the efficacy of propranolol for the treatment of IH was discovered, the successful utility of topical timolol, also a nonselective β-blocker, to treat small and superficial IH was demonstrated.[66–70] Not only inhibition of growth but also the promotion of regression has been observed with timolol treatment. Topical timolol is available in a 0.25% and 0.5% solution, as well as an extended release 0.5% (5 mg/mL) gel-forming solution. Frequency and method of application have varied from once daily under occlusion to twice daily without occlusion; 1 to 2 drops have typically been used. Although systemic absorption with ophthalmic use is known, data regarding percutaneous absorption are limited. However, it is reasonable to assume that use of timolol to an ulcerated IH or near mucosae would be associated with greater systemic absorption. Of note, its use in the treatment of ulcerated IH is currently under investigation in a controlled trial and should provide valuable information about the risk of systemic absorption and safety in this setting. Adverse effects of ophthalmic preparations of timolol in the pediatric population include bradycardia and bronchospasm, and contraindications for its use mirror those for systemic propranolol. In addition, apnea has been attributed to systemic absorption of ophthalmic timolol in 2 children.[71] As such, it has been suggested that timolol be used with caution in infants with a history of apnea or chronic lung disease and in premature infants less than 44 weeks corrected gestational age, as they are at additional risk of apnea of prematurity.[71] In the IH literature, timolol seems to be well-tolerated, but reports of sleep disturbances exist, suggesting that systemic absorption may occur.[69] As such, until further safety data are known, using similar caution with timolol use as with propranolol is prudent, particularly with ulcerated IH or near mucosae. Caregivers should be educated about potential adverse effects, which may indicate systemic absorption, and should be given specific instructions regarding the exact amount to be applied to avoid overdose.

## Corticosteroids

Systemic corticosteroids at a dose of 2 to 5 mg/kg/d (typically 2–3 mg/kg/d) have historically been the mainstay of therapy. Response to treatment is variable with 1 retrospective study reporting regression in one-third of cases, stabilization of growth in another third of cases, and minimal to no response in the final third of cases.[72] Adverse effects are common and include irritability, gastrointestinal upset, sleep disturbance, cushingoid facies, adrenal suppression, immunosuppression, hypertension, bone demineralization, cardiomyopathy, and growth retardation.[73] Catch-up growth occurs in most children once the corticosteroids are discontinued. The duration of treatment and approach to tapering corticosteroids are variable, as it depends the treatment response, age of the child, inherent growth characteristics of the IH, and complications of therapy. For example, younger infants tend to be treated longer (months) given their greater potential for IH growth, whereas older infants whose IH may be nearing the end of its proliferative phase would be less likely to need prolonged therapy. A prospective study of 16 infants evaluating the immunosuppressive effects of corticosteroids demonstrated that both lymphocyte cell numbers and function are affected. Because the levels of tetanus and diphtheria antibodies were not found to be protective in 11 and 3 of the patients, respectively, it has been recommended that patients who receive oral corticosteroids during the immunization period have these checked and additional immunizations provided if titers are not protective. In addition, prophylaxis with a combination of trimethoprim and sulfamethoxazole should be considered in infants to protect against *Pneumocystis* pneumonia (PCP) because there are reports of PCP in this setting.[74]

Intralesional and topical corticosteroids have also been reported to decrease the size or slow growth of IH.[73] Intralesional and topical corticosteroids are most effective for small and localized cutaneous hemangiomas. The efficacy of topical steroid is limited by the depth of its penetration compared with the depth of hemangioma involvement. Doses of intralesional triamcinolone should not exceed 3 to 5 mg/kg per treatment.[73] Repeated injections are often necessary to maintain response. Central retinal artery occlusion, believed to be the result of pressure exceeding systolic pressure during injection, has been reported in the treatment of periocular hemangiomas, limiting its use in this location.[73] Other complications related to intralesional corticosteroids include skin atrophy and necrosis, calcification, and rarely, adrenal suppression (dose-dependent).

## Vincristine

Vincristine has been reported to be effective in the treatment of IH and has historically been reserved for those IHs resistant to corticosteroids or in patients intolerant of corticosteroids. Single weekly doses of 1 to 1.5 mg/m$^2$ resulted in an improvement of all 9 patients, as reported by Enjolras and colleagues.[75–77] Constipation is the most common side effect, but neuromyopathy, most commonly presenting as foot drop, is a potentially serious side effect. Administration of vincristine requires placement of a central line; therefore, risks associated with this must be considered as well.

## Interferon

Recombinant interferon-$\alpha$, an inhibitor of angiogenesis, administered as a subcutaneous injection of 3 million units per square meter per day, has also been used successfully for the treatment of IH.[73] Side effects include flulike symptoms of fever, irritability, and malaise. Less commonly, transient neutropenia and liver enzyme abnormalities may develop. Spastic diplegia, irreversible in some cases, has also been a reported side effect. The development of spastic diplegia has been observed more frequently in infants treated at an earlier age, the time at which there is often greatest need for treatment. Consequently, its use is not recommended.

*Laser*

The pulsed dye laser (PDL) has been successfully used for vascular birthmarks, namely, capillary malformations or "port-wine stains" for years, and its efficacy in this setting is well-established. Controversy exists surrounding its use for the treatment of proliferating IH as adverse outcomes including ulceration and scarring have been described.[78] In addition, the use of PDL for intact IH is limited by the depth of the laser's penetration (1 mm). There are several reports and 2 prospective studies describing its benefit in the treatment of ulcerated hemangiomas in terms of both increasing reepithelialization and decreasing pain.[79,80] The mechanism for this is not well understood. The greatest consensus surrounding the use of the PDL for IH is in the treatment of residual telangiectases after involution, for which the PDL is most effective.

*Surgery*

Surgical excision may be an option for function-threatening or life-threatening hemangiomas when medical therapy fails or is not tolerated, but more commonly its role is for removal of residual fibrofatty tissue or correction of scarring after involution. Surgical correction may be pursued at an earlier age if it is clear that the child will ultimately need a procedure for the residual effects.

## REFERENCES

1. Kilcline C, Frieden IJ. Infantile hemangiomas: how common are they? A systematic review of the medical literature. Pediatr Dermatol 2008;25(2):168–73.

2. Kanada KM, Merin MR, Munden A, et al. A prospective study of cutaneous findings in newborns in the United States: correlation with race, ethnicity, and gestational status using updated classification and nomenclature. J Pediatr 2012;161(2):240–5.

3. Hemangioma Investigator Group, Haggstrom AN, Drolet BA, Baselga E, et al. Prospective study of infantile hemangiomas: demographic, prenatal, and perinatal characteristics. J Pediatr 2007;150(3):291–4.

4. Li J, Chen X, Zhao S, et al. Demographic and clinical characteristics and risk factors for infantile hemangioma: a Chinese case-control study. Arch Dermatol 2011;147(9):1049–56.

5. Drolet BA, Swanson EA, Frieden IJ, et al. Infantile hemangiomas: an emerging health issue linked to an increased rate of low birth weight infants. J Pediatr 2008;153(5):712 No-715.

6. Grimmer JF, Williams MS, Pimentel R, et al. Familial clustering of hemangiomas. Arch Otolaryngol Head Neck Surg 2011;137(8):757–60.

7. Walter JW, Blei F, Anderson JL, et al. Genetic mapping of a novel familial form of infantile hemangioma. Am J Med Genet 1999;82(1):77–83.

8. Drolet BA, Frieden IJ. Characteristics of infantile hemangiomas as clues to pathogenesis: does hypoxia connect the dots? Arch Dermatol 2010;146(11):1295–9.

9. North PE, Waner M, Mizeracki A, et al. A unique microvascular phenotype shared by juvenile hemangiomas and human placenta. Arch Dermatol 2001;137(5):559–70.

10. North PE, Waner M, Mizeracki A, et al. GLUT1: a newly discovered immunohistochemical marker for juvenile hemangiomas. Hum Pathol 2000;31(1):11–22.

11. Bischoff J. Progenitor cells in infantile hemangioma. J Craniofac Surg 2009;20(Suppl 1):695–7.

12. Barnes CM, Huang S, Kaipainen A, et al. Evidence by molecular profiling for a placental origin of infantile hemangioma. Proc Natl Acad Sci U S A 2005;102(52):19097–102.

13. Ritter MR, Reinisch J, Friedlander SF, et al. Myeloid cells in infantile hemangioma. Am J Pathol 2006;168(2):621–8.

14. Kleinman ME, Greives MR, Churgin SS, et al. Hypoxia-induced mediators of stem/progenitor cell trafficking are increased in children with hemangioma. Arterioscler Thromb Vasc Biol 2007;27(12):2664–70.

15. Khan ZA, Boscolo E, Picard A, et al. Multipotential stem cells recapitulate human infantile hemangioma in immunodeficient mice. J Clin Invest 2008;118(7):2592–9.

16. Dadras SS, North PE, Bertoncini J, et al. Infantile hemangiomas are arrested in an early developmental vascular differentiation state. Mod Pathol 2004;17(9):1068–79.

17. Boscolo E, Stewart CL, Greenberger S, et al. JAGGED1 signaling regulates hemangioma stem cell-to-pericyte/vascular smooth muscle cell differentiation. Arterioscler Thromb Vasc Biol 2011;31(10):2181–92.

18. Jinnin M, Ishihara T, Boye E, et al. Recent progress in studies of infantile hemangioma. J Dermatol 2010;37(4):283–98.

19. Greenberger S, Boscolo E, Adini I, et al. Corticosteroid suppression of VEGF-A in infantile hemangioma-derived stem cells. N Engl J Med 2010;362(11):1005–13.

20. Storch CH, Hoeger PH. Propranolol for infantile haemangiomas: insights into the molecular mechanisms of action. Br J Dermatol 2010;163(2):269–74.

21. Chang LC, Haggstrom AN, Drolet BA, et al. Growth characteristics of infantile hemangiomas: implications for management. Pediatrics 2008;122(2): 360–7.

22. Brandling-Bennett HA, Metry DW, Baselga E, et al. Infantile hemangiomas with unusually prolonged growth phase: a case series. Arch Dermatol 2008; 144(12):1632–7.

23. Drolet BA, Esterly NB, Frieden IJ. Hemangiomas in children. N Engl J Med 1999;341(3):173–81.

24. Chiller KG, Passaro D, Frieden IJ. Hemangiomas of infancy: clinical characteristics, morphologic subtypes, and their relationship to race, ethnicity, and sex. Arch Dermatol 2002;138(12):1567–76.

25. Haggstrom AN, Lammer EJ, Schneider RA, et al. Patterns of infantile hemangiomas: new clues to hemangioma pathogenesis and embryonic facial development. Pediatrics 2006;117(3):698–703.

26. Waner M, North PE, Scherer KA, et al. The nonrandom distribution of facial hemangiomas. Arch Dermatol 2003;139(7):869–75.

27. Haggstrom AN, Drolet BA, Baselga E, et al. Prospective study of infantile hemangiomas: clinical characteristics predicting complications and treatment. Pediatrics 2006;118(3):882–7.

28. Haggstrom AN, Beaumont JL, Lai JS, et al. Measuring the severity of infantile hemangiomas: instrument development and reliability. Arch Dermatol 2012; 148(2):197–202.

29. Chamlin SL, Haggstrom AN, Drolet BA, et al. Multicenter prospective study of ulcerated hemangiomas. J Pediatr 2007;151(6):684–9, 689–e1.

30. Shin HT, Orlow SJ, Chang MW. Ulcerated haemangioma of infancy: a retrospective review of 47 patients. Br J Dermatol 2007;156(5):1050–2.

31. Frank RC, Cowan BJ, Harrop AR, et al. Visual development in infants: visual complications of periocular haemangiomas. J Plast Reconstr Aesthet Surg 2010;63(1):1–8.

32. Al Dhaybi R, Superstein R, Milet A, et al. Treatment of periocular infantile hemangiomas with propranolol: case series of 18 children. Ophthalmology 2011; 118(6):1184–8.

33. Bilyk JR, Adamis AP, Mulliken JB. Treatment options for periorbital hemangioma of infancy. Int Ophthalmol Clin 1992;32(3):95–109.

34. Golitz LE, Rudikoff J, O'Meara OP. Diffuse neonatal hemangiomatosis. Pediatr Dermatol 1986;3(2):145–52.

35. Glick ZR, Frieden IJ, Garzon MC, et al. Diffuse neonatal hemangiomatosis: an evidence-based review of case reports in the literature. J Am Acad Dermatol 2012;67(5):898–903.

36. Dickie B, Dasgupta R, Nair R, et al. Spectrum of hepatic hemangiomas: management and outcome. J Pediatr Surg 2009;44(1):125–33.

37. Horii KA, Drolet BA, Frieden IJ, et al. Prospective study of the frequency of hepatic hemangiomas in infants with multiple cutaneous infantile hemangiomas. Pediatr Dermatol 2011;28(3):245–53.

38. Christison-Lagay ER, Burrows PE, Alomari A, et al. Hepatic hemangiomas: subtype classification and development of a clinical practice algorithm and registry. J Pediatr Surg 2007;42(1):62–7.

39. Huang SA, Tu HM, Harney JW, et al. Severe hypothyroidism caused by type 3 iodothyronine deiodinase in infantile hemangiomas. N Engl J Med 2000;343(3): 185–9.

40. Kulungowski AM, Alomari AI, Chawla A, et al. Lessons from a liver hemangioma registry: subtype classification. J Pediatr Surg 2012;47(1):165–70.

41. Orlow SJ, Isakoff MS, Blei F. Increased risk of symptomatic hemangiomas of the airway in association with cutaneous hemangiomas in a "beard" distribution. J Pediatr 1997;131(4):643–6.

42. O TM, Alexander RE, Lando T, et al. Segmental hemangiomas of the upper airway. Laryngoscope 2009;119(11):2242–7.

43. Perkins JA, Duke W, Chen E, et al. Emerging concepts in airway infantile hemangioma assessment and management. Otolaryngol Head Neck Surg 2009;141(2):207–12.

44. Girard C, Bigorre M, Guillot B, et al. PELVIS syndrome. Arch Dermatol 2006;142(7):884–8.

45. Stockman A, Boralevi F, Taieb A, et al. SACRAL syndrome: spinal dysraphism, anogenital, cutaneous, renal and urologic anomalies, associated with an angioma of lumbosacral localization. Dermatology 2007;214(1):40–5.

46. Drolet BA, Chamlin SL, Garzon MC, et al. Prospective study of spinal anomalies in children with infantile hemangiomas of the lumbosacral skin. J Pediatr 2010;157(5):789–94.

47. Iacobas I, Burrows PE, Frieden IJ, et al. LUMBAR: association between cutaneous infantile hemangiomas of the lower body and regional congenital anomalies. J Pediatr 2010;157(5):795–801.e1–7.

48. Frieden IJ, Reese V, Cohen D. PHACE syndrome. The association of posterior fossa brain malformations, hemangiomas, arterial anomalies, coarctation of the aorta and cardiac defects, and eye abnormalities. Arch Dermatol 1996;132(3):307–11.

49. Metry D, Heyer G, Hess C, et al. Consensus statement on diagnostic criteria for PHACE syndrome. Pediatrics 2009;124(5):1447–56.

50. Metry DW, Haggstrom AN, Drolet BA, et al. A prospective study of PHACE syndrome in infantile hemangiomas: demographic features, clinical findings, and complications. Am J Med Genet A 2006; 140(9):975–86.

51. Haggstrom AN, Garzon MC, Baselga E, et al. Risk for PHACE syndrome in infants with large facial hemangiomas. Pediatrics 2010;126(2):e418–26.

52. Hess CP, Fullerton HJ, Metry DW, et al. Cervical and intracranial arterial anomalies in 70 patients with

PHACE syndrome. AJNR Am J Neuroradiol 2010; 31(10):1980–6.

53. Siegel DH, Tefft KA, Kelly T, et al. Stroke in children with posterior fossa brain malformations, hemangiomas, arterial anomalies, coarctation of the aorta and cardiac defects, and eye abnormalities (PHACE) syndrome: a systematic review of the literature. Stroke 2012;43:1672–4.

54. Metz BJ, Rubenstein MC, Levy ML, et al. Response of ulcerated perineal hemangiomas of infancy to becaplermin gel, a recombinant human platelet-derived growth factor. Arch Dermatol 2004;140(7):867–70.

55. Frieden IJ. Addendum: commentary on becaplermin gel (Regranex) for hemangiomas. Pediatr Dermatol 2008;25(6):590.

56. Leaute-Labreze C, Dumas de la Roque E, Hubiche T, et al. Propranolol for severe hemangiomas of infancy. N Engl J Med 2008;358(24):2649–51.

57. Schiestl C, Neuhaus K, Zoller S, et al. Efficacy and safety of propranolol as first-line treatment for infantile hemangiomas. Eur J Pediatr 2011;170(4):493–501.

58. Sans V, Dumas de la Roque E, Berge J, et al. Propranolol for severe infantile hemangiomas: follow-up report. Pediatrics 2009;124(3):e423–31.

59. Schupp CJ, Kleber JB, Gunther P, et al. Propranolol therapy in 55 infants with infantile hemangioma: dosage, duration, adverse effects, and outcome. Pediatr Dermatol 2011;28(6):640–4.

60. Hogeling M, Adams S, Wargon O. A randomized controlled trial of propranolol for infantile hemangiomas. Pediatrics 2011;128(2):e259–66.

61. Zvulunov A, McCuaig C, Frieden IJ, et al. Oral propranolol therapy for infantile hemangiomas beyond the proliferation phase: a multicenter retrospective study. Pediatr Dermatol 2011;28(2):94–8.

62. Bagazgoitia L, Hernandez-Martin A, Torrelo A. Recurrence of infantile hemangiomas treated with propranolol. Pediatr Dermatol 2011;28(6):658–62.

63. Holland KE, Frieden IJ, Frommelt PC, et al. Hypoglycemia in children taking propranolol for the treatment of infantile hemangioma. Arch Dermatol 2010;146(7): 775–8.

64. Lawley LP, Siegfried E, Todd JL. Propranolol treatment for hemangioma of infancy: risks and recommendations. Pediatr Dermatol 2009;26(5):610–4.

65. Breur JM, de Graaf M, Breugem CC, et al. Hypoglycemia as a result of propranolol during treatment of infantile hemangioma: a case report. Pediatr Dermatol 2011;28(2):169–71.

66. Guo S, Ni N. Topical treatment for capillary hemangioma of the eyelid using beta-blocker solution. Arch Ophthalmol 2010;128(2):255–6.

67. Ni N, Langer P, Wagner R, et al. Topical timolol for periocular hemangioma: report of further study. Arch Ophthalmol 2011;129(3):377–9.

68. Moehrle M, Leaute-Labreze C, Schmidt V, et al. Topical timolol for small hemangiomas of infancy. Pediatr Dermatol 2012. [Epub ahead of print].

69. Chakkittakandiyil A, Phillips R, Frieden IJ, et al. Timolol maleate 0.5% or 0.1% gel-forming solution for infantile hemangiomas: a retrospective, multicenter, cohort study. Pediatr Dermatol 2012;29(1):28–31.

70. Oranje AP, Janmohamed SR, Madern GC, et al. Treatment of small superficial haemangioma with timolol 0.5% ophthalmic solution: a series of 20 cases. Dermatology 2011;223(4):330–4.

71. McMahon P, Oza V, Frieden IJ. Topical timolol for infantile hemangiomas: putting a note of caution in "cautiously optimistic". Pediatr Dermatol 2012;29(1): 127–30.

72. Enjolras O, Riche MC, Merland JJ, et al. Management of alarming hemangiomas in infancy: a review of 25 cases. Pediatrics 1990;85(4):491–8.

73. Barrio VR, Drolet BA. Treatment of hemangiomas of infancy. Dermatol Ther 2005;18(2):151–9.

74. Maronn ML, Corden T, Drolet BA. Pneumocystis carinii pneumonia in infant treated with oral steroids for hemangioma. Arch Dermatol 2007;143(9):1224–5.

75. Enjolras O, Breviere GM, Roger G, et al. Vincristine treatment for function- and life-threatening infantile hemangioma. Arch Pediatr 2004;11:99–107 [in French].

76. Fawcett SL, Grant I, Hall PN, et al. Vincristine as a treatment for a large haemangioma threatening vital functions. Br J Plast Surg 2004;57(2):168–71.

77. Boehm DK, Kobrinsky NL. Treatment of cavernous hemangioma with vincristine. Ann Pharmacother 1993;27(7–8):981.

78. Witman PM, Wagner AM, Scherer K, et al. Complications following pulsed dye laser treatment of superficial hemangiomas. Lasers Surg Med 2006;38(2): 116–23.

79. Morelli JG, Tan OT, Yohn JJ, et al. Treatment of ulcerated hemangiomas infancy. Arch Pediatr Adolesc Med 1994;148(10):1104–5.

80. David LR, Malek MM, Argenta LC. Efficacy of pulse dye laser therapy for the treatment of ulcerated haemangiomas: a review of 78 patients. Br J Plast Surg 2003;56(4):317–27.

# New Findings in Genodermatoses

Jonathan A. Dyer, MD[a,b],*

## KEYWORDS

- Genodermatoses • Genomic sequencing • Skin disease

## KEY POINTS

- New technologies are rapidly accelerating the rate of discovery in genetic skin diseases.
- Identification of the causative gene is the first step toward defining potential translational therapies.
- New discoveries continue, even for diseases such as epidermolysis bullosa or mendelian disorders of cornification (ichthyosis).
- Somatic mosaicism for mutations in genes of the PI3-AKT pathway explain a variety of overgrowth syndromes.
- Somatic mosaicism for mutations in genes of the RAS pathway leads to some forms of epidermal nevi suggesting these may be "mosaic RASopathies".

## INTRODUCTION

The pace of the study of inherited skin diseases is rapidly accelerating. Massively parallel (next-generation) sequencing technologies have created paradigm shifts in how these conditions are investigated. The time it takes to generate near-complete genetic data on an individual is now measured in days to weeks and the cost is decreasing rapidly. Advancement is ongoing and evolving third-generation sequencing technologies have generated speculation of generating a full human genome sequence overnight. The list of new techniques, fueled by the maturation of massively parallel DNA sequencing and bioinformatics technologies to handle the resultant data deluge, is continually growing, including linkage analysis, homozygosity mapping, case-control association, whole-genome genotyping, targeted resequencing, and whole-exome sequencing.[1] New technologies bring new challenges. The genetic causes of many inherited skin conditions are being rapidly elucidated,

leading to a deluge of genes and new data. Even for investigators in the field, keeping up with all of the new mutations and pathways at play is impractical. The subsequent deluge of "new genetic cause for disease X" articles being submitted to journals has led the Nature family of journals to publish new, more stringent guidelines for accepting articles reporting the genetic cause of a disease.[2] However, it is critical to realize that the identification of causative genes is just the beginning of the journey to understanding the pathomechanism of an inherited skin disease. This article highlights a few of the many new discoveries in inherited skin diseases from the past year.

## EPIDERMOLYSIS BULLOSA

A group of skin disorders characterized by skin fragility, blistering, and erosion, epidermolysis bullosa (EB) occurs because of inherited defects in structural proteins critical to maintaining cell structure and adhesion in the epidermis and

Funding sources: None.
Conflict of interest: None.
[a] Department of Dermatology, University of Missouri, 1 Hospital Drive, Room MA111D, Columbia, MO 65212, USA; [b] Department of Child Health, University of Missouri, 1 Hospital Drive, Room MA111D, Columbia, MO 65212, USA
* Department of Dermatology, University of Missouri, 1 Hospital Drive, Room MA111D, Columbia, MO 65212.
E-mail address: dyerja@health.missouri.edu

Dermatol Clin 31 (2013) 303–315
http://dx.doi.org/10.1016/j.det.2012.12.007
0733-8635/13/$ – see front matter © 2013 Elsevier Inc. All rights reserved.

derm.theclinics.com

dermoepidermal junction. Many of the EB subtypes exhibit great morbidity and some exhibit great mortality.

There are several exciting new developments in EB. Several recent reports have added to the understanding of EB subtypes, including the great range in severity that occurs in different forms of EB. A second patient was recently reported with a mild form of EB simplex caused by mutations in dystonin (DST; OMIM 113810), the gene encoding bullous pemphigoid antigen type 1 (BPAG1). The first patient with a DST mutation, long hypothesized as a potential cause of EB, was reported in 2010; however, the patient also had mutations in NOTCH3 (OMIM 600276) leading to neurologic features that were likely not related to the cutaneous phenotype. However, given the concomitant diagnoses it was difficult for investigators to determine what phenotypic findings were typical for BPAG1 mutations. In the newly reported patient (with a different BPAG1 mutation), neurologic features were absent and AR mutations in the DST gene led to a very mild EB simplex phenotype with blistering only with warmth or trauma.[3]

A case of lethal congenital EB resulted from mutations in the junction plakoglobin (JUP; OMIM 173325) gene encoding plakoglobin (PLG). PLG plays a critical role in desmosomal function via interaction with desmoplakin, which serves to tether intermediate filaments to the desmosomal plaque. PLG is also present in adherens junctions. Previously, JUP mutations had been detected in Naxos syndrome (OMIM 601214), which exhibits wooly hair, palmoplantar keratoderma, and arrhythmogenic heart disease.[4] The infant reported in this study exhibited severe skin fragility from birth with diffuse epidermal separation and massive transcutaneous water loss. The JUP mutation in this patient was unique and, instead of leading to a truncated plakoglobin protein as occurs in Naxos syndrome, led to complete PLG loss in the skin. Few desmosomes could be detected and those present were malformed. Because PLG plays a role in both desmosomal and adherens junction adhesion, its absence led to a complete loss of adhesion structures between keratinocytes.[5]

A new subtype of EB has been described in three patients with homozygous mutations in the integrin (ITG) α3 gene (OMIM 605025). ITGα6 (OMIM 147556) and ITGβ4 (OMIM 147557) mutations are known to cause subtypes of junctional EB (JEB) often associated with pyloric atresia (OMIM 226730) and, although phenotypic variability exists, many of these patients exhibit severe skin disease and die during infancy. Patients with integrin α3 mutations had significant multiorgan disease, including a congenital nephrotic syndrome with significant morbidity, and interstitial lung disease that is progressive and eventually lethal. Skin blistering was not a prominent feature in the immediate neonatal period and began after several months of age. Skin blistering worsened with time, with increasing fragility with trauma. Blistered areas healed slowly, with residual erythema but not scarring. The mucosa was free from lesions. Hairs were fine and sparse and, with time, onychodystrophy of the great toenails was noted as well as distal onycholysis of the fingernails. Respiratory distress or other pulmonary issues were typically the presenting complaint, with nephrotic syndrome and its resultant sequelae noted during laboratory evaluation for the respiratory problems. Ultrastructural studies did not correspond with any previously reported EB subtypes but showed disruption within the basement membrane zone.[6] Thus, an infantile onset progressive EB phenotype should prompt investigation for internal organ involvement.

A major source of mortality in patients with recessive dystrophic EB (RDEB) is metastatic squamous cell carcinoma. A newly published study investigates why cutaneous squamous cell carcinomas (cSCC) in patients with RDEB have a much higher rate of metastasis than standard cSCC or that seen in association with other inherited disorders such as xeroderma pigmentosum. The investigators hypothesized that type VII collagen deficiency created a permissive matrix environment for the growth and spread of cSCC. Increased type XII collagen, thrombospondin-1, and Wnt-5A were noted with deficiency of type VII collagen. Re-expression of normal type VII collagen decreased levels of these proteins, and reduced tumor cell invasion in culture and tumor growth in vivo.[7] Although the details of these interactions still must be clarified, this suggests that, if type VII collagen can be replaced in patients with RDEB, skin fragility and blistering can be affected and, possibly, the risk of cSCC and the permissive growth environment can be improved.

Revertant mosaicism, in which a secondary mutation occurs in a patient with an inherited disease that corrects or overcomes the primary inherited mutation, was considered a very rare event. Studies of non-Herlitz JEB (OMIM 226650) patients have shed greater light on the frequency of revertant mosaicism in these patients. Revertant mosaicism seems to be common in patients with generalized non-Herlitz JEB—possibly occurring in most patients. In patients with preexisting localized JEB, however, revertant lesions do not seem to be frequent. There does not seem to be a preference for which genetic repair mechanism is used. Such patients offer great promise as potential donors of their own reverted fibroblasts or keratinocytes for application to blistering areas as a form of natural gene therapy.[8]

Translation of the understanding of the underlying genetic causes of inherited skin disease into therapies has always been a major goal of research. Chronic ulcers often become a problem in EB patients and treating them can be challenging. Jonkman and colleagues[9] describe success using a punch grafting procedure using autologous donor skin for chronic ulcers in patients with laminin-332 deficient non-Herlitz JEB (OMIM 226650). Previous studies have described increased type VII collagen expression and skin adhesion in RDEB patients after injection with allogeneic fibroblasts; however, the mechanism of this increase was unclear.[10] A recent report notes increased cytokine expression after allogeneic fibroblast injection, including heparin binding–EGF-like growth factor (HB-EGF), which upregulates the patient's own COL7A1 expression.[11] The effect of recombinant HB-EGF on chronic EB ulcers has not been reported but is an obvious area for future study.

In the case of dystrophic EB, there have been several exciting developments focused on investigating and developing therapeutic approaches for the disease. Bone marrow–derived adult stem cells were known to play a role in maintenance of skin homeostasis; however, more recent work confirmed that these cells could generate and differentiate into skin cell types necessary for skin repair after wounding. This observation was taken to its translational conclusion with the report of a clinical trial of allogeneic bone marrow transplantation (BMT) in seven children with RDEB in 2010. Although the results of the successful BMTs were encouraging, with demonstration of detectable type VII collagen staining and clinical improvement in the patients, which lasted for more than 1 year after BMT, two of the seven children died due to complications from the BMT.[12] Newer trials are underway that use conditioning regimens of significantly reduced intensity. Induced pluripotent stem cells (iPSCs) can be generated from skin fibroblasts and can serve as a renewable source of autologous stem cells. They may also be differentiated into keratinocytes.[13] Initial methods of iPSC generation involved integration of viral transgenes that raised concerns that in vivo use could lead to tumor development. Currently, work is underway to develop methods of generating integration-free iPSCs. Another hurdle to the use of iPSCs is developing efficient and safe ways to correct the genetic defects present in patient-derived iPSCs. Efforts are underway to use customized zinc finger nucleases that are able to increase the incidence of homologous recombination at targeted mutation sites up to 10,000-fold. Alternatively, as noted previously, patients with revertant mosaic skin lesions offer a potential source of autologous-corrected iPSCs.[10] Direct replacement of type VII collagen using purified recombinant type VII collagen, topically and injected intravenously, is also under study. Previously, IV infusion of recombinant type VII collagen was reported to home to wounded skin and lead to functional anchoring fibril formation in a type VII collagen knockout mouse.[14] Recently, similar results were described in human RDEB skin grafted onto athymic nude mice.[15] An important caveat to these therapies is the concern for the potential development of antibodies against type VII collagen. Recent work suggests that patients with RDEB may have preexisting anti–type VII collagen antibodies, even when type VII collagen is not detectable in the skin. Although the source of these antibodies is not clear, one possibility is that many RDEB patients have subclinical patches of revertant fibroblasts or keratinocytes that make small amounts of type VII collagen that serve as a source for the antibody development (similar to the growing understanding of revertant mosaicism in non-Herlitz JEB). Currently, the clinical relevance of these antibodies is not known.

## ICHTHYOSES

The elucidation of the genetic causes of a variety of Mendelian disorders of cornification (MeDOC) has bolstered support for the bricks and mortar model of the epidermis.[16] Although the role of each individual component detected to date is not completely understood, as other players are discovered the interconnections between the elements become clearer. Again, this is allowing the development of pathomechanism-based therapies for these patients.

The genetic abnormalities underlying a form of lamellar ichthyosis found in golden retriever dogs led to the discovery of a new genetic cause of ichthyosis. The ichthyosis in the retrievers is similar to autosomal recessive congenital ichthyosis (ARCI) and occurs because of homozygous mutations in patatin-like phospholipase domain-containing protein 1 (PNPLA1; OMIM 612121). Although the specific function of PNPLA1 is unknown, it seems important for epidermal lipid barrier formation. On discovery of this mutation, the investigators screened ARCI patients without known mutations and found six patients from two families with PNPLA1 mutations. Affected patients could present as collodion babies and evolve into a mild-to-moderate nonbullous congenital ichthyosiform erythroderma. Erythema and keratosis involved the skin diffusely, including the flexures. A mild palmoplantar keratoderma was present and some patients had pseudosyndactyly of the second to third toes. Although acitretin therapy improved scaling, it worsened the erythema.[17]

The cause for a type of neuroichthyosis syndrome was identified in several Saudi families whose children who presented with a diffuse ichthyosis very similar to Sjögren-Larsson syndrome (SLS; OMIM 270200). However, the associated neurologic phenotype in these patients was more severe than SLS, with seizures, mental retardation, and significant spasticity. These patients had been diagnosed as having ichthyosis, spastic quadriplegia, and mental retardation (ISQMR; OMIM 614457), or pseudo-SLS. Patients can present with a collodion membrane at birth. All of these patients were profoundly developmentally delayed from infancy. Seizures began in the first months of life and were unresponsive to anti-epileptics. Bilateral inguinal hernias were noted. The ichthyotic skin changes were similar to SLS and often acrally accentuated. In these patients, AR mutations in the elongation of very long chain fatty acid-like 4 gene (ELOVL4; OMIM 605512), which encodes a very long chain fatty acid synthase, were detected. Heterozygous mutations in ELOVL4 cause macular degeneration in humans (autosomal dominant [AD] macular dystrophy or Stargardt disease 3; OMIM 600110). However, ocular findings in these patients were difficult to assess but seemed absent to mild. Very long chain fatty acids play important roles in cell membrane structure and in cell signaling.[18]

Historically, the peeling skin syndromes (PSSs) have been a poorly understood group of rare AR syndromes characterized by episodic to continual superficial skin peeling. Acral and generalized variants are recognized with subdivision of the generalized forms into inflammatory and noninflammatory subtypes. New genetic approaches have recently allowed characterization and clarification of several of these syndromes. Some years ago, transglutaminase 5 (OMIM 603805) mutations were discovered to be the cause of the acral PSS variant (OMIM 609796) that can mimic mild forms of EB simplex.[19] More recently, mutations in corneodesmosin (CDSN; OMIM 602593) were found to underlie the inflammatory variant of PSS (OMIM 270300) that is associated with allergies and significant atopic features.[20] Most recently, a large family with noninflammatory AR PSS (PSS type A) was studied using whole genome homozygosity mapping followed by whole-exome sequencing of a single proband. Using this approach, a homozygous missense mutation in the carbohydrate sulfotransferase 8 (CHST8; OMIM 610190) gene was detected. CHST8 encodes an N-acetylgalactosamine-4-O-sulfotransferase (GalNAc4-ST1) localized to the Golgi transmembrane and expressed in normal human epidermis. Cells expressing the mutant enzyme had decreased levels of total sulfated glycosoaminoglycans and the investigators postulate that increased turnover of the mutant enzyme was responsible. Additionally, expression levels of GalNAc4-ST1 increase in the upper epidermal layers, suggesting a role in epidermal differentiation.[21]

An AR subtype of ichthyosis termed exfoliative ichthyosis (OMIM 607936) shares some features with the PSS. Affected individuals develop dry, scaling skin diffusely over the body with peeling on the palms and soles. Using a combination of genetic approaches, including whole-genome homozygosity mapping, candidate-gene analysis, and deep sequencing, loss of function (LOF) mutations in cystatin A (OMIM 184600), a protease inhibitor, were determined to be the genetic cause of exfoliative ichthyosis. Two homozygous mutations, one a splice-site and the other a nonsense mutation were detected. Microscopic analysis revealed skin disruption at the basal or suprabasal epidermal layers. Further investigation suggests that a cell-cell adhesion defect exists when cystatin A is missing. This parallels the understanding of protease inhibitor function in the normal desquamation of the epidermis as revealed by Netherton syndrome (NS; OMIM 256500). In NS, deficiency of the serine protease inhibitor (OMIM 605010) allows overactive and ongoing epidermal protease activity to continually degrade the epidermal barrier, resulting in the cutaneous stigmata of NS, the desquamative elements of which may have clinical similarity with exfoliative ichthyosis and other variants of PSS.[22] A better understanding of the causes of these syndromes will enhance their clinical recognition and prevent misdiagnosis of affected patients. Also, given the role of the individual affected proteins in very specific sites of epidermal barrier function, detailed clinical and molecular study of patients with these individual disorders and with filaggrin deficiency may shed light on the exact mechanisms by which some epidermal barrier defects contribute to an inflammatory phenotype (atopic dermatitis; CDSN deficiency) while others do not.

In another promising example of bench to bedside translational research, the skin lesions of congenital hemidysplasia, ichthyosis, and limb defects (CHILD) syndrome (OMIM 308050), an X-linked dominant (XLD) disorder improved with topical therapy. CHILD syndrome is caused by defects in a key component of the cholesterol biosynthesis pathway, the NAD(P)H steroid dehydrogenase-like protein (OMIM 300275). Patients with CHILD syndrome exhibit chronic recalcitrant inflammatory segmental skin lesions, often hemilateral with associated ipsilateral limb defects. These lesions cause significant morbidity for patients and have not responded to standard systemic or topical therapies apart from sporadic reports of improvement with destructive or surgical interventions. Because the mammalian NAD(P)H steroid dehydrogenase-like protein defect leads to impaired cholesterol production, investigators first attempted topical application of cholesterol to the skin lesions to replace the deficiency, but there was no benefit. However, the addition of topical lovastatin to block overproduction of cholesterol precursors, in addition to topical cholesterol, led to significant improvement in one treated case with minimal side effects.[23]

## INFLAMMATORY AND/OR IMMUNOLOGIC SKIN DISEASES

Several recent studies have demonstrated the power of new genetic analysis strategies to identify genes of importance in cutaneous and systemic inflammatory pathways. One report describes two siblings of Lebanese descent from a consanguineous marriage with neonatal inflammatory skin and bowel disease (OMIM 614328) that developed skin lesions by the second day of life. These cutaneous lesions began as perioral and perianal erythema with fissuring and a generalized pustular rash that transitioned into psoriasiform erythroderma with periodic flares of erythema, scaling, and widespread pustules. Diarrhea began in the first week of life. In the neonatal period the diarrhea led to failure to thrive. It was bloody, clinically consistent with malabsorption, and worsened with flares in the cutaneous disease and with gastrointestinal infections. Compensatory mechanisms for the defect seem to exist in humans as there is some normalization of the gut phenotype with time. The children were prone to Staphylococcus aureus infections with recurrent blepharitis and otitis externa. Their hairs were short or broken and eyelashes and eyebrows were wiry and rough. Nail abnormalities were noted, including thickening with frequent paronychia due to recurrent candida and pseudomonal infections. The sister died at 12 years from parvovirus B19–associated myocarditis and the brother had asymptomatic left ventricular dilatation. Using single nucleotide polymorphism (SNP)-homozygosity mapping, the investigators detected three large regions of homozygosity. Probes from all exons in these regions of the genome were included on a capture array and exons from these regions in the affected brother were sequenced. After known SNPs were removed, a total of 22 unique SNPs were detected in coding regions. Parallel assessment of the data for insertion-deletion variations

detected a new deletion (4bp) in a disintegrin and metalloproteinase 17 (ADAM17; tumor necrosis factor α [TNF-α] converting enzyme [TACE]; OMIM 603639), that segregated with the disease in an AR manner. This mutation predicted a severely truncated protein.

Keratinocytes from the surviving sibling expressed ADAM10 (OMIM 602192), which cleaves some of the same substrates as ADAM17. Desmoglein 2 (DSG2; OMIM 125671) is a known direct target of both. Increased DSG2 expression was present in the patient's skin suggesting a role for ADAM17 in regulating DSG2 availability at cell junctions. DSG2 is the predominant DSG in cardiac myocytes and mutations in DSG2 are associated with arrhythmogenic and dilated cardiomyopathies. Abnormal DSG2 expression may be related to the cardiac findings noted in these siblings. Because ADAM17 encodes a TACE, abnormal TNF-α signaling would be predicted to result from ADAM17 mutations and PBMCs from the surviving sibling showed impaired TNF-α production after stimulation. The low level of TNF-α detected may be from low-level production via ADAM10. The investigators also note that lack of TNF-α may have contributed to the fatal outcome in the sister because it is known to be cardioprotective in acute myocarditis.[24]

A recent report elucidates the genetic cause of an AD cold urticarial syndrome (familial cold autoinflammatory syndrome 3; OMIM 614468). Affected patients develop cold urticaria with generalized cold exposure rather than by touching cold objects. Similarly, patients with this subtype of cold urticaria had negative skin testing with ice-cube and cold-water immersion but positive skin testing using evaporative cooling and generalized cold air exposure. Many patients developed additional features, including a common variable immunodeficiency (75%); a susceptibility to infections (56%), especially sinopulmonary; and autoimmune disorders (56%), such as thyroiditis. Some patients also developed granulomatous skin disease. The cold urticaria began early in life and was chronic. Abnormalities in patients included low IgM and IgA, low natural killer (NK) cells, decreased circulating CD19+ B cells, and IgA+ and IgG+ class-switched memory B cells. IgE was elevated in most patients. Antinuclear antibodies were present in 62%. Linkage analysis identified a single chromosomal region; however, whole-genome sequencing of one patient did not reveal any abnormalities. Analysis of a second family narrowed the linkage interval, allowing a candidate gene approach, which identified family-specific deletions in the PLCG2 gene (OMIM 600220), which encodes phospholipase Cγ2 (PLCγ2), a signaling molecule expressed in

B cells, NK cells, and mast cells. The disease-causing heterozygous deletions in PLCG2 occur in an autoinhibitory domain, leading to constitutive phospholipase activity and resulting in a gain of function (GOF) phenotype. Spontaneous degranulation below 20°C was noted in mast cells transfected with mutant PLCG2, a finding not present in controls. Also, these defects were temperature sensitive in B cells with enhanced signaling and cellular activation. The investigators propose the moniker PLCγ$_2$-associated antibody deficiency and immune dysregulation (PLAID) to identify this syndrome.[25]

The cause of various forms of chronic mucocutaneous candidiasis (CMC) syndromes and their causal interrelationships has been clarified greatly in several publications in the past year. Patients with CMC typically exhibit localized candida infections instead of systemic infection, due to defective cellular immunity. Defects in Th17-mediated immune function tend to result in fungal infections, reflecting the importance of Th17 cell function in the skin and/or mucosa. The pathway from fungal recognition to Th17 antifungal response involves several steps. Defects in these individual steps lead to various CMC syndromes. DECTIN1 (OMIM 606264) is a fungal pattern recognition receptor and fungal binding to dectin1 leads to signaling mediated by CARD9 (OMIM 607212). Defects in either can lead to CMC, semidominant (see later discussion) or AR in the case of dectin1 defects (OMIM 613108) and AR with CARD9 defects (OMIM 212050). In the case of DECTIN1, heterozygous carriers also showed increased *Candida* colonization and infections, though not at the level seen with CMC, suggesting a semidominant effect. Signal transducer and activator of transcription 3 (STAT3; OMIM 102582) plays a key role in Th17 cell differentiation and LOF in STAT3 impairs Th17 cell differentiation leading to AD hyperimmunoglobulin E syndrome (AD-HIES; OMIM 147060). Patients with AR-HIES (OMIM 243700) due to DOCK8 (OMIM 611432) mutations also exhibit impaired Th17 cell activity—albeit at a different point than that seen with STAT3 mutations. STAT1-dependent (OMIM 600555) pathways inhibit Th17 cell production and heterozygous mutations that result in GOF in STAT1 decrease Th17 cell number and activity, leading to AD CMC (OMIM 614162).[26] Interleukin 17 (IL-17) production is critical and mutations in the genes encoding this cytokine IL-17F (OMIM 606496) and its receptor IL-17RA (OMIM 605461) inhibit Th17 cell effector function and lead to CMC, AD (OMIM 613956), and AR (OMIM 613953), respectively.[27] The final step of antifungal immune response involves effective neutrophil function and impaired neutrophil production or activity can result in CMC, such as that seen with severe congenital neutropenia.[28]

Large genome wide association studies (GWAS) have been performed for a variety of multigenic inflammatory skin disorders. Psoriasis was at the forefront of this research and loci identified in these studies are now being better characterized. The identity of one of these loci, PSORS2 (OMIM 602723), has long been sought. Recent reports describe GOF mutations in caspase recruitment domain family member 14 (CARD14; OMIM 607211) as the PSORS2 gene. The GOF mutations in CARD14 lead to enhanced NF-kB activation. Identified through analysis of rare families with strong penetrance of psoriasis through multiple generations, examination of large numbers of psoriasis patients from multiple cohorts has identified a variety of CARD14 variants and is beginning to shed light on their relation to NF-kB activation and possibly other mechanisms involved in the generation of psoriatic lesions.[29,30]

## METABOLIC SYNDROMES

An enlightening study has expanded the spectrum of genetic causes for pseudoxanthoma elasticum (PXE; OMIM 264800) and shed further light on potential pathomechanisms of PXE lesion development. Generalized arterial calcification of infancy (GACI; OMIM 208000) is a well recognized caused of vascular calcification in children (the other being PXE) and is typically caused by homozygous mutations in ectonucleotide pyrophosphatase/phosphodiesterase 1 (ENPP1; plasma cell membrane glycoprotein PC-1; OMIM 173335), which generates pyrophosphate, a critical physiologic inhibitor of calcification. However, homozygous ENPP1 mutations could not be detected in all GACI patients and some were only heterozygous for ENPP1 mutations. The vascular findings in GACI overlap significantly with PXE, which is caused by mutations in ATP-binding cassette, subfamily C, member 6 (ABCC6; OMIM 603234). Examination of ABCC6 in 28 GACI patients with less than 2 ENPP1 mutations revealed 14 patients without ENPP1 mutations who had ABCC6 mutations (8 biallelic, 6 monoallelic). Additionally, three patients with biallelic ENPP1 mutations developed skin lesions typical for PXE. These results suggest GACI and PXE are at opposite ends of a similar phenotypic spectrum and show that ABCC6 mutations account for a significant subset of GACI cases.[31]

## OVERGROWTH SYNDROMES

Proteus syndrome (OMIM 176920) has long been a challenging entity of great interest to investigators because of its striking clinical findings and the hypothesis that John Merrick, the "Elephant Man," suffered from this syndrome. Recently, mosaic activating mutations in v-akt murine thymoma viral oncogene homolog 1 (Akt1; OMIM 164730) have been detected in patients meeting the discrete clinical criteria for Proteus syndrome. Characterized by progressive overgrowth of skin, connective tissue, brain, and other tissues, Proteus syndrome had long been hypothesized to represent a lethal mutation surviving by somatic mosaicism. In another example of the power of new DNA-sequencing technologies, investigators performed exome sequencing on DNA extracted from samples of abnormal and normal tissue in patients with Proteus syndrome. This detected a somatic activating mutation (c.49G->A, p.Glu17Lys) in the AKT1 oncogene. This encodes AKT1 kinase, which has been previously implicated in various cell functions such as proliferation and apoptosis. The investigators confirmed the presence of this mutation in a larger number of samples from patients with Proteus syndrome and AKT protein activation in lesional tissues. Of 29 subjects, activating mutations in AKT1 were found in 26. Thus, the previous hypothesis, that Proteus syndrome is caused by somatic mosaicism, was borne out. In this case it was due to activating AKT1 mutations. This likely explains past controversies regarding classification of these patients. Confusion was created when reports were published describing phosphatase and tensin homolog (PTEN; OMIM 601728) mutations in patients with Proteus syndrome. Other investigators in the field suggested that patients with PTEN mutations represented a separate segmental overgrowth syndrome similar to but distinct from Proteus syndrome in which PTEN mutations could not be detected. This PTEN-associated syndrome has been designated segmental overgrowth, lipomatosis, arteriovenous malformation, and epidermal nevus (SOLAMEN) syndrome by some investigators, although Happle[32] suggested the term type 2 segmental Cowden syndrome (T2SCS) because these patients carry a germline heterozygous PTEN mutation and their clinical findings result from somatic mosaic loss of heterozygosity (LOH) at the PTEN locus. Revealingly, LOF mutations in PTEN activate AKT1, and the direct linkage of these two proteins explains the overlapping, yet distinct, clinical findings in SOLAMEN and Proteus syndrome.

Another disorder long postulated to represent a lethal mutation surviving by somatic mosaicism, congenital lipomatous overgrowth with vascular, epidermal, and skeletal anomalies (CLOVES) syndrome, has also now been linked to the PI3K-AKT pathway. This rare sporadic overgrowth syndrome is not heritable. Affected patients exhibit asymmetric somatic hypertrophy as well as multiple organ anomalies. In a recent report, massively parallel sequencing was used to screen for somatic mosaic mutations in lesional tissues. Postzygotic activating mutations in phosphatidylinositol 3-kinase (PI3K), catalytic, alpha (OMIM 171834) were found in abnormal tissues from various embryonic origins, with mutant allele frequencies varying from 3% to 30%.[33] These same mutations, which result in increased PI3K, have been described in cancer. PI3K activation leads to Akt1 stimulation via phosphoinositide-dependent kinase 1 (PDK1; OMIM 605213) and this pathway is regulated by PTEN. Of interest to dermatologists are the keratinocytic epidermal nevi, which represent the epidermal overgrowth component of CLOVES. PIK3CA-activating mutations have previously been reported in isolated keratinocytic EN (see later discussion). The addition of CLOVES syndrome underscores that dysfunction of the PI3K-AKT pathway is common to several overgrowth syndromes. When limited to a single cell type, somatic mosaic lesions such as EN occur. However, if multiple cell lines are affected, a broader overgrowth syndrome may result.[34] Additionally, it suggests the hypothesis that activating mutations of PDK1 could lead to similar overgrowth syndromes.

## HAIR SYNDROMES

The genetic causes of inherited hair and nail defects are also yielding to investigation. Long known because of their striking phenotype, which often led to their inclusion in circus sideshows and speculation that their condition represented a form of atavism, patients with congenital generalized hypertrichosis (CGH) syndromes represent a diverse group of inherited conditions, all with striking, diffuse, overgrowth of hair. Inheritance is variable, with some forms exhibiting AD inheritance and others exhibiting XLD. Recent reports have identified some forms of CGH as genomic, rather than simply genetic, disorders; that is, they result from genomic changes instead of than simple point mutations. Previous studies have identified copy-number variations (CNVs; in this case either microdeletions or microduplications) on chromosome 17q24 in patients with AD CGH terminalis with or without gingival hyperplasia (OMIM 135400). Chromosome 8 rearrangements were detected in hypertrichosis universalis congenita—Ambras type (OMIM 145701).

Previously, linkage studies in two large Mexican families had identified a large region on the X chromosome linked to CGH. Using a large Chinese family with X-linked CGH (HTC2; OMIM 307150), recombination events allowed refinement of the disease locus to a critical region that overlapped with the areas reported from the Mexican families. Using a combination of high-resolution copy-number variation scan and targeted genomic sequencing, the investigators found an interchromosomal insertion on the X chromosome of a large piece of COL23A1 in affected members of the Chinese family. This insertion was just downstream of the SOX3 gene. On analysis of one of the Mexican families, a different, larger, insertion from another chromosomal region was identified inserted at the same palindromic site on the X chromosome. Because palindromic sequences are unstable and known to trigger genomic rearrangements, such as recurrent translocations and deletions, this palindromic X-chromosomal sequence likely mediates the interchromosomal insertions. The investigators suggested that these insertions could have introduced tissue-specific regulatory elements driving ectopic expression of SOX3 in follicles or their precursors with resultant abnormal hair patterning. Because some X-linked CGH pedigrees reported have had other syndromic associations, the investigators suggested different regulatory elements carried by different source chromosomal insertions in those families could result in the phenotypic variation.[35]

Cantu syndrome (OMIM 239850), also known as hypertrichotic osteochondrodysplasia, is a rare AD form of congenital hypertrichosis. Patients exhibit a triad of congenital hypertrichosis, cardiac defects, and distinctive coarse facial features. Cardiac defects include patent ductus arteriosus, cardiomegaly, cardiac hypertrophy, and pericardial effusion. Congenital macrosomia, macrocephaly, unusually deep palmoplantar creases, skeletal dysplasia, and recurrent respiratory infections are also reported. Whole exome sequencing of a patient and his parents led to the detection of heterozygous mutations in ATP-binding cassette, subfamily C, member 9 (ABCC9; OMIM 601439). Sequencing of ABCC9 in 15 additional cases of Cantu syndrome detected ABCC9 mutations in 13 of the 15. The two subjects in whom ABCC9 mutations could not be detected did not exhibit cardiac phenotypes. ABCC9 is part of an ATP-sensitive potassium channel complex and is widely expressed with variant splice forms. All mutations detected in Cantu syndrome patients affected both splice variants. These ATP-sensitive potassium channels couple the metabolic state of cells to their electrical activity. Four ABCC9 subunits are necessary to create a functional potassium channel and one defective subunit in the group will impair function of the channel, consistent with the dominant nature of the mutations in Cantu syndrome. Clinical overlap between the clinical findings of Cantu syndrome and those occurring in patients treated with minoxidil has been highlighted. Tellingly, minoxidil is a potassium-ATP channel agonist via direct binding of ABCC9 subunits. This confirms the prediction that ABCC9 mutations in Cantu syndrome cause channel opening. Knowing this, potassium-ATP channel antagonists may be tested for efficacy in Cantu syndrome. The investigators note that sulfonylurea antagonizes potassium-ATP channels and has been used successfully in patients with neonatal diabetes due to activating mutations in ABCC8.[36,37]

Just as the genetic cause of hypertrichosis syndromes is becoming clearer, additional causes of hereditary hypotrichosis are being identified. Hereditary hypotrichosis is a clinically and genetically heterogeneous group of inherited hair loss disorders often subdivided into syndromic and nonsyndromic forms. Hereditary hypotrichosis simplex (HHS; OMIMs 146520; 605389), in contrast to other nonsyndromic hereditary hypotrichosis, does not exhibit any hair shaft changes. HHS is typically subdivided into scalp limited and generalized forms and both AD and AR inheritance are described. Several genetic causes have been reported. In several unrelated Chinese families with an AD form of generalized HHS, exome sequencing detected a mutation in the RPL21 gene (OMIM 603636), encoding a ribosomal protein called L21. These patients had onset of hair loss around 2 to 6 months of age with progression over time. Near total scalp hair loss eventually resulted. Remaining hairs in patients would reach normal length but were dry, brittle, and slow growing. Most other body hair types were also affected, except beard hairs. Teeth, nails, and sweating were normal. Ribosomal protein L21 is a part of the 60S ribosomal subunit and is highly conserved. Apart from their role in protein synthesis, understanding is growing of the role of ribosomal proteins in cellular processes outside the ribosome itself. How defects in this ribosomal protein lead to ADHHS is not yet clear but is a topic for future studies.[38]

## NAIL SYNDROMES

The causes of inherited nail diseases, or onychogenodermatoses, have not been widely investigated. A recent study identified two consanguineous pedigrees with isolated nail dysplasia inherited in an AR fashion (nonsyndromic congenital nail disorder 10, (claw-shaped nails); OMIM 614157). The clinical findings included claw-shaped nails, onychauxis (nail thickening), and onycholysis (nail separation).

Some patients have been misdiagnosed as having pachyonychia congenita (OMIM 167200; OMIM 167210) and hidrotic ectodermal dysplasia (OMIM 129500) is also considered in the differential diagnosis.[15] A genome-wide SNP array was used to detect an overlapping homozygous region on the long arm of chromosome 8. Analysis of candidate genes from this highlighted region detected homozygous nonsense and missense mutations in FZD6 (OMIM 603409), encoding Frizzled 6, which belongs to a highly conserved membrane-bound Wnt receptor family involved in development and differentiation through a variety of pathways. Expression of the FZD6 missense mutation led to a shift in location of this receptor from the plasma membrane to lysosomes. The mutations described here seem to affect several Wnt-FZD pathways (canonical and noncanonical). Intact Wnt-FZD signaling is important for ectodermal appendage development, including nails. Disruption of this pathway causes a variety of conditions. For example, porcupine (PORCN; OMIM 300651), the gene defective in Goltz syndrome (focal dermal hypoplasia; OMIM 305600) is Wnt-signaling regulator. The FZD agonists R-spondin family (RSPO) member 4 (RSPO4; OMIM 610573) and RSPO1 (OMIM 609595) are defective in isolated anonychia congenita (OMIM 206800) and palmoplantar hyperkeratosis with true hermaphroditism (some with squamous cell carcinoma; OMIM 610644). Wnt10A (OMIM 606268) mutations cause odontoonychodermal dysplasia (OMIM 257980) and other ectodermal dysplasias such as Schöpf-Schulz-Passarge syndrome (OMIM 224750) and selective tooth agenesis 4 (OMIM 150400). LMX1B (OMIM 602575) and MSX1 (OMIM 142983), Wnt-associated transcription factors, play a role in patterning and nail bed formation and are mutated in nail-patella syndrome (OMIM 161200) and Witkop syndrome (OMIM 189500), respectively.[39,40]

## MOSAICISM

Mosaic skin disorders have long been attractive candidates for gene discovery because the patient's normal skin can serve as an ideal genetic control when compared with lesional tissue. With rapid DNA sequencing, the genetic causes of many mosaic skin lesions are being uncovered. The identification of activating mutations in the fibroblast growth factor receptor 3 (FGFR3; OMIM 134934) in nonsyndromic keratinocytic epidermal nevi (EN; OMIM 162900), suggested that some epidermal nevi represent mosaic activating mutations in known oncogenes.[41] Although the initial reports described FGFR3 mutations in isolated keratinocytic EN, a recent study describes a unique mutation in FGFR3 in a patient with a keratinocytic EN and associated syndromic features.[42]

In addition to FGFR3 mutations, subsequent reports described mutations in another known oncogene, phosphatidylinositol 3-kinase, catalytic, alpha (PIK3CA; OMIM 171834; see CLOVES syndrome above) in some nonsyndromic keratinocytic EN; however, these two defects were only responsible for a portion of EN cases.[43] The most recent addition to this list of oncogenes is HRAS (OMIM 190020), specifically the p.G13R mutation and, rarely, KRAS (OMIM 190070). Together, these account for approximately 40% of epidermal nevi.[44] The first report of RAS defects in a patient with an EN were HRAS mutations (p.G12S) detected in a middle-aged man with widespread EN and urothelial cell cancer.[45] Recently, somatic mosaic HRAS and KRAS mutations have been reported to cause nevus sebaceous.[46] This suggests that some forms of EN are essentially mosaic RASopathies.

Recently, porokeratotic eccrine and ostial duct nevi (PEODDN) were associated with mosaicism for mutations in GJB2 (OMIM 121011), the gene encoding connexin 26, which is defective in several syndromes, including keratitis-ichthyosis-deafness (KID; OMIM 148210) syndrome.[47] This finding is not unexpected because maternal mosaicism for GJB2 mutations has been reported in the mother of a child with KID syndrome. The mother presented with a widespread Blaschko-linear epidermal nevus that resembled a PEODDN. Parents of children with syndromes caused by GJB2 mutations should be examined for the presence of epidermal nevi because it could indicate underlying gonadal mosaicism and, thus, an increased recurrence risk of the GJB2-related condition with subsequent pregnancies.[48]

## CANCER SYNDROMES

The genetic cause of a new AD cancer syndrome was identified in a large family. Affected patients had a striking phenotype of telangiectasia, mild ectodermal dysplasia features (developmental anomalies of hair, teeth, and nails), and highly penetrant oropharyngeal cancer (cutaneous telangiectasia and cancer syndrome, familial; OMIM 614564). The candidate genomic region was mapped and a candidate gene approach identified a heterozygous missense mutation in the ataxia telangiectasia and Rad3-related gene (ATR; OMIM 601215), which plays a critical role in regulating genomic integrity. ATR coordinates and controls several mechanisms, including DNA replication origin firing, the stability of the DNA replication fork, cell cycle checkpoints, and DNA repair. The causative mutation occurs in a domain responsible for activating p53 and p53 activation was decreased in patient cells. Additionally LOH for the functional copy of the ATR gene was noted in cancer tissue from affected patients. AR loss of LOF mutations in ATR have been identified in Seckel syndrome (OMIM 21600), a developmental disorder not associated with malignancy.[49]

An AD familial keratoacanthoma syndrome (multiple self-healing epithelioma [MSSE]; Ferguson-Smith disease; OMIM 132800) resisted genetic analysis in the past. Though a specific region of chromosome 9q22.3 had been linked to the disease in 11 Scottish families, a lack of recombination events in the region limited further analysis and sequencing of positional candidate genes did not reveal causative mutations. With the increased throughput capacity of new generation sequencing technology, the investigators were able to evaluate a much larger region using exon capture and high throughput sequencing. This identified mutations in transforming growth factor beta receptor 1 (TGFBR1 or activin-receptor-like kinase 5; OMIM 190181), which was outside the previously suggested linkage region. Defects in TGF-β function are well known to lead to unrestricted cell growth. Missense mutations in TGFBR1 have also been implicated as a cause of AD Marfan syndrome (MFS)-like disorders, including Loeys-Dietz syndrome (LDS) 1A, OMIM 609192; LDS2A, OMIM 608967. Patients with these syndromes exhibit developmental anomalies in neurologic, skeletal and/or craniofacial, and (most importantly) cardiovascular systems but are not prone to cancer. Mutations in MSSE affect one of two regions of the protein; however, the net result of either is that no functional protein is produced. In cells heterozygous for the TGFBR1 mutation, the remaining wild-type allele is protective. However, tumors from MSSE patients exhibit LOH of the wild type TGFBR1 allele. This contrasts with MFS-related conditions in which TGFBR1 mutations result in increased TGF-β signaling instead of silencing it. How the tumors that arise in MSSE then self-resolve is not yet clear but is an area of active study.[50]

## SKIN-DEVELOPMENT SYNDROMES

Aplasia cutis congenita (ACC) has long been regarded as a spontaneous developmental disorder characterized by absence of skin at birth. Most commonly occurring on the scalp, it is often solitary. The cause of ACC is heterogeneous and a variety of conditions have been associated with its development. Adams-Oliver syndrome (AOS; OMIM 100300) is the association of ACC with terminal transverse limb defects. Most often sporadic, AOS is occasionally transmitted through families in an AD and/or AR fashion. Various additional associated defects have been reported, including cutis marmorata and cardiac and/or vascular abnormalities. There is wide variability in severity of the phenotype, from relatively mild and subtle limb defects and small areas of ACC to extremely morbid or even mortal defects, even within families. GWAS was used to study two kindreds with AD-AOS followed by a candidate gene and exome analysis of linked areas from a single patient. This led investigators to heterozygous mutations in a RhoGAP family member, RhoGTPase-activating protein 31 (ARHGAP31; OMIM 610911), which is also known as Cdc42 GTPase-activating protein (CdGAP) and which acts to downregulate both Cdc42 (OMIM 116952) and Rac1 (OMIM 602048). Patients in this kindred had scalp ACC and variable upper and/or lower limb defects, including short distal phalanges, partially absent fingers and/or toes, and syndactyly of the second and third toes. The investigators examined Arhgap31 expression in mouse embryos, which occurred in the distal tip of the limb buds during late stages of embryonic development. Arhgap31 expression was also noted in the mouse heart although cardiac anomalies were not seen in any of the affected patients in the study. The expression of Arhgap31 in limb buds, cranium, and early heart parallel the defects reported in AOS. A screen of additional AOS patients did not reveal others with Arhgap31 mutations; thus, it is a rare cause of AOS. The mutations present in ARHGAP31 truncate the C-terminus and result in downregulation of active Cdc42 suggesting the effect of the mutations is a dominant gain of function of Arhgap31. The C-terminus of these proteins typically interacts with the N-terminal RhoGAP domain to shield a constitutively active catalytic site and lack of the C-terminus likely leads to continuous exposure of the active site. The outcome of constitutive Cdc42 inactivation is disruption of the actin cytoskeleton and ARHGAP31 functions to control the temporal and spatial cytoskeletal remodeling and modulation necessary for cell shape maintenance and migration. In summary, a variety of reports suggest that Cdc42 and Rac1 play important roles in skin and limb development and the regulation of their activity by Arhgap31 explains how GOF mutations in this protein lead to phenotype of AOS.[51]

A second report confirms the importance of Cdc42 and Rac1 in AOS. In patients with AR AOS, mutations in dedicator of cytokine kinesis 6 (DOCK6; OMIM 614194) were detected after autozygome analysis and exome sequencing identified LOF mutations. DOCK6 is a known modulator of Cdc42 and Rac1. Specifically, it functions to increase the amounts of active Cdc42 and Rac1; thus, deficiency of DOCK6 would be predicted to lead to impaired activation of Cdc42 and Rac1, similar to that seen with the GOF mutations in Arh-GAP31.[52] These two studies shed light on the pathomechanism of AOS and also highlight the genetic heterogeneity of the condition. Clearly, defects in other members of this particular pathway or, perhaps, Cdc42 and Rac1 themselves could potentially lead to an AOS phenotype. Additionally, these findings generate the hypothesis that perhaps sporadic somatic mutations in these genes could lead to nonsyndromic localized ACC as a form of mosaicism. In this case, the undergrowth of the skin tissue would be the outcome of the somatic mosaicism instead of the overgrowth typical of EN. The limited expression of these genes to the specific body sites and time periods of embryogenesis that they demonstrate would explain the localized nature of ACC in patients carrying the germline mutation.

An intriguing AD adermatoglyphia syndrome (OMIM 136000), also known as immigration delay disease,[53] was investigated in a large family. Patients have a congenital absence of dermatoglyphs as well as reduced eccrine sweat gland number and overall sweating of the hands. The lack of dermatoglyphs led to problems for patients when fingerprints were required for identification, such as crossing international borders. Linkage and haplotype analysis was used to map the disease to a specific chromosomal region and a candidate gene approach identified SMARCAD1 (OMIM 612761) as a candidate gene. SMARCAD1 is a member of the SNF subfamily of a larger group of helicase proteins. Investigation of SMARCAD1 in the skin revealed the existence of a short, skin-specific (especially fibroblasts) isoform of SMARCAD1. Sequencing of SMARCAD1 from AD adermatoglyphia patients detected a heterozygous transversion that clearly segregated with the disease. This mutation disrupted a conserved donor splice site next to the 3 prime end of a noncoding exon present only in the skin specific short form of the gene, leading to aberrant splicing and poor short isoform RNA stability. How the skin-specific isoform functions in dermatoglyph or eccrine sweat gland development is not clear and a focus of ongoing study.[54]

## SUMMARY

Although this is a brief overview, it highlights a few of the discoveries in inherited skin diseases over the past 6 to 12 months. The rapid acceleration of data acquisition has allowed identification of many of the genetic causes of inherited skin diseases. However, the identification of a causative gene for a condition is simply the beginning. The genetic causes of some inherited skin diseases, such as RDEB, have been known for decades, yet it is only recently that treatments based on that knowledge seem to be inching closer to reality. With the rapid acceleration in the pace of genetic discovery, identification of causative genes will occur in days or weeks instead of months and, it is to be hoped, a similar contraction will occur in the time needed for that knowledge to lead to therapeutic interventions for patients. Additionally, the elucidation of the genetic causes of similar diseases and syndromes greatly enhances our understanding of how different pathways interact and contribute to normal and abnormal skin development and function. The promise of this greater understanding is the potential for development of new therapies, including new applications for existing drugs, to add to our armamentarium to treat these diseases. An exciting example is the use of suppression therapy to treat genetic diseases resulting from mutations that produce premature stop codons. Various agents, such as aminoglycoside antibiotics, have the ability to induce readthrough of premature stop codons and much effort is now going toward development of more efficient safer pharmacologic agents to do the same. Already reports exist describing positive outcomes in cell culture models for disorders such as ataxia-telangiectasia, and have progressed through animal models into Phase II human trials for hemophilia A and B, methylmalonic acidemia and Duchenne muscular dystrophy. Most excitingly Phase III clinical trials are underway for cystic fibrosis.[55]

It has been nearly 60 years since the discovery of the structure of DNA. From then until now our understanding and appreciation of inherited skin diseases has advanced greatly. However, the accelerating rate of scientific advancement suggests a new stage of inquiry in which identification of disease-causing mutations, that critical first step in understanding and investigation, will occur rapidly and not impede pursuing a deeper understanding of the origins and pathomechanisms of cutaneous diseases.

## REFERENCES

1. Mardis ER. A decade's perspective on DNA sequencing technology. Nature 2011;470(7333): 198–203.
2. Full spectrum genetics. Nat Genet 2011;44(1):1.
3. Liu L, Dopping-Hepenstal PJ, Lovell PA, et al. Autosomal recessive epidermolysis bullosa simplex due to loss of BPAG1-e expression. J Invest Dermatol 2012;132(3 Pt 1):742–4.
4. Petrof G, Mellerio JE, McGrath JA. Desmosomal genodermatoses. Br J Dermatol 2012;166(1):36–45.

5. Pigors M, Kiritsi D, Krumpelmann S, et al. Lack of plakoglobin leads to lethal congenital epidermolysis bullosa: a novel clinico-genetic entity. Hum Mol Genet 2011;20(9):1811–9.

6. Has C, Sparta G, Kiritsi D, et al. Integrin alpha3 mutations with kidney, lung, and skin disease. N Engl J Med 2012;366(16):1508–14.

7. Ng YZ, Pourreyron C, Salas-Alanis JC, et al. Fibroblast-derived dermal matrix drives development of aggressive cutaneous squamous cell carcinoma in patients with recessive dystrophic epidermolysis bullosa. Cancer Res 2012;72(14):3522–34.

8. Pasmooij AM, Nijenhuis M, Brander R, et al. Natural gene therapy may occur in all patients with generalized non-Herlitz junctional epidermolysis bullosa with COL17A1 mutations. J Invest Dermatol 2012; 132(5):1374–83.

9. Yuen WY, Huizinga J, Jonkman MF. Punch grafting of chronic ulcers in patients with laminin-332-deficient, non-Herlitz junctional epidermolysis bullosa. J Am Acad Dermatol 2012;68(1):93–97.e2.

10. Uitto J, Christiano AM, McLean WH, et al. Novel molecular therapies for heritable skin disorders. J Invest Dermatol 2012;132(3 Pt 2):820–8.

11. Nagy N, Almaani N, Tanaka A, et al. HB-EGF induces COL7A1 expression in keratinocytes and fibroblasts: possible mechanism underlying allogeneic fibroblast therapy in recessive dystrophic epidermolysis Bullosa. J Invest Dermatol 2011;131(8):1771–4.

12. Wagner JE, Ishida-Yamamoto A, McGrath JA, et al. Bone marrow transplantation for recessive dystrophic epidermolysis bullosa. N Engl J Med 2010; 363(7):629–39.

13. Itoh M, Kiuru M, Cairo MS, et al. Generation of keratinocytes from normal and recessive dystrophic epidermolysis bullosa-induced pluripotent stem cells. Proc Natl Acad Sci U S A 2011;108(21):8797–802.

14. Remington J, Wang X, Hou Y, et al. Injection of recombinant human type VII collagen corrects the disease phenotype in a murine model of dystrophic epidermolysis bullosa. Mol Ther 2009;17(1):26–33.

15. Abstracts of the Annual Meeting of the Society for Investigative Dermatology. May 9-12, 2012. Raleigh, North Carolina, USA. J Invest Dermatol 2012; 132(Suppl 1):S1–180 [abstract#419].

16. Elias PM, Williams ML, Feingold KR. Abnormal barrier function in the pathogenesis of ichthyosis: therapeutic implications for lipid metabolic disorders. Clin Dermatol 2012;30(3):311–22.

17. Grall A, Guaguere E, Planchais S, et al. PNPLA1 mutations cause autosomal recessive congenital ichthyosis in golden retriever dogs and humans. Nat Genet 2012;44(2):140–7.

18. Aldahmesh MA, Mohamed JY, Alkuraya HS, et al. Recessive mutations in ELOVL4 cause ichthyosis, intellectual disability, and spastic quadriplegia. Am J Hum Genet 2011;89(6):745–50.

19. Cassidy AJ, van Steensel MA, Steijlen PM, et al. A homozygous missense mutation in TGM5 abolishes epidermal transglutaminase 5 activity and causes acral peeling skin syndrome. Am J Hum Genet 2005;77(6):909–17.

20. Oji V, Eckl KM, Aufenvenne K, et al. Loss of corneodesmosin leads to severe skin barrier defect, pruritus, and atopy: unraveling the peeling skin disease. Am J Hum Genet 2010;87(2):274–81.

21. Cabral RM, Kurban M, Wajid M, et al. Whole-exome sequencing in a single proband reveals a mutation in the CHST8 gene in autosomal recessive peeling skin syndrome. Genomics 2012;99(4):202–8.

22. Blaydon DC, Nitoiu D, Eckl KM, et al. Mutations in CSTA, encoding Cystatin A, underlie exfoliative ichthyosis and reveal a role for this protease inhibitor in cell-cell adhesion. Am J Hum Genet 2011;89(4): 564–71.

23. Paller AS, van Steensel MA, Rodriguez-Martin M, et al. Pathogenesis-based therapy reverses cutaneous abnormalities in an inherited disorder of distal cholesterol metabolism. J Invest Dermatol 2011; 131(11):2242–8.

24. Brandl K, Tomisato W, Beutler B. Inflammatory bowel disease and ADAM17 deletion. N Engl J Med 2012; 366(2):190.

25. Ombrello MJ, Remmers EF, Sun G, et al. Cold urticaria, immunodeficiency, and autoimmunity related to PLCG2 deletions. N Engl J Med 2012;366(4):330–8.

26. van de Veerdonk FL, Plantinga TS, Hoischen A, et al. STAT1 mutations in autosomal dominant chronic mucocutaneous candidiasis. N Engl J Med 2011; 365(1):54–61.

27. Puel A, Cypowyj S, Bustamante J, et al. Chronic mucocutaneous candidiasis in humans with inborn errors of interleukin-17 immunity. Science 2011; 332(6025):65–8.

28. Engelhardt KR, Grimbacher B. Mendelian traits causing susceptibility to mucocutaneous fungal infections in human subjects. J Allergy Clin Immunol 2012;129(2):294–305.

29. Jordan CT, Cao L, Roberson ED, et al. Rare and common variants in CARD14, encoding an epidermal regulator of NF-kappaB, in psoriasis. Am J Hum Genet 2012;90(5):796–808.

30. Jordan CT, Cao L, Roberson ED, et al. PSORS2 is due to mutations in CARD14. Am J Hum Genet 2012;90(5):784–95.

31. Nitschke Y, Baujat G, Botschen U, et al. Generalized arterial calcification of infancy and pseudoxanthoma elasticum can be caused by mutations in either ENPP1 or ABCC6. Am J Hum Genet 2012;90(1):25–39.

32. Happle R. Type 2 segmental Cowden disease vs. Proteus syndrome. Br J Dermatol 2007;156(5):1089–90.

33. Kurek KC, Luks VL, Ayturk UM, et al. Somatic Mosaic Activating Mutations in PIK3CA Cause CLOVES Syndrome. Am J Hum Genet 2012;90:901–8.

34. Lindhurst MJ, Sapp JC, Teer JK, et al. A mosaic activating mutation in AKT1 associated with the Proteus syndrome. N Engl J Med 2011;365(7):611–9.

35. Zhu H, Shang D, Sun M, et al. X-linked congenital hypertrichosis syndrome is associated with interchromosomal insertions mediated by a human-specific palindrome near SOX3. Am J Hum Genet 2011;88(6):819–26.

36. Harakalova M, van Harssel JJ, Terhal PA, et al. Dominant missense mutations in ABCC9 cause Cantu syndrome. Nat Genet 2012;44(7):793–6.

37. van Bon BW, Gilissen C, Grange DK, et al. Cantu Syndrome Is Caused by Mutations in ABCC9. Am J Hum Genet 2012;90(6):1094–101.

38. Zhou C, Zang D, Jin Y, et al. Mutation in ribosomal protein L21 underlies hereditary hypotrichosis simplex. Hum Mutat 2011;32(7):710–4.

39. Frojmark AS, Schuster J, Sobol M, et al. Mutations in Frizzled 6 cause isolated autosomal-recessive nail dysplasia. Am J Hum Genet 2011;88(6):852–60.

40. Naz G, Pasternack SM, Perrin C, et al. FZD6 encoding the Wnt receptor frizzled 6 is mutated in autosomal-recessive nail dysplasia. Br J Dermatol 2012;166(5):1088–94.

41. Hafner C, van Oers JM, Vogt T, et al. Mosaicism of activating FGFR3 mutations in human skin causes epidermal nevi. J Clin Invest 2006;116(8):2201–7.

42. Ousager LB, Bygum A, Hafner C. Identification of a novel S249C FGFR3 mutation in a keratinocytic epidermal naevus syndrome. Br J Dermatol 2012; 167(1):202–4.

43. Hafner C, Lopez-Knowles E, Luis NM, et al. Oncogenic PIK3CA mutations occur in epidermal nevi and seborrheic keratoses with a characteristic mutation pattern. Proc Natl Acad Sci U S A 2007;104(33): 13450–4.

44. Hafner C, Toll A, Gantner S, et al. Keratinocytic epidermal nevi are associated with mosaic RAS mutations. J Med Genet 2012;49(4):249–53.

45. Hafner C, Toll A, Real FX. HRAS mutation mosaicism causing urothelial cancer and epidermal nevus. N Engl J Med 2011;365(20):1940–2.

46. Groesser L, Herschberger E, Ruetten A, et al. Postzygotic HRAS and KRAS mutations cause nevus sebaceous and Schimmelpenning syndrome. Nat Genet 2012;44(7):783–7.

47. Easton JA, Donnelly S, Kamps MA, et al. Porokeratotic eccrine nevus may be caused by somatic connexin26 mutations. J Invest Dermatol 2012;2(9): 2184–91.

48. Titeux M, Mendonca V, Decha A, et al. Keratitis-ichthyosis-deafness syndrome caused by GJB2 maternal mosaicism. J Invest Dermatol 2009;129(3): 776–9.

49. Tanaka A, Weinel S, Nagy N, et al. Germline mutation in ATR in autosomal-dominant oropharyngeal cancer syndrome. Am J Hum Genet 2012;90(3): 511–7.

50. Goudie DR, D'Alessandro M, Merriman B, et al. Multiple self-healing squamous epithelioma is caused by a disease-specific spectrum of mutations in TGFBR1. Nat Genet 2011;43(4):365–9.

51. Southgate L, Machado RD, Snape KM, et al. Gain-of-function mutations of ARHGAP31, a Cdc42/Rac1 GTPase regulator, cause syndromic cutis aplasia and limb anomalies. Am J Hum Genet 2011;88(5): 574–85.

52. Shaheen R, Faqeih E, Sunker A, et al. Recessive mutations in DOCK6, encoding the guanidine nucleotide exchange factor DOCK6, lead to abnormal actin cytoskeleton organization and Adams-Oliver syndrome. Am J Hum Genet 2011;89(2):328–33.

53. Burger B, Fuchs D, Sprecher E, et al. The immigration delay disease: adermatoglyphia-inherited absence of epidermal ridges. J Am Acad Dermatol 2011; 64(5):974–80.

54. Nousbeck J, Burger B, Fuchs-Telem D, et al. A mutation in a skin-specific isoform of SMARCAD1 causes autosomal-dominant adermatoglyphia. Am J Hum Genet 2011;89(2):302–7.

55. Keeling KM, Bedwell DM. Suppression of nonsense mutations as a therapeutic approach to treat genetic diseases. Wiley Interdiscip Rev RNA 2011;2(6): 837–52.

# Pediatric Photosensitivity Disorders

Omar Pacha, MD, Adelaide A. Hebert, MD*

## KEYWORDS

- Photosensitivity • Pediatric • Dermatology • Albinism • Photoallergy • Sunburn • Photodistribution
- Photoprotection

## KEY POINTS

- Photodermatoses are rare in the pediatric population but should be suspected when the history and clinical picture are consistent with a light-induced origin.
- Underlying causes of photodermatoses may include genetic predisposition, metabolic disorders, immunosuppression, or medication use.
- Photodermatoses may become evident as early as the newborn period, particularly with certain disorders triggered by phototherapy for hyperbilirubinemia.
- As in adults with sunlight-induced photodermatoses, children may be impacted by seasonal influences and certain wavelengths that increase their risk of sensitivity.
- Photoprotection, such as sunscreens, photoprotective clothing, and films on windows, may be important recommendations in pediatric patients predisposed to photodermatoses.

## INTRODUCTION

Photosensitivity disorders in childhood are rare, with the notable exception of overexposure as sunburn, and therefore require a more circumspect approach. Practitioners who treat children are key players in identifying and managing the many photosensitivity disorders that rarely present in childhood. A classic photodistribution of skin findings may suggest photosensitivity, but a correct diagnosis depends on a detailed history correlated with clinical findings. The role of the physician is not only to identify and treat these disorders but also to counsel patients and their families on specific light avoidance, photoprotection, and, in a few cases, major lifestyle adjustments. Many photosensitivity disorders require a multidisciplinary approach, with involvement of a dermatologist to coordinate appropriate care.

## INITIAL PRESENTATION

Distribution is the most classic unifying feature of photodermatitis. Eruptions are usually confined to light-exposed areas, most prominently on the nose and cheeks, posterior neck, and extensor surfaces of the upper extremities. Spared areas include those of the body normally covered with clothing, and anatomically shaded areas such as the scalp, anterior neck, and flexor surfaces. Examination of doubly covered areas such as the buttocks, and the chest in the case of female patients, can be especially helpful in identifying less-obvious cases of photosensitivity, because many fabrics are weakly photoprotective. After sun exposure, signs and symptoms of phototoxicity can begin anywhere from a few minutes to several hours later, and then peak within several hours to a few days. Therefore, even nonimmediate exposure is suspect as a cause.

The authors have no relevant financial interests to disclose.
Department of Dermatology, The University of Texas Medical School-Houston, 6655 Travis Street, Houston, TX 77030, USA
* Corresponding author. Department of Dermatology, The University of Texas Medical School-Houston, 6655 Travis Street, Suite 980, Houston, TX 77030.
E-mail address: Adelaide.A.Hebert@uth.tmc.edu

Dermatol Clin 31 (2013) 317–326
http://dx.doi.org/10.1016/j.det.2012.12.008
0733-8635/13/$ – see front matter © 2013 Published by Elsevier Inc.

## CLASSIFICATIONS: PHOTOTOXICITY VERSUS PHOTO ALLERGY

Most photosensitivity disorders can be described as either phototoxic or photoallergic; clinical characteristics suggest that even the idiopathic disorders probably fit one of these definitions. Phototoxicity occurs when a chromophore absorbs radiation, which in turn leads to a mechanism of tissue reactivity through excitation of that chromophore.[1] This process is distinct from the direct tissue damage that occurs with infrared and ionizing radiation. The action spectrum for photosensitivity falls within ultraviolet to visible electromagnetic radiation; individual chromophores are excited by specific ranges of wavelength.[2] The archetypal characteristics of acute phototoxicity are erythema, edema, and possible vesicle or bulla formation, followed by hyperpigmentation (tanning) and desquamation (peeling) secondary to melanin stimulation and cell death, respectively.[3]

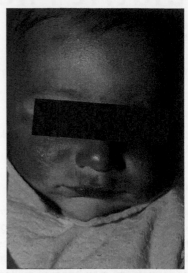

Fig. 2. A phototoxic reaction in an infant on medication that increased his risk of sunburn.

## PHOTOTOXIC REACTIONS
### Sunburn

Sunburn is the most common phototoxic reaction (Figs. 1 and 2). Ultraviolet B (UVB) (290–320 nm) radiation elicits most of the response, although ultraviolet A (UVA) radiation may account for a small percentage of the observed erythema and is more implicated in the production of tans.[3] Individual susceptibility is most dependent on epidermal melanin content. As with all phototoxicity, sunburn is augmented by

- Increased ambient temperature

- Increased hydration of the stratum corneum from humidity and swimming
- Occlusion by adhesive bandages (which may be confused with contact sensitivity to the adhesive)[4]
- Increased elevation
- Increased reflected surfaces, such as water or snow[5,6]

The clinical presentation of sunburn is the same as for acute phototoxicity (ie, erythema and edema followed by desquamation, and finally hyperpigmentation). These manifestations can be painful and their clinical presence disconcerting. Treatment, however, is limited once symptoms have arisen. Pain control with oral nonsteroidal anti-inflammatory drugs and, in those with severe and extensive damage, oral steroids and topical steroids may be considered. For most, supportive treatment with over-the-counter pain management and frequent application of topical emollients is sufficient.

Prevention is key and identification of patients who have a predisposition to sunburn is useful. The most practical recommendations include daily sunscreen and protective clothing in fair children who are innately more prone to burning, and appropriate sunscreen application for those less likely to burn but with exceptionally high sun exposure. As a rule, the American Academy of Dermatology recommends daily use of sunscreens with an SPF of 30 or higher for all individuals.[7] Most people apply sunscreen in insufficient quantity and too infrequently to get the labeled protection.[8] Recent regulation in the United States will limit the

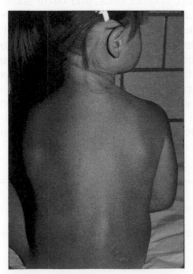

Fig. 1. Sunburn in a fair skinned child.

rating of sunscreens to SPF 50+ and change terminology with regard to use while swimming. The use of the term *broad spectrum* will be permitted for products that are also able to provide UVA protection.[9]

## Phytophotodermatitis

Phytophotodermatitis results from contact with plant extracts containing furocoumarins (psoralens) and subsequent activation of these chromophores by ultraviolet radiation. Citrus fruits, especially lemons, limes, and mangoes, and many common weeds contain these topically photosensitizing chemicals. The cutaneous reaction is typical of phototoxicity, but lesions are usually well demarcated and may demonstrate dramatic erythema and hyperpigmentation. Common presentations are the upper lip from drinking citrus beverages, the hands from handling culprit weeds, and the lower legs from contact with certain grasses. Bizarre streaks may appear secondary to dripping liquid. Dermatitis bullosa striata pratensis, or meadow dermatitis, is a phytophotodermatitis characterized acutely by linear vesicle formation and subsequent hyperpigmentation on exposed legs from contact with meadow grass.

Photoallergy is much less common than phototoxicity. Endogenous or exogenous haptens are activated by light, usually in the UV range. Contact photoallergies are typically type IV delayed hypersensitivity reactions, which are mediated by T cells. The resulting eruptions appear as papular to eczematous lesions in light-exposed areas.[1]

## PHOTOALLERGIC REACTIONS

Solar urticaria is an immunoglobulin E (IgE)–mediated hypersensitivity reaction to a photoallergen.[10] Two types of solar urticaria exist. In one, specific IgE is generated against a photoinduced cutaneous allergen caused by a specific wavelength. In the other, abnormal immunoglobulin is created that reacts with a normal chromophore.[11] In this rare entity, erythema, urticaria, and pruritus develop on skin exposed to light for as little as a few minutes. Wheals wane a few hours after they develop.[12] Histamine or other cellular mediator release probably causes this reaction,[13] and shock has occurred subsequent to large surface area exposures. The action spectrum differs with individual cases, and can extend from the UV range into visible light. Repeated exposure leads to a hardening phenomenon. In addition to photoprotection, antimalarials[14] and nonsedating antihistamines[15] have been used with some success.

## DISORDERS OF ENDOGENOUS CHROMOPHORE PRODUCTION

The porphyrias are a group of disorders of heme synthesis that result in the abnormal production of tetrapyrrole heme precursors, or porphyrinogens. Porphyrins, the oxidized product of these precursors, are potent photosensitizers. The action spectrum of the porphyrins ranges from 400 to 405 nm (the Soret band) to visible red (600–650 nm).[16] The relationship between sunlight and disease in erythropoietic protoporphyria (EPP) and erythropoietic porphyria (EP) is usually obvious. In these porphyrias of bone marrow origin, exposure results in acute painful stinging of the skin. In contrast, variegate porphyria and porphyria cutanea tarda (PCT) are associated with a more chronic photosensitivity.[17]

Autosomal dominantly inherited EPP is the most common erythropoietic porphyria, with an average age at presentation of 4 years. Patients may have no trouble with sunlight at all, or experience discomfort during exposure that persists approximately 24 hours.[17] Symptoms are accompanied by the development of erythema and edema in the photodistribution pattern of the face, neck, and backs of the hands, usually without vesicle formation. Chronic exposure leads to waxy scarring over these areas and furrowed, linear scars radiating from around the mouth.[18]

Congenital erythropoietic porphyria, or Günther disease, is a rare autosomal recessive disorder that presents in infancy or early childhood. The first sign may be inconsolable crying during and after sun exposure. As with EPP, erythema and edema develop in the characteristic photodistribution; however, vesicle and bulla formation are common. Rupture and healing of bullae result in erosions and scarring. If repeated exposure is not avoided, scarring and mutilation of facial features and fingers ensues. Affected skin develops scleodermoid changes and hypertrichosis. Soluble porphyrins cause red to purplish discoloration of the teeth and reddish discoloration of the urine that fluoresce under a Wood lamp. Although EPP usually causes a mild hemolytic anemia, the associated anemia may be severe.[18]

PCT is the most common porphyria, affecting 1 in approximately every 25,000 people. This condition is inherited in an autosomal dominant pattern, and usually does not present until the third or fourth decade. Familial cases of PCT, however, can present in the first decade of life.[16] Onset is typically insidious, and relationship to sun exposure is difficult to establish. Exposed skin, especially the dorsa of the hands, becomes thin and fragile. Intermittently, vesicles and bullae form and slowly heal to leave atrophic scars and milia. Chronic changes also include facial hypertrichosis and scarring alopecia.[17] The association of PCT with human immunodeficiency virus and hepatitis C has not been reported in children, although many reports exist for adults.

Variegate porphyria (VP) is also autosomal dominantly inherited, and has an increased incidence in Dutch South Africans (Afrikaners). Clinically, VP is almost indistinguishable from PCT. This variant usually presents after puberty, and is characterized by acute attacks similar to acute intermittent porphyria. Gastrointestinal manifestations of these attacks include constipation, nausea and vomiting, and colic that may resemble an acute abdomen. Neuropsychiatric symptoms vary from peripheral neuropathy to psychosis or seizures.[19]

Assessment of plasma porphyrin level and the porphyrin fluorescence spectrum confirms a diagnosis of porphyria. A pediatric hematologist should be involved to help manage anemia in the case of the EPs, and iron overload in the case of PCT. Management of VP will require both an experienced neurologist and a nutritionist. Beta-carotene may benefit patients with EP, EPP, or VP, whereas antimalarials have been used with success in PCT.[20,21] More recently, afamelanotide, a melanocyte-stimulating hormone, has shown promise, at least in EPP.[22]

Porphyrin-related cutaneous sequelae may also arise in otherwise healthy neonates as a result of blue light phototherapy in those predisposed because of jaundice. Newborns with erythroblastosis fetalis are treated with blue light phototherapy to accelerate bilirubin breakdown, and these breakdown products include porphyrins. These photosensitizers occasionally produce a clinical picture similar to the syndromes mentioned earlier, with purpuric patches, bullae, and erythema appearing in the light-exposed areas, and dramatic sparing of shielded ones. This condition is named *transient porphyrinemia of the newborn*.[23]

## MELANIN DEFICIENCY SYNDROMES

Albinism is a group of disorders unified by abnormalities in melanin synthesis. Ten types (I–VII, plus subtypes of I and VI) of oculocutaneous albinism are described. A different interruption in the synthesis of tyrosine to melanin occurs in each type. The 2 most common are tyrosinase-negative (type I) and tyrosinase-positive (type II).[24] Enzymatic evaluation can be performed through analysis of freshly harvested hair bulbs. Skin color may vary from milky white to dark brown depending on the variant type and race of the

patient, but patients will always appear lighter than their unaffected first-degree relatives.[25] The use of contact lenses with opaque artificial irises can offer some photoprotection while improving visual acuity.[26] All individuals with albinism are more susceptible to sunburn and are at increased risk for actinic changes and the development of cutaneous malignancies later in life.

Other diseases in which melanin is deficient also predispose to decreased tolerance of ultraviolet radiation. In phenylketonuria, the enzyme system that oxidizes phenylalanine to tyrosine is deficient. Without tyrosine as a substrate, melanin production is reduced, leading to hypopigmentation of the skin, hair, and eyes. Patients with pigment-losing disorders, such as vitiligo, piebaldism, pityriasis alba, and other varieties of leukoderma, also have variable resistance to ultraviolet light.

Hermansky-Pudlak syndrome is a group of heterogeneous rare autosomal recessive disorders that cause oculocutaneous albinism and lisosomal storage deficiency. Many patients may be of Puerto Rican heritage, with 1:1800 people having the syndrome, making it the most common single gene disorder in Puerto Rico.[27] These patients may experience blindness, easy bruisability, and prolonged bleeding. They eventually progress to pulmonary fibrosis and granulomatous colitis, which ordinarily is the cause death.[28]

## DISORDERS OF CELLULAR REPAIR

In some heritable diseases, a deficiency of repair mechanisms that respond to ultraviolet-damaged tissue is responsible for observed photosensitivity. Acquired disorders of cellular repair are secondary to vitamin deficiency. In the absence of other abnormalities, cutaneous chromophores in these diseases are normal.

## XERODERMA PIGMENTOSUM

Xeroderma pigmentosum (XP) is an autosomal recessive, degenerative disease generated by abnormal repair of DNA damaged by ultraviolet radiation and environmental mutagens (**Figs. 3** and **4**).[29] The disease is categorized into 7 known complementation groups, assigned A through G. Each group has a specific deficit of DNA excision repair, and therefore cells of different complementation groups, if fused in culture, can reach almost normal levels of DNA repair.[30]

The most common XP disease in the United States is complementation group C. Photophobia, photosensitivity, and pigment changes manifest themselves in the first few years of life. Exposed areas show acute erythema after ultraviolet light

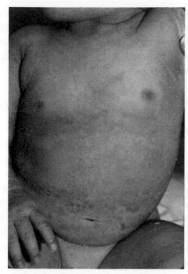

Fig. 3. Xeroderma pigmentosum in early phase.

irradiation, and subsequent dark, dense freckling. Repeated exposures lead to the chronic changes for which the syndrome is named: dry, atrophic, hyperpigmented skin. Actinic changes including keratoses develop in childhood, with the median age for the first nonmelanoma skin cancer occurring at 8 years. The risk of developing cutaneous carcinomas and melanoma is 1000 times greater than that of the normal population.[31]

Internal malignancies are also common, occurring 10 to 20 times more frequently in XP. The anterior, ultraviolet-exposed structures of the eye are affected as frequently as the skin. Acute exposure causes photophobia, but chronic insult to the eye results in severe keratitis, corneal opacification, and vascularization. Melanoma may arise from the iris in the anterior chamber of the eye. Atrophic scarring of the eyelids may lead to entropion or ectropion.

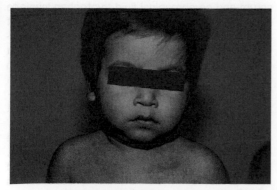

Fig. 4. Xeroderma pigmentosum in the early stages.

Neurologic manifestations are seen in approximately 30% of cases, and may present in early infancy through the second decade of life. Findings range from mild to severe hyporeflexia, progressive mental retardation, sensorineural deafness, and seizures. The most severe described variant is De Sanctis-Cacchione syndrome, which includes the features of XP with microcephaly and progressive mental deterioration.

The simplest neurologic screening of all patients should include audiometry and deep tendon reflexes. Routine laboratory tests do not contribute to the diagnosis; however, in all cases, cells demonstrate abnormal excision repair in culture after ultraviolet irradiation. Complementation group typing is accomplished using the fibroblasts from a fresh skin biopsy transported in microbial transport medium. The Armed Forces Institute of Pathology in Washington, DC performs UV survival and unscheduled DNA synthesis assays in addition to complementation testing. Currently, clinical trials are underway to investigate T4N5, a topical preparation containing a prokaryotic DNA repair enzyme in a liposomal vehicle. Areas treated with this experimental drug show fewer DNA cyclobutyl pyrimidine dimers than control sites in patients with XP.[32,33]

## BLOOM SYNDROME

Bloom syndrome is a rare autosomal recessive disorder usually found in individuals of Ashkenazi Jewish descent.[34] Short stature, increased risk of malignancy, and immunodeficiency of varying severity characterize the syndrome.[35] At the cellular level, an increase is seen in the number of sister chromatid exchanges and chromosomal breaks, which is now understood to be a deficiency in a RecQ helicase, similar to Rothmund-Thomson syndrome and is described in more detail in that section.[36] The disorder typically presents in the first few months of life as a butterfly pattern of erythema and subsequent telangiectasia formation on the face after the infant's first exposure to sunlight. Cheilitis and poikiloderma may develop after repeated ultraviolet insult.

Immunodeficiency ranges from subclinical to severe. Levels of IgA, IgG, or IgM may be inadequate, and cellular immunity may be weakened.[37] Severe ear infections may be recurrent and lead to hearing deficits. Infants must be vigilantly watched for the development of gastrointestinal infections, which can be life-threatening. Immunity generally improves with age, but recurrent pneumonias are a common cause of death.[38] Leukemia is the most common malignancy presenting in childhood; carcinomas, including those of the skin, usually do not occur until adulthood.[38] Intelligence is unaffected, and 82% of affected persons reach 20 years of age.[39]

## COCKAYNE SYNDROME

Cockayne syndrome is a rare autosomal recessive disorder characterized by short stature, subcutaneous fat loss, and progressive neurologic degeneration.[40] Recognizable physical characteristics include microcephaly with sunken eyes, a thin nose, and large ears. The trunk is short, the extremities are long, and hands and feet are large.[34,41] Radiographically, cranial thickening is evident. Ultraviolet radiation leads to excessive sister chromatid exchange and cell destruction. Although some DNA repair mechanisms are intact, ultraviolet exposure suppresses DNA synthesis.[31] Unlike Bloom syndrome, no increased incidence of malignancy is seen with Cockayne syndrome. Photosensitivity is often the presenting sign of disease but is not a universal finding in all cases. Short exposures to sunlight result in exaggerated sunburn response, including erythema, edema, and vesicle formation. Hyperpigmentation, scarring, and telangiectasias result from chronic exposure. Mental retardation is universal and may be profound.[40] Neurologic functions progressively deteriorate, causing death by the second or third decade; many patients die before 10 years of age.

## ROTHMUND-THOMSON SYNDROME

Rothmund-Thomson syndrome is also a rare entity inherited in an autosomal dominant pattern. Individual findings vary by case, but major characteristics include short stature, skeletal abnormalities, abnormal hair growth, and cataracts.[42] Recently, mutations in RecQ helicases have been linked to Rothmund-Thomson syndrome. Apparently these helicases suppress illegitimate recombination, which leads to the DNA recombination that is characteristic of this disease.[43] Affected persons have both normal immunity and intelligence but are predisposed to the development of malignancy, including osteosarcoma at sites of skeletal abnormality[44] and skin cancers.

Cutaneous changes typically begin in the first 3 to 6 months, manifesting as erythematous patches over the cheeks, which may vesiculate. These patches progress to involve the forehead, pinnae, neck, dorsa of the hands, extensor surfaces of the arms, lower legs, and buttocks. This acute phase of the disease is self-limiting, and may last from a few months to several years.[42] The role of light exposure in the pathogenesis of the syndrome is not completely clear. Acute photosensitivity is rare, and although lesions are most prominent in exposed areas, the doubly covered buttocks are commonly involved. In the absence of malignancy, prognosis is good.

## DISORDERS OF TRYPTOPHAN METABOLISM

Pellagra is an acquired chronic disorder usually seen in association with a diet deficient in quality protein, specifically lacking the essential amino acid tryptophan. Although rare in the United States, pellagra may be seen among poor people who depend on corn as a dietary staple, such as Central Americans, and in individuals with absorptive disorders.[45] Corn is rich in phenylalanine, which is a competitive inhibitor of tryptophan transport.

Pellagra is often characterized by the 3 Ds: dermatitis, diarrhea, and dementia. A fourth D is often added—death—which may be sudden and unheralded.[46]

Skin lesions usually appear as a clearly demarcated erythematous eruption resembling sunburn over areas exposed to sunlight. Lesions are typically symmetric and may be associated with pruritus and burning. The dorsa of the hands are most commonly affected, but lesions also present on the forearms, face, and around the neck (Casal necklace). Erythema may evolve to bulla formation and subsequent ulceration. Brownish pigmentation of the sloughing epidermis occurs, which reveals pink skin underneath. Oral manifestations include angular cheilitis, a swollen "beef red" tongue, and nonspecific mouth sores.

The clinical picture of pellagra is mirrored in the rarer diseases of tryptophan deficiency. Hartnup disease is an autosomal recessive defect of the system responsible for neutral amino acid transport in the jejunum and renal tubule.[47] The result is a loss of amino acids in the stool and urine. Treatment with oral tryptophan ethyl ester, a lipid-soluble derivative of the amino acid, can return serum and cerebrospinal fluid tryptophan levels to normal.[48] Hydroxykynureninuria is a deficiency of kynureninase, an enzyme essential in the metabolism of tryptophan to niacin. These children exhibit psychomotor retardation and episodic ataxia in addition to photosensitivity.

## IDIOPATHIC PHOTODERMATOSES

Polymorphous light eruption (PMLE) is one of the most common photosensitivity disorders (**Figs. 5–7**). Women are more commonly affected, and initial presentation is in the first 2 decades. As the name implies, PMLE may present in a variety

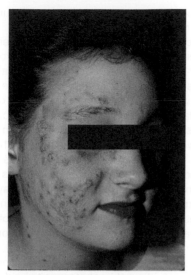

Fig. 5. Polymorphous light eruption in a child with American Indian extraction.

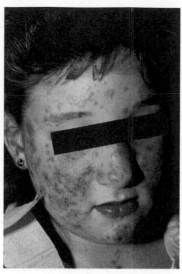

Fig. 7. Facial papules and erosions of polymorphous light eruption.

of appearances, but each case typically has only a single morphology. The most common clinical presentation is an eczematous eruption similar to a photo drug reaction or atopic dermatitis. Other morphologic types include a papular or vesicular eruption and plaque dermatitis.[49] Eruptions should be exclusively limited to sun-exposed areas such as the face, posterior neck, a "V" pattern on the chest, and limb extensor surfaces. Lesions occur 1 to 2 days after sun exposure and, in the absence of repeated exposure, resolve in 1 to 2 weeks. Chronic exposure causes persistence of the lesions, and a "hardening" effect, or increased

tolerance to sunlight, occurs.[50] PMLE begins in the spring and begins to remit in the late summer as tolerance builds. Class II topical steroids may be of benefit in acute eruptions. Regimens commonly used in adults, such as oral corticosteroids, antimalarials, and PUVA, are not appropriate in most pediatric cases (Figs. 8–10).

Actinic prurigo is an autosomal dominant photodermatitis that occurs almost exclusively in individuals of Native American ancestry, including many Hispanics. UVA and possibly UVB trigger the cutaneous response. Research has shown an association of actinic prurigo with certain HLA

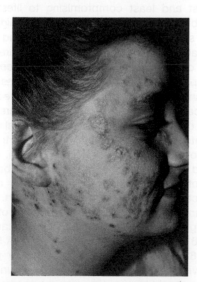

Fig. 6. Polymorphous light eruption with atrophic scarring on the face in a child of American Indian extraction.

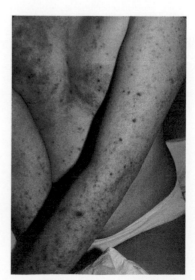

Fig. 8. Polymorphous light eruption on the arms of a female of American Indian extraction.

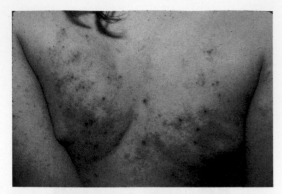

Fig. 9. Papules and erosions on the chest of a girl with polymorphous light eruption. This photo illustrated that the eruption can extend to non sun exposed areas.

types. The disease is classified by either early or late onset; 45% of patients have onset of the disease from infancy to 9 years of age.[51] Early onset (before 20 years of age) is associated with a greater incidence of cheilitis and ocular involvement.[51] The eruptions of actinic prurigo resemble chronic eczematous PMLE but are severely pruritic. Often the presentation is that of both an acute and chronic dermatitis, especially in pediatric patients. Cheilitis involves the upper or lower lips, and may be the only lesion present.[52] Scleral injection, tearing, and ocular pruritus are seen in almost half of the cases in Mexico.[53] Type I topical corticosteroids have been shown to clear lesions in 10 days.[54] UVB and PUVA may induce tolerance, and long-acting antihistamines can improve pruritus. Thalidomide is used with success in Mexico[55] and Colombia.[56] Early-onset actinic prurigo has a better long-term prognosis than the

late-onset type, with improvement occurring in the later teenage years.

Hydroa vacciniforme is a rare photosensitivity disorder distinguished by vesicle (hydroa) formation in sun-exposed areas that heals with pox-like ("vacciniforme") scarring.[57] Tense, deep-seated vesicles on an erythematous base develop 1 to 2 days after exposure. Blisters umbilicate and crust as they heal. The average age of onset is 6 years, with 90% of cases appearing by 16 years of age.[58] Prurigo aestivalis, a probable milder variant of hydroa vacciniforme, presents as pruritic erythema and vesicles a few hours to days after sun exposure. Hydroa vacciniforme and prurigo aestivale may respond to beta-carotene or antimalarials but usually remit spontaneously by the later teenage years.

The lag time between sun exposure and eruption in these idiopathic photosensitivity disorders implies a photoallergic response. However, no immunologic abnormalities have been revealed. In contrast to lupus erythematosus, PMLE has no observed immunoglobulins at the dermal-epidermal junction. Delayed cell-mediated hypersensitivity has been postulated to account for the late response.

## PHOTOPROTECTION

Reduction of light exposure is paramount in the management of all photosensitivity disorders. Psychological and socioeconomic factors make complete avoidance of sunlight difficult; however, many steps can be taken to decrease the amount of unnecessary irradiance. The approach that is simplest and least compromising to lifestyle is the habitual use of a broad-spectrum, high-SPF topical sunscreen on all potentially exposed areas. Physical sunblocks, such as zinc oxide, are available in colors and skin tones to be more cosmetically appealing. Other opaque sunscreens, such as titanium dioxide, are often combined with chemical ultraviolet-absorbing agents. Care in selecting clothing will also provide a practical means of photoprotection. Parents should be told, as a rule of thumb, to choose tightly woven, darker colored fabrics (such as denim). Hats or baseball caps offer some shading of the face, and in some cases gloves may need to be worn. A few companies manufacture lines of photoprotective clothing especially for children (Sun Precautions, Inc., 2815 Wetmore Avenue, Everett, WA 98201; 1-800-882-7860). In patients with ocular photosensitivity, ultraviolet-protective wraparound sunglasses should be worn.[59]

Some photosensitivity diseases respond to treatment with oral sunscreens. Beta-carotene

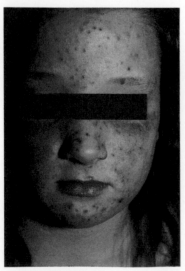

Fig. 10. Papules and excoriations on the face of a girl with polymorphous light eruption.

absorbs only visible light in the 360 to 500 nm range, which can be of benefit in certain porphyrias.[60] This provitamin relies on its ability to reduce oxygen radicals generated by photoexcited porphyrins, not ultraviolet absorption, for its effect.[61] Antimalarial agents may increase skin pigmentation but do not protect against sunburn. Omega-3 polyunsaturated fatty acids have been reported to reduce the sunburn response, possibly by reducing prostaglandin E2 levels.[62]

At home, windows can be covered with Lexan film to reduce ultraviolet transmission. Indoor lighting is a potential source of ultraviolet radiation that can be lessened with the use of shades and special bulb filters. Screens that affix with suction cups are available for use on the rear side windows of a car. Patients should try to avoid peak sunlight hours; to the extreme, some families of children affected with XP have rearranged their normal daytime activities to the night hours.

## SUMMARY

Diagnosis and management of these often rare photodermatoses is challenging. However, with careful history, occasional phototesting, and thoughtful physical examination, a diagnosis can be made. Clinical suspicion is important and stems from knowledge of these diseases and their presentations and recognition that exposure can be substantially separated temporally and often with other systemic signs and symptoms. Knowledge of these diseases is important to avoid much suffering, skin damage, cancer, and mortality.

## REFERENCES

1. Epstein JH. Phototoxicity and photoallergy in man. J Am Acad Dermatol 1983;8:141–7.
2. Gaspari AA. Mechanisms of resolution of allergic contact dermatitis. Am J Contact Dermat 1996;7:212–9.
3. Cavallo J, DeLeo VA. Sunburn. Dermatol Clin 1986; 4:181.
4. Epstein JH. Phototoxicity and photoallergy. Semin Cutan Med Surg 1999;18:274–84.
5. Levine GM, Harber LC. The effect of humidity on the phototoxic response to 8-methoxypsoralen in guinea pigs. Acta Derm Venereol 1969;49:82.
6. Owens DW, Knox JM. Influence of heat, wind, and humidity on ultraviolet radiation injury. Natl Cancer Inst Monogr 1978;(50):161.
7. AAD website on sunscreens. Available at: http://www.aad.org/media-resources/stats-and-facts/prevention-and-care/sunscreens. Accessed November 8, 2011.
8. Moloney FJ, Collins S, Murphy GM. Sunscreens: safety, efficacy and appropriate use. Am J Clin Dermatol 2002;3:185–91.
9. Available at: http://www.fda.gov/Drugs/Development ApprovalProcess/DevelopmentResources/Over-the-CounterOTCDrugs/StatusofOTCRulemakings/ucm072134.htm. Accessed November 8, 2011.
10. Hasei K, Ichihashi M. Solar urticaria. Determinations of action and inhibition spectra. Arch Dermatol 1982; 118:346.
11. Botto NC, Warshaw EM. Solar urticaria. J Am Acad Dermatol 2008;59:909–20.
12. Horio T, Yoshioka A, Okamoto H. Production and inhibition of solar urticaria by visible light exposure. J Am Acad Dermatol 1984;11:1094–9.
13. Hawk JL, Eady RA, Challoner AV, et al. Elevated blood histamine levels and mast cell degranulation in solar urticaria. Br J Clin Pharmacol 1980;9:183.
14. Epstein JH, Vandenberg JJ, Wright WL. Solar urticaria. Arch Dermatol 1963;88:135.
15. Diffey BL, Farr PM. Treatment of solar urticaria with terfenadine. Photodermatol 1988;5:25.
16. Harber LC, Bickers DB. Photosensitivity diseases, principles of diagnosis and treatment. Toronto: BC Decker; 1988.
17. Cohen PR, DeLeo VA. Disorders of porphyrin metabolism genetic disorders of the skin. Chicago: Mosby-Year Book; 1990.
18. Poh-Fitzpatrick MB. The erythropoietic porphyrias. Dermatol Clin 1986;4:291.
19. Corey TJ, DeLeo VA, Christianson H, et al. Variegate porphyria. Clinical and laboratory features. J Am Acad Dermatol 1980;2:36–43.
20. Mathews-Roth MM, Pathak MA, Fitzpatrick TB, et al. Beta-carotene as a photoprotective agent in erythropoietic protoporphyria. N Engl J Med 1970;282:1231–4.
21. Sand Petersen C, Thomsen K. High-dose hydroxychloroquine treatment of porphyria cutane tarda. J Am Acad Dermatol 1992;26:614–9.
22. Harms J, Lautenschlager S, Minder CE, et al. An alphamelanocyte-stimulating hormone analogue in erythropoietic protoporphyria. N Engl J Med 2009; 360(3):306–7.
23. Paller AS, Eramo LR, Farrell EE, et al. Purpuric phototherapy-induced eruption in transfused neonates: relation to transient porphyrinemia. Pediatrics 1997;100:360–4.
24. King RA, Summers CG. Albinism. Dermatol Clin 1988;6:217.
25. Hoppenjans WB, Fu JJ, Nordlund JJ. Albinism. In: Demis DJ, editor. Clinical dermatology. 24th edition. Philadelphia: Lippincott-Raven; 1997. p. 1. Unit. 11–26.
26. Burger DS, London R. Soft opaque contact lenses in binocular vision problems. J Am Optom Assoc 1993; 64:176.
27. Witkop CJ, Nuñez BM, Rao GH, et al. Albinism and Hermansky-Pudlak syndrome in Puerto Rico. Bol Asoc Med P R 1990;82:333.
28. Gahl WA, Brantly M, Kaiser-Kupfer MI, et al. Genetic defects and clinical characteristics of

patients with a form of oculocutaneous albinism (Hermansky–Pudlak syndrome). N Engl J Med 1998;338:1258–65.

29. Kraemer KH, Lee MM, Scotto J. Xeroderma pigmentosum: cutaneous, ocular, and neurologic abnormalities in 830 published cases. Arch Dermatol 1987; 123:241.

30. Copeland NE, Hanke CW, Michalak JA. The molecular basis of xeroderma pigmentosum. Dermatol Surg 1997;23:447–55.

31. Leal-Khouri S, Hruza GJ, Hruza LL, et al. Management of a young patient with xeroderma pigmentosum. Pediatr Dermatol 1994;11:72–5.

32. Zahid S, Brownell I. Repairing DNA damage in xeroderma pigmentosum: T4N5 lotion and gene therapy. J Drugs Dermatol 2008;7:405.

33. Yarosh D, Klein J, Kibitel J, et al. Enzyme therapy of xeroderma pigmentosum: safety and efficacy testing of T4N5 liposome lotion containing a prokaryotic DNA repair enzyme. Photodermatol Photoimmunol Photomed 1996;12:122–30.

34. Pesce K, Rothe MJ. The premature aging syndromes. Clin Dermatol 1996;14:161–70.

35. Mays SR, Hebert AA. Bloom's syndrome. In: Demis DJ, editor. Clinical dermatology. 24th edition. Philadelphia: Lippincott-Raven; 1997. p. 3. Unit. 7–59.

36. LaRocque JR, Stark JM, Oh J, et al. Interhomolog recombination and loss of heterozygosity in wild-type and Bloom syndrome helicase (BLM)-deficient mammalian cells. Proc Natl Acad Sci U S A 2011; 108:11971.

37. Weemaes CM, Bakkeren JA, Haraldsson A, et al. Immunological studies in Bloom's syndrome. A follow-up report. Ann Genet 1991;34(3–4):201–5.

38. German JC. Bloom's syndrome. Dermatol Clin 1995; 13:7–18.

39. German J. Bloom syndrome: a mendelian prototype of somatic mutational disease. Medicine (Baltimore) 1993;72:393–406.

40. Soffer D, Grotsky HW, Rapin I, et al. Cockayne syndrome: unusual neuropathological findings and review of the literature. Ann Neurol 1979;6:340–8.

41. Goldsmith LA. Genetic skin diseases with altered aging. Arch Dermatol 1997;133:1293.

42. Garzon MC, DeLeo VA. Photosensitivity in the pediatric patient. Curr Opin Pediatr 1997;9:377.

43. Xu X, Liu Y. Dual DNA unwinding activities of the Rothmund–Thomson syndrome protein, RECQ4. EMBO J 2009;28:568–77.

44. Drouin CA, Mongrain E, Sasseville D, et al. Rothmund-Thomson syndrome with osteosarcoma. J Am Acad Dermatol 1993;28:301–5.

45. Lanska DJ. Stages in the recognition of epidemic pellagra in the United States: 1865-1960. Neurology 1996;47:829–34.

46. Dumitrescu C, Lichiardopol R. Particular features of clinical pellagra. Rom J Intern Med 1994;32:165.

47. Galadari E, Hadi S, Sabarinathan K. Hartnup disease. Int J Dermatol 1993;32:904.

48. Jonas AJ, Butler IJ. Circumvention of defective neutral amino acid transport in Hartnup disease using tryptophan ethyl ester. J Clin Invest 1989;84:200.

49. Willis I. Polymorphous light eruptions. In: Demis DJ, editor. Clinical dermatology. 24th edition. Philadelphia: Lippincott-Raven; 1997. Unit 19–3.

50. Van Praag MC, Boom BW, Vermeer BJ. Diagnosis and treatment of polymorphous light eruption. Int J Dermatol 1994;33:233–9.

51. Lane PR, Hogan DJ, Martel MJ, et al. Actinic prurigo: clinical features and prognosis. J Am Acad Dermatol 1992;26:683–92.

52. Birt AR, Hogg GR. The actinic cheilitis of hereditary polymorphic light eruption. Arch Dermatol 1979;115: 699.

53. Hojyo-Tomoka T, Vega-Memije E, Granados J, et al. Actinic prurigo: an update. Int J Dermatol 1995;34:380–4.

54. Lane PR, Moreland AA, Hogan DJ. Treatment of actinic prurigo with intermittent short-course topical 0.05% clobetasol 17-propionate: a preliminary report. Arch Dermatol 1990;126:1211.

55. Londoño F. Thalidomide in the treatment of actinic prurigo. Int J Dermatol 1973;12:326–8.

56. Saul A, Flores O, Novales J. Polymorphous light eruption: treatment with thalidomide. Australas J Dermatol 1976;17:17–21.

57. Halasz CL, Leach EE, Walther RR, et al. Hydroa vacciniforme: induction of lesions with ultraviolet A. J Am Acad Dermatol 1983;8:171–6.

58. McGrae JD, Perry HO. Hydroa vacciniforme. Arch Dermatol 1963;87:618.

59. American Academy of ophthalmology. Sunglasses. Available at: http://www.aao.org/eyecare/tmp/ Sunglasses.cfm. Accessed November 11, 2012.

60. Pathak MA, Fitzpatrick TB, Greiter F, et al. Preventive treatment of sunburn, dermatoheliosis, and skin cancer with sun-protective agents. Dermatology in General Medicine 1993;4:1689–717.

61. Hebert AA. Photoprotection in children. Adv Dermatol 1993;8:309.

62. Rhodes LE, Durham BH, Fraser WD, et al. Dietary fish oil reduces basal and ultraviolet B-generated PGE2 levels in skin and increases the threshold to provocation of polymorphic light eruption. J Invest Dermatol 1995;105:532–5.

# Spitz Nevi
## A Bridge Between Dermoscopic Morphology and Histopathology

Miryam Kerner, MD[a,1], Natalia Jaimes, MD[b,1],
Alon Scope, MD[c], Ashfaq A. Marghoob, MD[a,*]

## KEYWORDS

- Pediatric • Dermoscopy • Spitz nevi

## KEY POINTS

- Spitz nevi often display at least 1 of the dermoscopic melanoma-specific structures.
- The most common melanoma-specific structures seen in Spitz nevi are atypical network, negative network, crystalline structures, atypical dots and globules, streaks, blue-white veil overlying a palpable portion of the lesion, atypical blotch, and atypical vascular structures.
- The dermoscopic patterns most commonly associated with Spitz nevi are starburst, negative network, and thickened dark reticular, globular, and homogeneous patterns.
- Spitz nevi may evolve from one pattern to another during longitudinal monitoring. For example, some globular Spitz nevi may evolve into a starburst pattern and then into a homogeneous pattern before entering the phase of senescence or involution.
- Spitz nevi manifesting a multicomponent pattern cannot be differentiated from melanoma based solely on the clinical and dermoscopic morphology of the lesion.

## INTRODUCTION

Few benign melanocytic lesions encountered in clinical practice elicit the level of angst, confusion, and controversy as that generated by lesions within the so-called spectrum of Spitz nevi. Sophie Spitz first described these benign "epithelioid and spindle cell" melanocytic neoplasms in her seminal publication in 1948.[1] She observed that these lesions were most prevalent in childhood, and despite displaying histopathologic features that overlapped with melanoma, they usually exhibited a biological behavior commonly associated with benign neoplasms. Based on the aforementioned characteristics, these tumors were termed "benign juvenile melanomas." Although the term "benign juvenile melanoma" is an oxymoron, it does somehow convey the conundrum faced by physicians when confronted by such lesions: Is the neoplasm truly benign? Could it represent a malignancy masquerading as a benign tumor? Is it a tumor with a higher propensity for developing

Conflict of Interest: None.

Some of the wording and text may be similar to an article on Spitz nevi that was edited by Dr Marghoob for the second edition of the *Atlas of Dermoscopy* and a review article on dermoscopy written by the authors and submitted to the *Journal of Pediatric Dermatology*. Some of the images have been or will be published but Dr Marghoob retains the copyright on the images.

[a] Department of Dermatology, Memorial Sloan-Kettering Cancer Center, New York, NY, USA; [b] Dermatology Service, Universidad Pontificia Bolivariana; Aurora Skin Cancer Center, Medellín, Colombia, USA; [c] Department of Dermatology, Sheba Medical Center and Sackler School of Medicine, Tel Aviv University, Tel Aviv, Israel
[1] These authors contributed equally to this work.
* Corresponding author. Memorial Sloan-Kettering Cancer Center, 800 Veterans Memorial Highway, 2nd Floor, Hauppauge, NY 11788.
E-mail address: marghooa@mskcc.org

Dermatol Clin 31 (2013) 327–335
http://dx.doi.org/10.1016/j.det.2012.12.009
0733-8635/13/$ – see front matter © 2013 Elsevier Inc. All rights reserved.

melanoma? The advent of in vivo diagnostic instruments such as dermoscopy and confocal microscopy, as well as molecular diagnostic techniques have helped, to some extent, ease clinicians' anxieties for a subset of Spitz nevi. However, for most "Spitzoid" lesions, the aforementioned questions remain unanswered and thus they are almost as disconcerting today as they were more than 6 decades ago. To complicate matters, the introduction of sentinel lymph node biopsies has even perpetuated the paradoxic notion that Spitz nevi somehow straddle 2 worlds: the benign and the malignant. This notion is based on observations that the regional sentinel lymph node in patients with Spitz nevi not uncommonly display aggregates of melanocytes with cytologic features akin to those seen in Spitz nevi. It is presently speculated that these aggregates of melanocytes in regional nodes reflect a process of passive drainage of dermal melanocytes via the lymphatics. The term "benign metastasis" sometimes used to describe this phenomenon is yet another oxymoron, and its use should be discouraged based on current understanding of biology of benign versus malignant neoplasms.

What is recurrently underscored in studies of Spitz nevi is that their clinical and histopathologic morphology often overlaps with melanoma. While Spitz nevi are benign neoplasms that do not result in widespread metastasis and death, their biology and natural history remain to be fully

elucidated. Their etiology, rate of growth, and factors inducing senescence and involution remain active areas of research. Evidence is slowly accumulating that a subset of Spitz nevi, specifically those with a starburst pattern, has a predictable pattern of growth (**Figs. 1** and **2**).[2,3] In addition, it has been documented that Spitz nevi can involute.[4] That said, it is clear that aggressive biological behavior of a subset of Spitzoid lesions, particularly those displaying rapid growth and/or lymph node involvement, does occur and can cause alarm. Based on the information currently available on Spitz nevi, management decisions often seem to be propelled by the low pretest probability of developing melanoma in children compared with adults. Thus, pediatric dermatologists are often more inclined toward conservative monitoring of Spitz nevi in children, whereas dermatologists dealing with Spitz nevi in adults often prefer to biopsy these lesions.

## DERMOSCOPIC MORPHOLOGY OF SPITZ NEVI

Dermoscopy-based studies have revealed a set of morphologic features that can help clinicians identify Spitz nevi. In addition, dermoscopy has been used to longitudinally monitor Spitz nevi, providing a unique opportunity to observe the biological nature of these lesions. Knowledge of the dermoscopic structures and patterns commonly encountered in Spitz nevi, together with understanding of their growth dynamics, can inform the decision

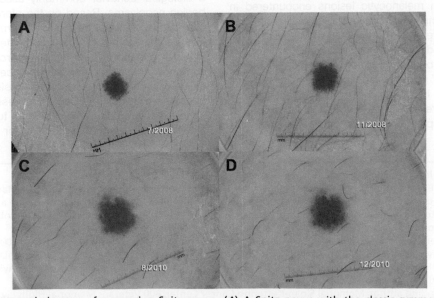

**Fig. 1.** Dermoscopic images of a growing Spitz nevus. (*A*) A Spitz nevus with the classic symmetric starburst pattern. This pattern indicates that the lesion will enlarge, usually symmetrically, and thus it represents radial growth phase of the Spitz nevus as confirmed by the follow-up image (*B*). Once the lesion enters senescence the streaks are no longer visible and the lesion will stop enlarging, as can be seen in (*C*) and (*D*).

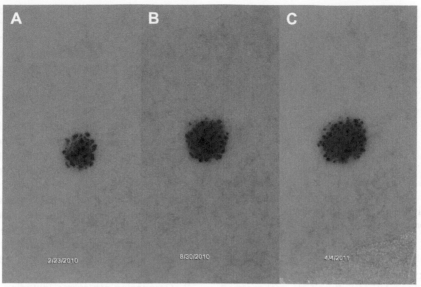

**Fig. 2.** Dermoscopic images of a growing Spitz nevus. (*A*) A Spitz nevus with a globular pattern. As demonstrated in the follow-up images (*B*) and (*C*), the globular pattern can evolve into a starburst pattern with peripheral tiered globules.

whether to biopsy or monitor. Clinically Spitz nevi can be pigmented or nonpigmented, and can appear as flat or raised lesions. Dermoscopically Spitz nevi can display melanoma-specific structures; however, unlike melanoma, these structures tend to be distributed in a symmetric and organized manner within the lesion.

## Dermoscopic Structures

1. *Atypical (irregular) network* consists of a network with increased variability in the thickness and color of the lines and/or increased variability in the size of the holes of the network (**Fig. 3**). It can be black or dark brown with

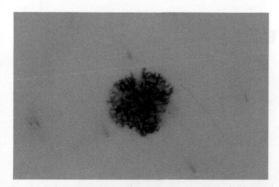

**Fig. 3.** Spitz nevus manifesting an atypical thickened network. This Spitz nevus displays a reticular pattern, characterized by an atypical, black, thickened network. The black color of the network often corresponds with the presence of melanin in the stratum corneum.

a subtle blue-white veil, and it may end abruptly at the periphery of the lesion. The lines of the network correspond to melanin in the keratinocytes and/or melanocytes along the rete ridges, and the holes correspond to the suprapapillary plates. The thickened network often attests to confluent junctional nests of melanocytes. A peculiar type of network with a black reticulated appearance, described as superficial black network, has been observed in approximately 11% of biopsied Spitz nevi. Histopathologically this black network corresponds to focal areas of pigmented parakeratosis.[5]

2. *Negative network*, also known as reticular depigmentation or inverse network, consists of serpiginous hypopigmented interconnecting lines that surround elongated and irregularly shaped curvilinear brown globular structures. The exact histologic correlate of negative network remains to be elucidated, but likely corresponds to bridging of adjacent rete ridges or to large pigmented dermal nevomelanocytic nests in the papillary dermis. Spitz nevi are more likely to harbor a negative network that is symmetrically distributed within the lesion (**Fig. 4**), whereas melanoma is more likely to display an eccentric and/or heterogeneous negative network.

3. *Crystalline structures*, also known as shiny white lines or streaks, consist of short, bright white lines, often oriented orthogonal to each other, which can only be seen with polarized

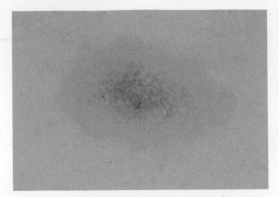

**Fig. 4.** Spitz nevus with negative network pattern. Spitz nevi with this pattern are difficult to differentiate from melanoma based on dermoscopic morphology alone.

dermoscopy (**Fig. 5**). This structure is believed to correspond to an altered stromal matrix.[6] In Spitz nevi, dense collagen and sclerotic stroma, either in the papillary dermis or interspersed among neoplastic cells, is frequently found.[7] In a dermoscopic-histopathologic correlation study, Spitz nevi with crystalline structures possessed a higher degree of fibroplasia than Spitz nevi without crystalline structures.[7]

4. *Atypical dots and globules* consist of dots and/or globules of differing size, shape, and/or color (**Fig. 6**). These dots and globules correlate with nests of melanocytes that vary in size, shape, and depth.[8]

5. *Peripheral streaks* are brown or black radial projections at the periphery of the lesion extending from the tumor toward the surrounding normal skin. Such streaks can present as pseudopods (**Fig. 7**A), which have small knobs at their distal tips, or as radial streaming (see **Fig. 7**B), which lack these knobs. Streaks correspond to confluent junctional nests of melanocytes at the periphery of the lesion and reflect the radial growth phase of the Spitz nevus.[9]

6. *Blue-white veil over raised areas* consists of a confluent blue pigmentation with an overlying white ground-glass haze. The blue-white veil in Spitz nevi often has a homogeneous hue and is located symmetrically within the lesion (**Fig. 8**A), whereas in melanoma the blue-white veil often presents with differing hues and is asymmetrically distributed. On histopathology, the blue-white veil corresponds to aggregates of pigmented melanocytes in the dermis, in combination with compact orthokeratosis overlying the epidermis (see **Fig. 8**C).

7. *Regression structures* including scar-like depigmentation and peppering/granularity, which correlate with fibrosis and melanophages, respectively, are rarely, if ever, seen in Spitz nevi. Mones and Ackerman[10] reported that histopathologically "Spitz nevi never undergo regression in the manner of melanoma, as manifested by destruction of neoplastic melanocytes in the papillary dermis and epidermis." Similarly, dermoscopic and confocal microscopic studies have reported absence of regression structures in Spitz nevi.[11]

8. *Atypical vessels* consisting of dotted and/or serpentine vessels are common in Spitz nevi, especially in the nonpigmented variant (**Fig. 9**).[12,13]

9. *Blotch* is defined as a dark-brown to black, usually homogeneous area of pigment that obscures one's ability to see underlying

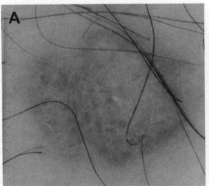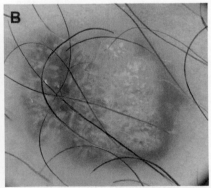

**Fig. 5.** Rapidly growing nodule on the leg of a young adult. This lesion proved to be a Spitz nevus by histopathology. Image (*A*) is acquired using nonpolarized light and (*B*) with polarized dermoscopy. As shown in the images, crystalline structures can only be visualized with polarized dermoscopy (*B*). Biopsy remains the only way to diagnose such clinically dynamic and morphologically atypical Spitz tumors.

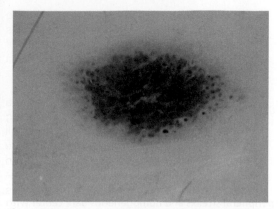

Fig. 6. Spitz nevus displaying a globular pattern with globules of varying size, shape, and color. The blue-white veil present in the center of this lesion is a common finding in Spitz nevi. The blue color is due to the presence of melanin in the deep dermis.

dermoscopic structures. Blotch is due to dense melanin pigmentation at the stratum corneum and/or epidermis. Although in Spitz nevi blotches tend to be symmetrically distributed (see **Fig. 8A**), in the atypical variant they can be off-center and can simulate a melanoma (**Fig. 10**).

10. *Peripheral brown structureless areas* consist of light-brown areas without any discernible structures, located at the periphery of the lesion, corresponding to flattening of the dermo-epidermal junction with proliferation of single melanocytes with pagetoid spread.[8,14] Similar to regression structures, these peripheral structureless areas are rarely seen in Spitz nevi.

Histopathologically, Spitz nevi are junctional or compound nevi revealing a symmetric silhouette with relatively dense cellularity. The junctional nests of Spitz nevi are often large with vertical orientation or a confluence of adjacent nests resulting in irregularly shaped masses (see **Fig. 8C**). These findings can be correlated with the atypical globules and/or the negative network seen under dermoscopy. The pigmented spindle cell nevi, also known as Reed nevi, reveal melanocytes that are usually arranged in large nests and are characteristically positioned closely together, often fusing to form large and irregularly shaped aggregates along the dermo-epidermal junction.[8] This confluence of junctional nests may correlate with dermoscopically identified negative network and atypical globules.

## Dermoscopic Patterns

Considering the distribution of dermoscopic structures within the lesion, recognizable patterns manifested in Spitz nevi have emerged. Contrary to melanoma, dermoscopic patterns in Spitz nevi exhibit symmetry in the distribution of dermoscopic colors and structures.

Colors present in Spitz nevi tend to be distributed symmetrically. Colors can range from whitish-pink and brown to blue or black, depending on the amount and depth of melanin pigment and/or vessels in the lesion.

The dermoscopic patterns observed in Spitz nevi include starburst, globular, reticular, negative network, homogeneous, and atypical patterns. The starburst, globular, and atypical patterns are the most common dermoscopic patterns seen in surgically excised Spitz nevi (**Fig. 11**).[15]

### Starburst pattern

More than 50% of biopsied pigmented Spitz nevi present with the starburst pattern. Under

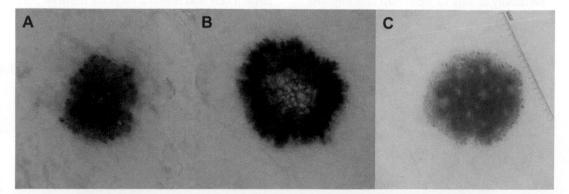

Fig. 7. The starburst pattern in a Spitz nevus can present with 1 of 3 morphologies. (*A*) Spitz nevus with starburst pattern composed of pseudopods. (*B*) Spitz nevus with starburst pattern composed of radial streaming. This lesion also has central dark homogeneous pigmentation with crystalline structures and a blue-white veil. (*C*) Spitz nevus with starburst pattern composed of peripheral tiered globules. ([*B*] *Courtesy of* Dr Adam Korzenko MD, Stony Brook, NY, USA.)

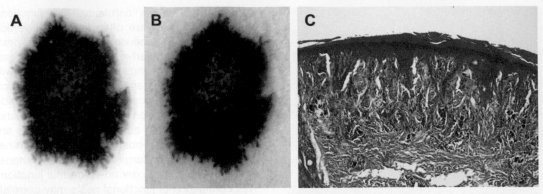

Fig. 8. (*A*) Spitz nevus with starburst pattern composed of peripheral streaks and homogeneous dark center with blue-white veil, which is more conspicuous under nonpolarized dermoscopy. (*B*) The same Spitz nevus under polarized dermoscopy, which permits the visualization of crystalline structures in the center. (*C*) Histopathology of this lesion reveals compact orthokeratosis in the overlying epidermis and melanin in the dermis, both of which are responsible for the blue-white veil seen under nonpolarized dermoscopy (*A*).

dermoscopy, the starburst pattern consists of dark homogeneous pigmentation with peripheral streaks around the entire perimeter of the lesion, arranged in a symmetric fashion. The starburst pattern is named as such because it conjures up an image, in our mind, of an exploding star (see **Figs. 1**A, B, **7**, **8**A, B, and **11**).

Variants of the starburst pattern:

1. *Starburst pattern composed of streaks.* This pattern can be formed by pseudopods (see **Fig. 7**A) or radial streaming (see **Fig. 7**B). The pigmented center of Spitz nevi with a starburst pattern composed of streaks is usually blue-gray or brown-black in color, and is often associated with a blue-white veil (see **Figs. 7**B and 8A). It is not uncommon to visualize crystalline structures within the starburst pattern (see **Fig. 8**B). The starburst pattern has a diagnostic sensitivity of 96% for Spitz nevi (see **Fig. 7**B).[16]

2. *Starburst pattern composed of multiple rows of peripheral globules.* This pattern consists of tiered globules at the periphery of the lesion (see **Fig. 7**C). Though reminiscent of the pattern of peripheral globules seen in growing Clark nevi, the pattern in Spitz nevi consists of several rows of globules, as opposed to that in Clark nevi, which tend to exhibit a single row of peripheral globules.

### Globular pattern

The globular pattern in Spitz nevi consists of globules of varying size, shape, and/or color (see **Figs. 6** and **11**). Colors include brown, black, and/or blue-gray. These globules tend to be distributed throughout the lesion, with prominence of central gray-blue pigmentation with a blue-white veil. Approximately 22% of biopsied Spitz nevi manifest a globular pattern.[17] Spitz nevi with a globular pattern can also reveal a negative network.

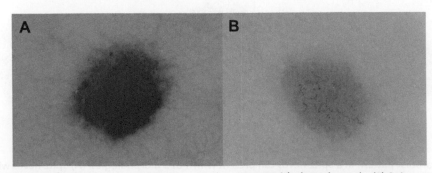

Fig. 9. (*A*) Spitz nevus displaying a homogeneous vascular pattern with dotted vessels. (*B*) Spitz nevus displaying atypical vessels including dotted and serpentine vessels. Spitz nevi manifesting a polymorphic vascular pattern (2 or more vascular morphologies) are impossible to be differentiated from melanoma based on dermoscopic morphology alone.

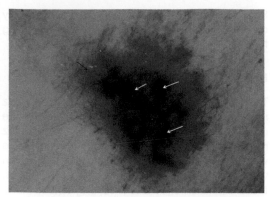

**Fig. 10.** Spitz nevus displaying an asymmetric multi-component pattern, with multiple off-center blotches and focal streaks (*arrows*). Without a biopsy this pattern is difficult to differentiate from melanoma.

## Homogeneous pattern

The homogeneous pattern is characterized by a diffuse homogeneous color throughout the lesion.

Variants of the homogeneous pattern:

1. *Pigmented homogeneous pattern.* This type of Spitz nevus can be darkly pigmented, manifesting a diffuse dark-brown to black-bluish color, and can be accompanied by a reddish hue at the periphery (**Fig. 12**). The homogeneous pigmented pattern has been proposed to represent the senescent phase of some Spitz nevi.[4]

2. *Nonpigmented homogeneous pattern.* This pattern can present as lesions with a homogeneous pink color without any discernible vascular structures, or with a visible vascular pattern (see **Figs. 9** and **11**). This pattern is frequently encountered in classic Spitz nevi seen on the face of children. In homogeneous pink Spitz nevi, it is not uncommon to see dotted vessels under dermoscopy (see **Figs. 9**A and **11**). On occasion a polymorphic vascular pattern consisting of dotted and serpentine vessels can be seen, making it impossible to differentiate it from melanoma without a biopsy (see **Fig. 9**B).[12,13] Pink variant of Spitz nevi is a common pattern seen in children. Unfortunately, melanomas that develop in children also tend to be amelanotic and nodular, making the differentiation between the amelanotic Spitz nevus and amelanotic melanoma impossible based on primary morphology alone.[18] That said, suspected pink Spitzoid lesions in children that have no documented history of change argue against the diagnosis of nodular melanoma.[19]

## Negative network pattern

This pattern consists of a homogeneous and symmetrically arranged negative network (see **Figs. 4** and **11**). Spitz nevi presenting with a negative network pattern are difficult to differentiate from melanoma based on dermoscopic morphology

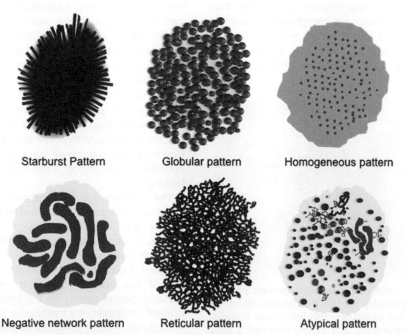

Starburst Pattern        Globular pattern        Homogeneous pattern

Negative network pattern        Reticular pattern        Atypical pattern

**Fig. 11.** Schematics of dermoscopic patterns commonly seen in Spitz nevi.

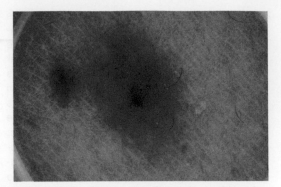

**Fig. 12.** Spitz nevus with homogeneous pattern, manifesting a diffuse brown color in the center accompanied by a reddish hue at the periphery.

alone. However, documented stability of the lesion will speak in favor of the lesion being a Spitz nevus.

### Reticular pattern

The reticular pattern consists of a network that may appear atypical because of the presence of a black, thickened network (see **Figs. 3** and **11**) that can have a black or blue-gray coloration. A specific type of network associated with Spitz nevi has been termed "superficial black network," which is due to the presence of excessive amounts of melanin in the stratum corneum. This black pigment can often be diminished or removed by tape stripping.[5]

### Atypical or multicomponent pattern

The colors and structures within Spitz nevi can be arranged in an asymmetric distribution, thus making the dermoscopic morphology resemble that of melanoma (see **Figs. 10** and **11**; **Fig. 13**). Based on dermoscopic morphology it is impossible to differentiate these asymmetric multicomponent

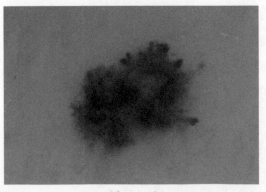

**Fig. 13.** Spitz nevus with a multicomponent pattern, displaying asymmetry in the distribution of colors and dermoscopic structures. This lesion was biopsied to rule out melanoma, and biopsy revealed a Spitz nevus.

Spitz nevi from melanoma. These dermoscopically challenging Spitz nevi often prove to be challenging for pathologists as well.

## DERMOSCOPIC EVOLUTION OF SPITZ NEVI

The various dermoscopic patterns seen in Spitz nevi may represent a cross-sectional view of the different stages of the natural evolution of Spitz nevi. It has been documented that a Spitz nevus with a starburst pattern predicts that the lesion will undergo symmetric radial growth and once these lesions enter senescence, they tend to manifest a homogeneous or reticular pattern (see **Fig. 1**).[2–4,20] In addition, it has been observed that some Spitz nevi can initially manifest a globular pattern, evolving into a symmetric starburst pattern with tiered globules (see **Fig. 2**).[3] Although the long-term longitudinal natural history of Spitz nevi remains largely unknown, evidence is starting to emerge that the final stage in the natural evolution of Spitz nevi is complete involution.[4]

## SUMMARY

Although Spitz nevi remain a clinical conundrum, some inroads have been made in our understanding regarding their dermoscopic morphology and natural evolution. Dermoscopy has allowed us to identify patterns that are highly predictive of a Spitz nevus, as exemplified by the starburst pattern. Based on the low pretest probability of a melanoma arising in a child and the high diagnostic sensitivity of the starburst pattern for a Spitz nevus, some clinicians are opting to monitor these lesions instead of resorting to a biopsy. Digital monitoring has in turn shed light on the natural evolution of the starburst-patterned Spitz nevus. It has been shown that these starburst-type lesions are Spitz nevi in their active radial growth phase and that once they enter senescence they manifest a homogeneous or reticular pattern, with some eventually involuting. However, for the other patterns of Spitz nevi, information regarding their natural evolution is lacking.

The options for management of the classic symmetric starburst Spitz nevi in children remain biopsy and monitoring. In all other Spitzoid lesions, in particular pink lesions with polymorphic vascular pattern, the diagnosis of a melanoma remains a possibility. For adults, most clinicians are of the opinion that Spitz nevi should be excised, based mainly on the knowledge that the pretest probability for melanoma is higher in older individuals. Future longitudinal follow-up of Spitz nevi will likely change our views, and contribute to creating clear guidelines for monitoring versus excision of lesions showing a Spitzoid morphology on dermoscopy in both children and adults.

## ACKNOWLEDGMENTS

The authors thank Dr Adam Korzenko for providing **Fig. 7**B.

## REFERENCES

1. Spitz S. Melanomas of childhood. Am J Pathol 1948; 24:591–609.
2. Argenziano G, Agozzino M, Bonifazi E, et al. Natural evolution of Spitz nevi. Dermatology 2011; 222:256–60.
3. Nino M, Brunetti B, Delfino S, et al. Spitz nevus: follow-up study of 8 cases of childhood starburst type and proposal for management. Dermatology 2009;218:48–51.
4. Argenziano G, Zalaudek I, Ferrara G, et al. Involution: the natural evolution of pigmented Spitz and Reed nevi? Arch Dermatol 2007;143:549–51.
5. Argenziano G, Soyer HP, Ferrara G, et al. Superficial black network: an additional dermoscopic clue for the diagnosis of pigmented spindle and/ or epithelioid cell nevus. Dermatology 2001;203: 333–5.
6. Requena C, Requena L, Kutzner H, et al. Spitz nevus: a clinicopathological study of 349 cases. Am J Dermatopathol 2009;31:107–16.
7. Botella-Estrada R, Requena C, Traves V, et al. Chrysalis and negative pigment network in Spitz nevi. Am J Dermatopathol 2012;34:188–91.
8. Mooi WJ. Spitz nevus and its histologic simulators. Adv Anat Pathol 2002;9:209–21.
9. Scope A, Gill M, Benveuto-Andrade C, et al. Correlation of dermoscopy with in vivo reflectance confocal microscopy of streaks in melanocytic lesions. Arch Dermatol 2007;143:727–34.
10. Mones JM, Ackerman AB. "Atypical" Spitz's nevus, "malignant" Spitz's nevus, and "metastasizing" Spitz's nevus: a critique in historical perspective of three concepts flawed fatally. Am J Dermatopathol 2004;26:310–33.
11. Pellacani G, Longo C, Malvehy J, et al. In vivo confocal microscopic and histopathologic correlations of dermoscopic features in 202 melanocytic lesions. Arch Dermatol 2008;144:1597–608.
12. Argenziano G, Zalaudek I, Corona R, et al. Vascular structures in skin tumors: a dermoscopy study. Arch Dermatol 2004;140:1485–9.
13. Kilinc Karaarslan I, Ozdemir F, Akalin T, et al. Eruptive disseminated Spitz naevi: dermatoscopic features. Clin Exp Dermatol 2009;34:e807–10.
14. Busam KJ, Barnhill RL. Pagetoid Spitz nevus. Intraepidermal Spitz tumor with prominent pagetoid spread. Am J Surg Pathol 1995;19:1061–7.
15. Ferrara G, Argenziano G, Soyer HP, et al. The spectrum of Spitz nevi: a clinicopathologic study of 83 cases. Arch Dermatol 2005;141:1381–7.
16. Yadav S, Vossaert KA, Kopf AW, et al. Histopathologic correlates of structures seen on dermoscopy (epiluminescence microscopy). Am J Dermatopathol 1993;15:297–305.
17. Argenziano G, Scalvenzi M, Staibano S, et al. Dermatoscopic pitfalls in differentiating pigmented Spitz naevi from cutaneous melanomas. Br J Dermatol 1999;141:788–93.
18. Gupta D, FI, Cordoro K, et al. Evidence for modification of the ABCDE criteria for pediatric melanoma. J Am Acad Dermatol 2012;66:AB1 AAD poster abstract 5407.
19. Liu W, Dowling JP, Murray WK, et al. Rate of growth in melanomas: characteristics and associations of rapidly growing melanomas. Arch Dermatol 2006; 142:1551–8.
20. Pizzichetta MA, Argenziano G, Grandi G, et al. Morphologic changes of a pigmented Spitz nevus assessed by dermoscopy. J Am Acad Dermatol 2002;47:137–9.

# Procedural Pediatric Dermatology

Brandie J. Metz, MD

## KEYWORDS

• Dermatology • Pediatric • Dermatologic procedures • Infants • Children • Anesthesia

## KEY POINTS

- Performing dermatologic procedures in infants and children presents multiple challenges and requires knowledge of age-specific development.
- Timing of surgical intervention is a key aspect in optimizing surgical outcome.
- Knowledge of the risks and benefits of general anesthesia can help the physician to determine when a procedure is best performed under general anesthesia.
- Staged excision and purse string excision may result in smaller, more acceptable scars for certain large congenital nevi or hemangiomas.
- A few special techniques can help the dermatologist create a more pleasant experience for pediatric patients and their families.

Performing dermatologic procedures in infants and children presents multiple challenges. Children are not simply smaller versions of adults. Each age has its own unique set of challenges. Young children are unable to understand the necessity of a procedure and may be unwilling to cooperate. As children get older, they become more difficult to restrain during a procedure. For these reasons, procedures that are simple to perform in adults can be extremely challenging to perform in children.

An understanding of pediatric developmental milestones is essential to providing optimal dermatologic care of the pediatric patient. This article combines the author's experiences with data from the literature to provide guidance for performing dermatologic procedures in children. Additionally, the surgical approach to a few specific types of birthmarks is addressed.

## GENERAL APPROACH TO PEDIATRIC PATIENTS

Many factors influence pain, including age, fear and anxiety, cognitive development, and past experiences. Inadequate pain control has significant negative implications for children, including long-term consequences regarding their reactions to later painful events and acceptance of subsequent health care interventions. Therefore, an approach to pediatric patients that makes them as comfortable as possible and minimizes pain is crucial.

A few easy techniques can help to make children more comfortable both before and during dermatologic procedures:

- Sit at or below the level of the child; this is less intimidating than having a physician standing or sitting above the child.
- Include the child in the conversation rather than addressing only the parents. The child will feel more respected and is more likely to believe and trust what is being said.
- Explain the procedure thoroughly in an unthreatening manner. It is important to use terms that describe the impending events while avoiding words that conjure painful images, such as "shot," "needle," or "prick." Try to describe what the procedure will feel like. For instance, with injections, a pinch will be felt followed by warmth. Once this is over, nothing should be felt. There should be no surprises.

Funding Sources: None.
Conflict of Interest: None.
Pediatric Dermatology of Orange County, 3500 Barranca Parkway, Suite 230, Irvine, CA 92606, USA
E-mail address: bmetz@pedsdermoc.com

Dermatol Clin 31 (2013) 337–346
http://dx.doi.org/10.1016/j.det.2012.12.011

derm.theclinics.com

- Most importantly, do not lie. If a child is told that a procedure will not hurt and it does, trust of that physician (and perhaps other physicians) will be compromised in the future.

The postoperative approach can also help improve the experience for the patient and parents. Praise the child, no matter how poorly the procedure went. Rewards, such as stickers and lollipops, facilitate a selective memory; the child focuses on the reward rather than the painful procedure. Physicians and parents should be reassured that nearly all children bounce back once they realize that the procedure is over.

## PARENTAL PRESENCE

Conflicting views and practices exist regarding whether parents should be present at the time of their child's medical procedure. Although this has not been studied specifically in the setting of pediatric dermatology procedures, it has been reviewed in the setting of childhood immunizations, venipuncture, induction of anesthesia, lumbar puncture, and bone marrow aspiration. The results of a systematic review revealed no evidence of increased technical complications when a parent was present. Although parental presence may not have a clear, direct influence on child distress and behavioral outcomes, there are potential advantages to parental presence (**Box 1**). Most importantly, reported parental satisfaction was higher when they were present during the procedure.[1]

The practice of the author is usually to have the parents present unless they specifically ask not to be. It can be reassuring to the patient to have a parent sitting at the head of the table, providing a hand to hold. When a parent is present, it is important to ensure that they are seated in a chair with a back. A parent who is standing or who is seated on a rolling stool is more likely to faint

### Box 1
### Disadvantages and advantages to parental presence during pediatric dermatologic procedures

*Disadvantages*

- Increased parental anxiety
- Increased physician/staff anxiety

*Advantages*

- Elimination of separation anxiety (which begins to develop around 9 months of age)
- Decreased anxiety in child
- Increased parental satisfaction

and require the physician's attention to be directed away from the patient.

## POSITIONING THE PATIENT

Trays should be covered both before and after a procedure, hiding from the patient's view the intimidating instruments (before a procedure) and blood-soaked gauze after a procedure. The surgical field should be strategically draped so that the child does not see the surgical field. This also allows the physician to inject the local anesthetic without the patient seeing the needle.

Toddlers are often particularly anxious about dermatologic procedures, and they are more difficult to restrain than younger infants because of their size and strength. A "toddler wrap" or swaddle is an effective way to restrain a child and maintain a sterile field (**Fig. 1**). To accomplish this, a blanket or sheet should be placed under the child and then wrapped around both arms, with the end tucked under the far arm. Then the other side should be wrapped back around the child and the end secured underneath the child. This secure wrap can be used for skin biopsies and small excisions on the midsection of the body, arms, and legs by leaving the affected body part unwrapped.[2] The nurse or medical assistant can then hold the affected body part so that the patient is stable during the procedure. As a general rule, the parents should never be enlisted to hold the child. That way, the parent remains the "rescuer" in the child's eyes.

## DISTRACTION TECHNIQUES

A portable DVD player is an inexpensive and simple way to provide distraction during procedures. If children begin watching a movie before anesthetic injection, they tend to be less nervous about the impending procedure. This distraction is also useful during the procedure, lengthening the time that children are able, or willing, to sit still.

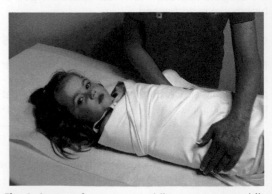

**Fig. 1.** Image of a proper "toddler wrap" or swaddle.

A tablet computer is slightly more expensive, but can be loaded with movies, puzzles, games, TV shows, and cartoons. In conjunction with a subscription to a streaming video service, this can provide endless options for patients of all ages as a method of distraction during dermatologic procedures.[3]

## INJECTION TECHNIQUES

The simple insertion of a needle has been shown to be one of the most frightening and distressing medical procedures for children. In a survey of 119 children, 65 thought a "shot" or "needle" represented life's most painful experience.[4] Various techniques can be used to reduce the stress and pain associated with local anesthetic injection (Box 2).[5]

The pain associated with the infiltration of buffered lidocaine has been shown in multiple studies to be less than the pain associated with infiltration of unbuffered lidocaine. The magnitude of the pain decrease associated with buffered lidocaine was larger when the solution contained epinephrine.[6] However, the concentrations of both lidocaine and epinephrine decrease once sodium bicarbonate is added. Both lidocaine and epinephrine maintain greater than 90% concentration 2 weeks after buffering when stored at 0°C to 4°C (32°F–39°F). Proper refrigeration permits batch buffering of lidocaine with epinephrine and storage for up to 2 weeks.[7] Because infiltration of cold lidocaine is more painful, the buffered lidocaine should be warmed by placing the syringe in warm water immediately before injection.

## TOPICAL ANESTHETICS

Administration of topical anesthetics can help minimize the pain and anxiety associated with anesthetic injection and other painful procedures, such as intralesional injections and laser treatments. Many dosage forms exist, providing clinicians with options for various circumstances.

---

Box 2
Techniques to decrease injection-related pain

- Use counterstimulatory methods (pinching an adjacent area).
- Infiltrate the local anesthetic deep.
- Use small (30-gauge) needles.
- Buffer and warm the lidocaine.
  - 1 mL of 8.4% sodium bicarbonate (1 mEq/mL) per 10 mL of 1% lidocaine
- Infiltrate anesthetic slowly.

---

The most commonly used topical anesthetics are those in cream formulations. Eutectic mixture of local anesthetics (EMLA) is a mixture of lidocaine and prilocaine. EMLA is available with a prescription, and should be applied, under occlusion, 1 hour before the procedure.[8] Methemoglobinemia is a well-documented potential complication of prilocaine-containing creams. EMLA should only be applied to small areas, and should be used with caution in children younger than 3 years because of the incomplete maturation of the NADH-methemoglobin reductase sytem.[9]

Liposomal 4% lidocaine (LMX) is available over the counter. The recommended application is 30 minutes before the procedure. Although occlusion is not required for maximum efficacy, LMX is also usually applied under occlusion to avoid a mess. LMX does not contain prilocaine, and therefore has no risk of causing methemoglobinemia.

Several novel delivery systems for topical anesthetics have been introduced in the past few years. The Synera (Nuvo Research, Inc, Ontario, Canada) is a lidocaine and tetracaine patch with a built-in heating element. Applied 30 minutes before a procedure, this patch provides local anesthesia for superficial dermatologic procedures, such as shave biopsies, electrodessication, and injections.[10]

## NONANESTHETIC TECHNIQUES FOR PAIN REDUCTION

Ethyl chloride, although not a local anesthetic, can safely provide cutaneous analgesia in children when it is impractical to wait for a topical anesthetic preparation to take effect. Vapocoolant sprays provide transient skin anesthesia within seconds of application via evaporation-induced skin cooling. They also can be reapplied as needed with no systemic toxicity and no risk of methemoglobinemia. Published clinical trials support their use in children 3 years of age and older.[11]

Oral sucrose solution is currently commonly used in neonatal intensive care units and for circumcisions, and is used by some pediatricians for immunizations. An article in the March/April 2010 issue of Pediatric Dermatology reported the use of an oral sucrose solution for pain relief in infants who were undergoing steroid injections into hemangiomas.[12] This 24% solution of sucrose is administered 2 minutes before the procedure, either through placing it on the anterior tip of the tongue or dipping a pacifier into the solution. The sucrose may work through activation of sites in the brain that decrease pain perception, or it may cause the release of chemicals that cause babies to have less feeling of pain. In addition to hemangioma steroid injections, oral sucrose solution could be used by dermatologists for biopsies and laser treatments in infants younger than 1 year.

## TIMING OF SURGERY

The timing of surgical intervention is a key aspect in optimizing surgical outcome, and is typically a joint decision between the patient's parents and the physician. Parents often ask about a "window of opportunity" in timing a procedure, and whether missing this window could adversely affect outcome. Although no hard and fast rules exist regarding when is the best time to perform surgery, several factors affect the decision. The main factors include anatomic location, the physical activity level of the child, and psychological effects on the patient if the procedure is delayed.

Smaller benign lesions favor waiting until adolescence, when a procedure can be performed with local anesthesia. Lesions that favor excision during infancy include medium or large lesions on the trunk or limbs, a large nevus sebaceus on the scalp, and lesions located in cosmetically sensitive areas.

The following scenarios demonstrate the decision-making process when determining the best timing of surgical intervention in children.

1. A medium or large lesion on the trunk may be easier to excise in an infant, when "baby fat" is still present, than in a more muscular teenager, in whom tension on the wound would be greater and scars more likely to stretch.
2. A large nevus sebaceus can be easily excised during infancy, when the scalp is thinner and has much more "give," than during adolescence, when it might require staged procedures or a flap.
3. Because tension on a wound on the limb of an infant not yet walking would be less than that on the limb of an ambulating toddler, the optimal time to remove lesions requiring excision on the lower extremity is before 10 months of age, before walking begins. If a procedure must be performed in an older toddler, waiting until the walking becomes much more stable is advised.
4. If the family desires removal, consideration should be given to excising a congenital nevus on the face before preschool age. At this age, children become aware of others' comments and their self-esteem may suffer from such comments.

## GENERAL ANESTHESIA

No set rules exist about the age at which procedures can be performed with local anesthesia.

Elective procedures can often be delayed until preadolescent or adolescent years to avoid risks of general anesthesia. However, general anesthesia should be considered when a procedure is necessary but a child is too young to fully cooperate with local anesthesia. General anesthesia is also recommended for cases of vascular malformations requiring multiple laser treatments to avoid exposing the child to repeated painful procedures.

The American Society of Anesthesiologists states that the risk of an anesthetic complication for a healthy child is 1:20,000 to 80,000 or less.[13] Several factors determine the risk of anesthesia in pediatric patients:

- Age: the highest-risk period is the first month of life. Several studies extend this to the first year of life.
- Nature of the procedure: emergency procedures have an approximately a 3-fold increase in risk versus elective procedures.

A 2005 retrospective review of 881 procedures performed on 269 patients by 6 pediatric dermatologic surgeons or laser surgeons at 2 institutions evaluated the risks of general anesthesia specifically for pediatric dermatologic procedures. Approximately 5% of patients experienced nausea or emesis. Otherwise, no serious adverse events occurred.[14] A 2010 study of 681 procedures in 226 patients undergoing pediatric dermatologic surgery reported no anesthesia-related complications.[15]

The following factors likely contribute to the safety of general anesthesia for pediatric dermatologic procedures:

- Short procedure duration
- Elective basis
- Healthy patients
- Anesthesiologists/anesthetists trained in pediatric anesthesia
- Anesthesia administered in children's hospitals

A French survey found an increased morbidity associated with pediatric surgical cases attended by anesthesiologists who cared for fewer than 200 children a year, further suggesting improved outcomes when procedures were performed by pediatric anesthesiologists.[16]

### New Data on Effects of General Anesthesia

Newer data on general anesthesia and the developing brain are causing anesthesiologists and surgeons to reevaluate the effects of general anesthesia on children. The concern arises from animal studies suggesting that anesthetic drugs may cause apoptosis, and that if this occurs during a critical period of brain development, it may correlate with later behavioral disturbances. These data raise concerns that general anesthesia given to infants and young children may induce similar problems.[17]

A recent study exposed newborn rhesus monkeys to ketamine anesthesia for 24 hours. The cognitive function of these animals, compared with controls, was assessed at 7 months of age. It took all of the monkeys some time to learn tasks, for which they received food rewards, but after 3 months the control animals begin to outpace the ketamine-exposed animals. Additionally, the ketamine-exposed animals never caught up with the development of the control monkeys. The authors concluded that these findings are proof that (ketamine) anesthesia exposure at a young age can alter important cognitive functions substantially and permanently.[18]

Other primate studies, in which newborn rhesus monkeys were exposed to ketamine anesthesia, suggest that the duration of anesthesia may contribute to apoptosis. In one study, monkeys exposed to ketamine anesthesia for 3 hours did not have increased levels of neuronal cell death, whereas monkeys exposed to ketamine anesthesia for 9 or 24 hours showed a significant increase in neuronal cell death in the frontal cortex.[19]

The largest study in children is a cohort study of 5357 children: 4764 with no anesthesia exposure and 593 with exposure before age 4 years. Results showed no difference in the incidence of learning disabilities between children who had a single anesthesia exposure early in life and those who had none, but children with 2 or 3 exposures to anesthesia were more likely to have a learning disability. However, these results do not conclusively prove that the anesthesia exposures were the cause of the learning disabilities, because it is highly possible that children who need multiple procedures may have other illnesses that confound the results.[20]

Another study compared identical twins younger than 3 years and classified them as concordant exposed, concordant not exposed, or discordant (one exposed, one not exposed). The incidence of learning disability was not different in the discordant twins.[21]

Several ongoing prospective studies are further evaluating the effects of anesthesia on children. The relevance of animal data to humans remains unknown, but a panel of experts, convened by the US Food and Drug Administration in March 2011, concluded that "at this time, the evidence is not yet conclusive enough to support warning parents of potential risk."[22]

## OPTIMIZING SCARS

Postoperative activity restrictions are challenging to enforce in the pediatric population but are critical to cosmetic outcome. The following are tips to improve healing and optimize the outcome of surgical scars.

- "Oversew": increase the number of dermal sutures, especially if the wound is near a joint or other area of frequent movement.
- Use a few permanent sutures, such as clear polypropylene (Prolene, Ethicon), when placing the deep sutures.
- Running subcuticular sutures can be left in place longer than 2 weeks without the risk of "track marks" from epidermal sutures.
- A running subcuticular Monocryl closure with buried knots can be used in areas of high tension and left in place indefinitely.
- Because postoperative discomfort is minimal, children forget that they underwent a procedure; therefore, bulky, exaggerated dressings can serve as a reminder to restrict activity.
- Occlusive silicone gel bandages, applied at least 12 hours a day, usually at night, for 3 months can help to flatten scars or prevent raised scars.[23]

## SURGICAL MANAGEMENT OF SPECIFIC LESIONS
### Nevus Sebaceus

Nevus sebaceus of Jadassohn is a common benign congenital lesion that occurs primarily on the scalp or face. These lesions present as round or oval, pink to orange, waxy, hairless plaques on the scalp, or linear plaques on the face. Lesions are usually solitary and vary in size from a few millimeters to several centimeters. Histologically, a nevus sebaceus consists of sebaceous glands, ectopic apocrine glands, and immature hair structures. Lesions tend to grow proportionally with patients. At puberty, they commonly become thicker and more verrucous as a result of hormonal stimulation of the sebaceous glands within them.

Surgical excision has traditionally been recommended out of concern for the development of secondary malignant neoplasms within these lesions. However, recent literature has shown that the actual rate of basal cell carcinoma (BCC) within nevus sebaceus is actually low, approximately 0.8%. This decreased rate of BCC is likely the result of better knowledge of the histology of adnexal

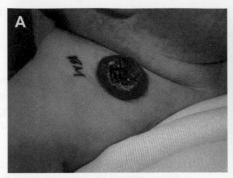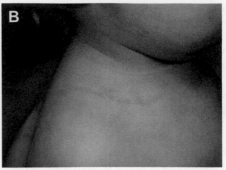

**Fig. 2.** (*A*) This hemangioma was likely to have redundant skin after involution and a scar from the ulceration. Because eventual surgical revision was inevitable, the decision was made to excise this hemangioma. (*B*) The resulting scar is shown 8 months after excision and primary closure.

tumors, and perhaps because of more frequent excision for cosmetic reasons.[24] This low risk of malignant transformation is thought to exist primarily later in adulthood, although a BCC arising within a nevus sebaceus in a 10-year-old boy was recently reported.[25] Benign tumors, such as syringocystadenoma papilliferum and trichoblastoma, are more common, ultimately occurring in 10% to 15% of lesions.

Nevus sebaceus do not always have to be excised, but excision should be discussed and considered in infancy if the lesion is large and cosmetically disfiguring, it develops suspicious tumors within the nevus, or is symptomatic.

Most teenagers will ultimately prefer a scar on the scalp than a bumpy raised birthmark. This fact, along with the small risk of tumor development,

justifies removal when desired by the patient or family. The best approach for a small nevus sebaceus is likely surgical excision in preadolescence under local anesthesia. Some large, cosmetically disfiguring lesions may be excised under general anesthesia in infancy or the toddler years.

## SURGICAL MANAGEMENT OF HEMANGIOMAS
### When to Consider Excision of Hemangiomas

Hemangiomas of infancy, because they are benign lesions that spontaneously involute, rarely require surgical intervention. In a retrospective analysis of hemangiomas, only approximately 3% of hemangiomas were managed with surgical excision.[26] When contemplating excision of a hemangioma, it is helpful to consider whether resection is inevitable. The most common indication for early surgical intervention would likely be a pedunculated hemangioma located on a cosmetically sensitive area, such as the face, which is predicted to leave fibrofatty tissue requiring eventual surgical

**Fig. 3.** In a purse-string closure, the edge of the circular wound is drawn together by a single running suture. Gathering the suture apposes the wound margin.

> **Box 3**
> Technique for purse-string excision of a hemangioma
>
> - Only the skin that is unalterably changed by the hemangioma is removed.
> - The edge of the circular wound is drawn together by a single running suture (see **Fig. 3**).
> - The suture is gathered to appose the wound margin.
> - If a small opening remains, a gauze wick, Gelfoam, or 1 to 2 simple interrupted sutures should be placed in the direction of relaxed skin tension lines.

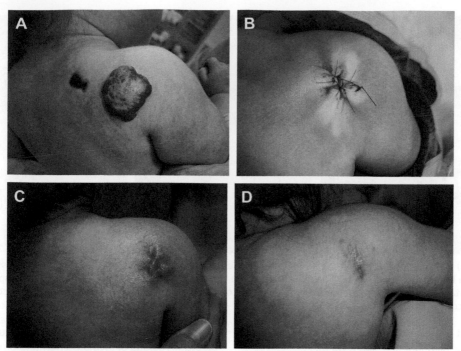

**Fig. 4.** (*A*) Hemangioma shown before excision. (*B*) Patient immediately postoperatively, with a purse-string closure and a few simple interrupted sutures to approximate the epidermis. (*C*) Patient at suture removal 2 weeks later. Parents should be advised that this scar will flatten and improve with time. (*D*) Patient at 3 months postoperatively. Her parents were satisfied with this scar and decided not to pursue a second procedure to linearize the scar.

excision. In this scenario, early surgical excision is likely to result in the same scar as excision after involution, thus sparing a child the psychosocial impact of having a disfiguring hemangioma. Other reasons include ulceration projected to induce a scar greater than a surgical scar (**Fig. 2**), severe refractory pain and discomfort from ulceration, or an easily resectable lesion failing to respond to medical therapy.

## Purse-String Excision of Hemangiomas

Hemangiomas can be excised in an elliptical fashion and closed with a primary linear closure. For large lesions, however, this may result in long scars or scars under a high amount of tension. Circular excision and purse-string closure offers an alternative surgical approach to hemangiomas requiring excision, and often represents a good option because the original lesion is circular (**Fig. 3**). The technique for purse-string closure is outlined in **Box 3**.[27]

Parents must be warned that the immediate postoperative appearance is not the final appearance of the wound. A few weeks are needed for the radial ridges to flatten. As this occurs, circular scars have a tendency to become ovoid (**Fig. 4**). After several months, the decision must be made

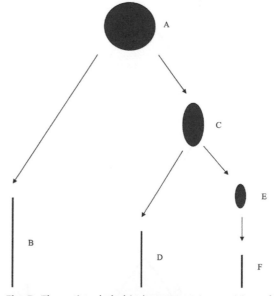

**Fig. 5.** The rationale behind a purse-string excision of a circular lesion, such as a hemangioma. If a lesion (A) is excised as an ellipse with primary linear closure, it results in a linear scar (B). If excised as a circle and then closed with a purse-string closure, it results in an oval scar (C). This scar can then be excised in a second stage to create a shorter linear scar (D). Alternatively, further purse-string closures can be performed to result in a smaller oval (E) or linear scar (F).

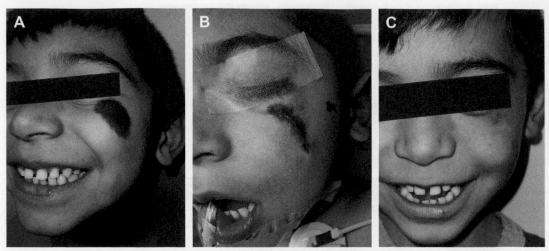

**Fig. 6.** (*A*) Five-year-old boy with a medium-sized congenital nevus on the face. A single-staged excision would result in a long scar under high tension, which would be likely to cause ectropion. (*B*) This lesion was approached with a 2-staged excision. Patient is shown before the second stage. (*C*) Patient is shown 1 month after completion of the second-stage excision.

to accept the small ovoid scar or consider another circular or elliptical excision (**Fig. 5**).

## Laser Treatment of Hemangiomas

The surgical management of hemangiomas also includes a pulsed dye laser. Accepted indications

for laser treatment of hemangiomas include telangiectatic residua of involuted hemangiomas and to accelerate healing and decrease pain in ulcerated hemangiomas.

Because pulsed dye laser has a short depth of penetration and was developed for treating capillary malformations, it is most effective in treating

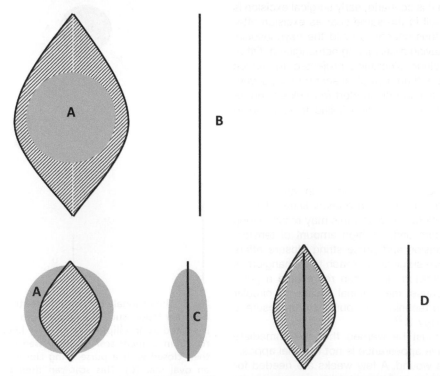

**Fig. 7.** A single-staged elliptical excision of a lesion (A) results in a linear scar (B). In a staged excision, the lesion (A) is partially removed, resulting in a scar surrounded by the residual lesion (C). The remainder of the lesion is then excised in a second procedure, resulting in a shorter final scar (D).

superficial lesions. It will not necessarily arrest the proliferation or speed the involution of the deeper dermal component of hemangiomas.

A recent report suggests that pulsed dye laser treatment may be able to counteract the rapid proliferation if undertaken early and performed at regular 2- to 3-week intervals.[28] Other authors, however, caution against the use of pulse dye laser in the treatment of proliferative hemangiomas, citing the potential risk of ulceration and scarring. However, most of these studies citing risk of scarring were reported before the availability of the dynamic cooling device. More severe ulcerations were noted with higher fluences.[29] In contrast with port wine stains, which can tolerate higher fluences with repeated treatments, hemangiomas should be treated with relatively low fluences. A more recent review evaluating the outcomes of hemangiomas treated with the most current laser technology had a much lower (1%) risk of ulceration.[30]

### Staged Excisions of Medium-Sized Congenital Nevi

The management of congenital melanocytic nevi (CMN) must take into consideration the risk of malignancy, the psychosocial distress to the child caused by the birthmark, and the potential morbidity associated with the surgery. The clinical judgment of the dermatologist and parental opinion are the main determinants in the management CMN. A cost analysis suggests that surgical excision ultimately costs the same as continued long-term follow-up of the nevus.[31]

When excision is necessary or desired and primary closure of a defect is not possible, 3 main options are available for wound closure: grafting, tissue expanders, and staged excision. Staged excision is an excellent option for medium-sized congenital nevi that are not amenable to excision in a single procedure (Fig. 6). In a staged excision, portions of a lesion are sequentially excised to produce a shorter scar under less tension (Fig. 7). The timing of staged excisions is critical. Enough time should elapse between stages for the tension on the wound to relax, but it should not be long

enough for a scar to spread or hypertrophy (Box 4). The ideal interval between stages is generally 6 to 8 weeks.

## SUMMARY

Performing dermatologic procedures in pediatric patients presents many challenges. The use of topical anesthetics and careful attention to injection technique can minimize injection-related pain. Knowledge of the risks and benefits of general anesthesia can help physicians determine when a procedure is best performed under general anesthesia. Although performing dermatologic procedures in children requires more preparation than performing the same procedures in adults, dermatologists can create a more pleasant experience for the patient and family by using a few special techniques.

## REFERENCES

1. Piira T, Sugiura T, Champion GD, et al. The role of parental presence in the context of children's medical procedures: a systematic review. Child Care Health Dev 2005;31(2):233–43.
2. Lyon VB, Palmer CM, Wagner AM, et al. Toddler wrap for abdominal biopsy or excision. Pediatr Dermatol 2008;25(1):109–11.
3. Lacuiere DA, Courtman S. Use of the iPad in paediatric anaesthesia. Anaesthesia 2011;66(7):629–30.
4. Rice LJ. Needle phobia: an anesthesiologist's perspective. J Pediatr 1993;122(5 Pt 2):S9–13.
5. Arndt KA, Burton C, Noe JM. Minimizing the pain of local anesthesia. Plast Reconstr Surg 1983;72:676–9.
6. Cepeda MS, Tzortzopoulou A, Thackrey M, et al. Adjusting the pH of lidocaine for reducing pain on injection. Cochrane Database Syst Rev 2010;(12): CD006581.
7. Larson PO, Ragi G, Swandby M, et al. Stability of buffered lidocaine and epinephrine used for local anesthesia. J Dermatol Surg Oncol 1991;17(5):411–4.
8. Buckley MM, Benfield P. Eutectic lidocaine/prilocaine cream. A review of the topical anaesthetic/analgesic efficacy of a eutectic mixture of local anaesthetics (EMLA). Drugs 1993;46(1):126–51.
9. Raso SM, Fernandez JB, Beobide EA, et al. Methemoglobinemia and CNS toxicity after topical application of EMLA to a 4-year-old girl with molluscum contagiosum. Pediatr Dermatol 2006;23(6):592–3.
10. Sawyer J, Febbraro S, Masud S, et al. Heated lidocaine/tetracaine patch (Synera, Rapydan) compared with lidocaine/prilocaine cream (EMLA) for topical anaesthesia before vascular access. Br J Anaesth 2009;102(2):210–5.
11. Cohen Reis E, Holubkov R. Vapocoolant spray is equally effective as EMLA cream in reducing

> **Box 4**
> **Tips for successful staged excision in children**
>
> - Take as much of the lesion during the first stage as possible
> - Do not wait too long between stages; the scar will spread or hypertrophy and the benefit of staging the excision will be lost.

immunization pain in school-aged children. Pediatrics 1997;100(6):E5.

12. Sorell J, Carmichael C, Chamlin S. Oral sucrose for pain relief in young infants with hemangiomas treated with intralesional steroids. Pediatr Dermatol 2010;27(2):154–5.

13. Chen BK, Eichenfield LF. Pediatric anesthesia in dermatologic surgery; when hand-holding is not enough. Dermatol Surg 2001;27:1010–8.

14. Cunningham BB, Gigler V, Wang K, et al. General anesthesia for pediatric dermatologic procedures: risks and complications. Arch Dermatol 2005;141(5):573–6.

15. Juern AM, Cassidy LD, Lyon VB. More evidence confirming the safety of general anesthesia in pediatric dermatologic surgery. Pediatr Dermatol 2010; 27(4):355–60.

16. Auroy Y, Ecoffey C, Messiah A, et al. Relationship between complications of pediatric anesthesia and volume of pediatric anesthetics. Anesth Analg 1997;84(1):234–5.

17. Hays SR, Deshpande JL. Newly postulated neurodevelopmental risks of pediatric anesthesia. Curr Neurol Neurosci Rep 2011;11(2):205–10.

18. Paule MG, Li M, Allen RR, et al. Ketamine anesthesia during the first week of life can cause long-lasting cognitive deficits in rhesus monkeys. Neurotoxicol Teratol 2011;33(2):220–30.

19. Zou X, Patterson TA, Divine RL, et al. Prolonged exposure to ketamine increases neurodegeneration in the developing monkey brain. Int J Dev Neurosci 2009;27(7):727–31.

20. Wilder RT, Flick RP, Sprung J, et al. Early exposure to anesthesia and learning disabilities in a population-based birth cohort. Anesthesiology 2009;110(4): 796–804.

21. Bartels M, Althoff RR, Boomsma DI. Anesthesia and cognitive performance in children: no evidence for a causal relationship. Twin Res Hum Genet 2009; 12(3):246–53.

22. Kuehn BM. FDA considers data on potential risks of anesthesia use in infants, children. JAMA 2011; 305(17):1749–50, 1753.

23. Mustoe TA, Gurjala A. The role of the epidermis and the mechanism of action of occlusive dressings in scarring. Wound Repair Regen 2011;19(Suppl 1): S16–21.

24. Cribier B, Scrivener Y, Grosshans E. Tumors arising in nevus sebaceus: a study of 596 cases. J Am Acad Dermatol 2000;42(2 Pt 1):263–8.

25. Altaykan A, Ersoy-Evans S, Erkin G, et al. Basal cell carcinoma arising in nevus sebaceous during childhood. Pediatr Dermatol 2008;25(6):616–9.

26. Kim HJ, Colombo M, Frieden IJ. Ulcerated hemangiomas: clinical characteristics and response to therapy. J Am Acad Dermatol 2001;44(6):962–72.

27. Mulliken JB, Rogers GF, Marler JJ. Circular excision of hemangioma and purse-string closure: the smallest possible scar. Plast Reconstr Surg 2002;109(5): 1544–54.

28. Chapas AM, Geronemus RG. Our approach to pediatric dermatologic laser surgery. Lasers Surg Med 2005;37(4):255–63.

29. Witman PM, Wagner AM, Scherer K, et al. Complications following pulsed dye laser treatment of superficial hemangiomas. Lasers Surg Med 2006;38: 116–23.

30. Rizzo C, Brightman L, Chapas AM, et al. Outcomes of childhood hemangiomas treated with the pulsed-dye laser with dynamic cooling: a retrospective chart analysis. Dermatol Surg 2009;35(12):1947–54.

31. Roldan FA, Hernando AB, Cuadrado A, et al. Small and medium-sized congenital nevi in children: a comparison of the costs of excision and long-term follow-up. Dermatol Surg 2009;35(12):1867–72.

# The Role of Psychiatry and Psychology Collaboration in Pediatric Dermatology

Michael Perry, MD[a], William C. Streusand, MD[b,c,d],*

## KEYWORDS

• Collaborative • Psychosomatic • CBT • Atopic dermatitis • Acne • Scratching

## KEY POINTS

- Situational stress and other emotional conditions are linked to several pediatric dermatologic conditions.
- This link can be a factor in the skin condition itself or contribute to self-image distress from having a skin condition.
- Treatment alliances are best with patients and their family if the treating doctors do not dichotomize into a part etiology that is "emotional" or a part etiology that is "physical."
- Pediatric dermatologists should establish collaborative relationships with qualified mental health practitioners to evaluate and treat comorbid psychological issues and assist in the behavioral interventions that optimize treatment outcomes.

It has long been accepted that certain emotional states can become evident in ones skin.[1] For example, a person flushes when embarrassed, and the extremities become cold when one becomes stressed. In the past decade or so, it has become accepted that there is a unique dialogue between one's psyche and one's skin. Beyond transient states of emotion, the skin and mind interact in many disease states that are just now being studied. In some psychopathological states in which the skin is clearly involved, such as trichotillomania, delusional parasitosis, and dermatitis artefacta, treatment goals are primarily psychiatric. In other disease states, treatment options and goals are not so clear. In conditions that cause emotional stress, such as alopecia and urticaria, treatment of the physical ailment can alleviate the psychological burden caused by the disease. Other disease states, such as atopic dermatitis (AD), psoriasis, and acne, among others, can be exacerbated and alleviated by psychogenic factors. In these states, in which research suggests there exist interplay between the mind and the body; treatment options are not so straightforward. These states certainly not only lead to a degree of emotional unrest but also can be caused or exacerbated by the stress and other psychological factors.

Although intellectually, medical professionals find it easy to reject a rigid assertion of a mind-body dichotomy philosophy, practical medical language is riddled with its implication. Often psychiatric consultation services are posed the question "is the condition real or is it psychiatric?" A pejorative tone is struck with the labeling of a condition as psychogenic. Pediatricians and pediatric subspecialists are trained to diligently pursue a differential diagnosis and then rule out those that do not match up, leaving the correct diagnosis that should imply a best course of action for treatment.

a The University of Texas Medical Branch, 301 University Boulevard, Galveston, TX 77555, USA; b Collaborative Care, Child, Adolescent, & Adult Psychiatry, 5910 Courtyard Dr, Suite 220, Austin, TX 78731, USA; c Department of Educational Psychology, University of Texas at Austin, George I. Sanchez Building, 5th Floor, Suite 504, 1 University Station D5800 Austin, TX 78712, USA; d CollaboraCare for Kids, 1600 West 38th Street, Suite 306 Austin, TX 78731, USA
* Corresponding author. 5910 Courtyard Drive, suite 220, Austin, TX 78731.
E-mail address: drstreusand@collaboracare.com

Dermatol Clin 31 (2013) 347–355
http://dx.doi.org/10.1016/j.det.2012.12.012
0733-8635/13/$ – see front matter © 2013 Elsevier Inc. All rights reserved.

When this process turns up no objective findings, often the parents are then told the symptoms are psychiatric, and a mental health consultation is ordered.

Pediatricians naturally feel that their skill set is exhausted, and one needs to logically bring in an expert from a different skill set, a psychiatrist. The patient is then handed over to the new clinician, leaving parents and patient often feeling disbelieved or abandoned, angry, and dissatisfied with care.

Parents naturally are advocates for their children getting quality medical care and relief of symptoms where often a "stress" or psychological component is the last thing on their minds, and any suggestion of psychological or psychiatric interventions is met with indifference, distain, or overt hostility. They may seek more expert opinions from centers with larger reputations, leading to many costly and nonproductive workups.

Perhaps it is best to try and rid one's vocabulary of terms such as psychosomatic and introduce the notion that many skin symptoms have a stress component either in cause or in effect from the beginning of a new evaluation. Introducing a mental health professional as an embedded member of the treatment team from day one of the evaluation has often produced a higher level of acceptance and satisfaction. It is critically important that the pediatrician/pediatric subspecialists and mental health professional stay engaged and be willing to consider emotional and physical causes and manifestations from the initiation of an evaluation.

In the adult literature, such states are fairly well studied. However, research among children (ages 0–18 years) is lacking. Furthermore, psychocutaneous disorders can pose a large developmental obstacle during the adolescent years when the individual begins to develop a distinct sense of self. Behavioral and environmental factors can affect not only the disease process itself but also the treatment programs a young patient can follow.

In children and adolescents, disease states and treatment regimes can also place a burden on caregivers.[2,3] Furthermore, research suggests that dysfunction in a child's home environment can further affect certain psychocutaneous disorders.[4–6] Therefore, effective treatment should not only be aimed at the physical and the psychological but also fit within the context of a child's family structure and overall home environment.

Research by Jafferany and colleagues[7–9] suggests that there is a significant need for education in psychocutaneous disorders from the perspective of both dermatologists and psychiatrists.

Fried[10] believes that psychocutaneous research medicine has come of age and that treatment should include what they term a "skin-emotion" specialist. In caring for a child, pediatricians would certainly need to be a part of this mix as well.

This article builds on the work done by Czyzewski and Lopez[11] by identifying those pediatric psychocutaneous disorders in which clinical psychiatry would be beneficial in management of the disease. The authors use current literature to examine certain disease processes and explore the interplay between a child's psyche and skin within the framework of mind-body interaction. Furthermore, they explore the impact these disease states have on the individual, the child's family, and development of the self. Finally, the authors make recommendations for treatment and identify further areas needing research.

## THE IMPACT ON THE INDIVIDUAL

Dermatologic ailments account for 15% to 20%[12] of visits to family practices, yet the effect of these conditions is only partially appreciated. Skin conditions can seem insignificant or surface-level nuisance. However, they can have profound effects on the individual patient. As a significant portion of one's physical presentation to the world, the skin plays a role in determining one's identity. When there is a pathologic condition that affects one's skin, it can alter the perception of the self, especially for children.

AD, an inflammatory skin condition, presents unique problems for the developing child. It affects between 15% and 20% of children and accounts for 2.7% of all concerns presenting to family physicians.[12] In an infant, AD can affect skin sensation and emotional development through altered parent/child bonding, which depends on physical contact in the early years.[13] AD is known to interfere with sleeping patterns, causing insomnia due to discomfort, and research has shown increased levels of psychological disturbance in patients with AD compared with controls.[12]

According to Saunes,[14] in the comprehensive, population-wide Young-HUNT study, there is "a strong and consistent association between mental distress and AD." Further, the psychological burden of this disease can manifest itself as "headache and neck or shoulder pain" in both boys and girls.[15] "However, for adolescents with AD, the association between symptoms and mental distress was stronger for boys than for girls."[15] Reporting of symptoms varied with sex and age, with the 17- to 19-year age group reporting more symptoms than the younger, 13- to

16-year age group. However, girls reported more mental distress symptoms across the board than boys.[15] As the investigators mention, this is somewhat expected, as adolescence is a fragile period of life when feeling good and looking good are both paramount goals but increasingly fleeting for the developing teen.

It is accepted that stress can cause exacerbations of AD and that states of emotional unrest can precipitate outbreaks.[13,16] It has been theorized that the hypothalamic-pituitary-adrenal (HPA) axis is involved in the mind-body interaction between stress and symptoms of AD via increased blood cortisol levels.[17–19] Asfar and colleagues[17] found that children with AD do not, in fact, have more anxiety or higher levels of cortisol than control groups. However, they also postulate that the severity of symptoms associated with AD can cause increased anxiety.

Similarly, acne is another dermatopathological disorder with effects that extend beyond the skin. Depending on the source, the prevalence of acne among children is 30% to 100%, with 93.3% of 16- to 18-year olds affected.[12,20,21] However, most health care professionals address only the physical ailments without addressing the full impact of the condition. In fact, individuals with acne suffer social, psychological, and emotional sequelae that are great as those reported by patients with chronic disabling asthma, epilepsy, diabetes, back pain, or arthritis on questionnaires.[22,23] Only patients with cardiac disease reported higher impairment. The most well-studied psychiatric impact of acne is its association with teenage depression and anxiety, largely due to the social impact of the disease.[24–28] However, this is not true across the board and the impact of acne, as with all skin conditions from person to person, which is why treatment strategies should be tailored to the individual as discussed later.

Summarizing the impact of acne beyond the physical, Sulzberger and Zaidens[29] claim "there is probably no single disease which causes more psychic trauma, more maladjustment between parents and children, more general insecurity and feeling of inferiority and greater sums of psychic suffering than does acne vulgaris."[12] It has also been found that acne impairs a child's quality of life, mood, and overall self-esteem.[30] Gathering together multiple studies relying on teen questionnaires, Dunn and colleagues[30] demonstrated acne having between moderate to severe effects on teens' quality of life. According to Niemeier and colleagues,[31] acne's impact on one's quality of life leads to greater levels of depression and anxiety. A similar effect was found on an individual's self-esteem, with girls being the most affected by facial lesions.

Acne also has effects on an individual's mood. Rapp and colleagues[32] demonstrated that anger is a significant factor in both quality of life and satisfaction with treatment among acne sufferers. Furthermore, emotional upset can also happen during the course of acne. Psychiatric comorbidity is also frequently encountered in the presence of acne. Picardi and colleagues[33] found a high degree of psychological comorbidity (>30%) among acne sufferers. With a higher degree of depression among those with acne, it is important to assess suicidal ideation during patient encounters. Furthermore, the number of patients who actually seek treatment of acne far underestimates those who actually suffer from the disorder.[31] In addition, with the high degree of psychiatric comorbidity, acne sufferers may have psychiatric disorders "hidden" behind their acne. Therefore, a psychiatric assessment may be needed.[31]

Similar to AD, the relationship between stress and acne is complex, with each affecting and exacerbating the other. In a somewhat older study, Lorenz and colleagues[34] demonstrated within days of a stressful interview where anger was intentionally induced, an exacerbation of acne was observed.[31] As has been shown, the presence of acne is undoubtedly a stressor for many children. Furthermore, stress can increase acne severity. During times of stress in a child's life, for example, during high school or university examinations, there is a higher correlation with increased acne severity.[35] The exact relationship between acne and stress is yet to be elucidated, but hormone production, inflammatory neuropeptides, and increased sebum production have all been suggested.[35]

Another chronic skin condition frequently linked to life stressors is psoriasis, the inflammatory, hyperproliferative disorder that can severely affect patient's daily lives. The effect of the disease seems to decrease as patients age[14,36]; therefore, the most severe symptoms should be expected in children. The link between stress and exacerbations of psoriasis is not disputed. However, the mechanism by which emotional stress can exacerbate psoriasis is unclear. Some have proposed that dysregulation of the hypothalamic-pituitary axis could be the key.[37] It is postulated that altered cortisol levels in patients with psoriasis modulating the HPA axis can lead to increased outbreaks. Decreased and increased cortisol levels have been found in patients with psoriasis.[37] Therefore, the causal link between stress and outbreaks seems unclear, and more research elucidating this connection is needed.

Bilgic and colleagues[21] examined the relationship between psoriasis, depression, and anxiety and the effect on the quality of life in children. Study and control groups were divided according to age into 2 groups, 8 to 12 years and 13 to 18 years, in an attempt to account for the psychological effect of puberty. Using a series of questionnaires, the investigators found that younger children with psoriasis are more affected by psychological factors than teenagers and that teenage measures are not sensitive enough to fully account for the impact of psoriasis. This study corresponds with similar findings in adults. The investigators expected to find an increased level of psychological impact among teens, but this was not observed, prompting the need for further research.

Evers and colleagues[37] found that "daily stressors" may alter cortisol levels at "moments of high stress." Furthermore, patients with persistently high levels of stressors had lower average blood cortisol levels. This finding suggests that the HPA axis is hypoactive in these individuals. This finding has also been seen in patients with stress-related disorders such as chronic pain and chronic fatigue, suggesting an overall downregulation of the HPA axis leading to hypocortisolism. Hypocortisolism is also seen in patients with a history of high level of childhood stressors. Evers and colleagues[37] theorized that these patients may be particularly susceptible to the effect of stress on their psoriasis. Richards and colleagues[36] found similar results in patients with stress-responsive psoriasis. They postulate that such patients are primed for exacerbations to their condition by altered HPA axis responses to stress.

Patients seem to believe that there is a link between stress and psoriasis flares. Heller and colleagues[38] have dubbed those who believe emotional stress exacerbates their condition "stress responders," and the prevalence of such ranges from 37% to 78%. Stress seems to affect not only the severity of outbreaks but also the duration for symptom resolution. Evers and colleagues[37] found that greater than half of all patients with psoriasis report, albeit retrospectively, an increase in stress before an outbreak.

History is also important in those with psoriasis, as there seems to be a correlation between childhood trauma/stressors and psoriasis. Simonic and colleagues[39] found negative life experiences at all periods of childhood development. However, the investigators found no correlations between the severity of psoriatic outbreaks and childhood trauma. Those affected with psoriasis did not significantly differ in the number of past positive experiences compared with control groups. This finding suggests a yet-to-be-elucidated relationship between past stress, aside from current stressors, and outbreaks of psoriasis.

## IMPACT ON THE HOME AND SOCIAL FUNCTIONING

Beyond the psychological makeup of the individual, a child's social environment can have a profound impact on the progression of dermatopathology. As an exterior organ, the skin becomes integral to a growing child's identity and plays a role not only in self-esteem but also in the way one relates to others. Diseases such as AD, psoriasis, and acne prospectively affect the way an individual interacts with their environment; so also, one's social background can alter the progression of such diseases. For example, Poot and colleagues[40] found that past family dysfunction played a role in the development and exacerbations of psoriasis, alopecia, and AD. In a multicentric case-control study, the investigators constructed the family trees of patients with these conditions and found that those in the experimental groups had "three times the risk of having moderate family dysfunction compared with controls." Severity of dysfunction was assessed, and compared with controls, those in the experimental groups had "16 times the risk of having a severe family dysfunction," associated with their disease. Although this study was conducted on adults, many of those studied reported prior family dysfunction occurring since childhood.

In a small study, Langan and colleagues[28] demonstrated a link between exacerbations of AD and a damp environment, heat, and stress. Bockelbrink and colleagues[4] showed that home environment stressors, such as divorce/separation of parents and serious illness or death of a family member can influence the risk of a child developing AD.

Furthermore, a child's skin disorder can also place increasing demands on the caregiver. Balkrishnan and colleagues[19] found that the burden of having a child with AD affects the family and primary caregiver in 3 principle ways: the burden of caring for a child with AD causes caregivers to believe their child's case is severe, the increased worry about covering the cost of care for the child, and in coordination, increased use of supplemental, "nonmedical services." Although the researchers agree this was a preliminary study, and much more work is needed to fully elucidate the burden placed on a child's family in the care of AD, it does begin to reveal the impact such a disease can have beyond the individual patient.

Similarly, having AD can have a profound impact on the way a patient interacts with his or her environment. Evers and colleagues[13] found that, compared with controls, patients with AD and psoriasis believed that their disease greatly affected their daily lives in the form of increased fatigue, feelings of helplessness, a perception of less acceptance among peers, and, therefore, less social support. Such feelings, the researchers believed, contributed to the overall psychological distress caused by the disease. For the purposes of this article, such increased distress could then exacerbate the disease itself, as explained earlier, in the case of more severe outbreaks and a longer time to resolution. Although this study was conducted on adults, it is reasonable to believe such feelings affect children to a similar, if not greater, degree. All these contributed to an overall decreased quality of life for patients with AD.

Not only can the stress of the home environment affect the progression and exacerbation of the disease but the disease itself can cause stressors on those in the home. Faught and colleagues[2] showed that mothers of young children with AD had higher stress scores than parents of normal children and parents of children with chronic diseases such as diabetes and deafness. Overall stress on the caregivers was comparable to those with children suffering from chronic diseases requiring constant management such as enteral feeding or Rhett Syndrome.[2] Maternal stress levels were also correlated with the severity of the child's disease, with more severe cases having higher scores.

Fennessy and colleagues[3] found that disturbance in children with AD is profound. This disease shows a reverse class gradient, with children in higher classes more affected than those in low. Sleep disturbance was the primary sequelae of the disease, which the investigators postulated could account for the other observed disturbances of "irritability, lack of concentration, inability to participate in leisure activities," and an overall decline in normal function.[3,41] Other studies the investigators cite point to increased "clinginess" and fear in infants with AD.[3]

Fennessy and colleagues[3] also found that mothers caring for children with AD reported a similar pattern of sleep disturbance as children, as the disease affects the overall quality of life for families as well as patients. Furthermore, families of children with AD faced financial hardships in the form of "loss of income because of time off work, traveling costs to clinics, childcare costs for siblings, specialist clothing, bedding, and equipment."[3]

Similarly, patients with psoriasis often have a degree of past social dysfunction of extra personal stressors that play a role in the development of their disease. Poot and colleagues[40] demonstrated a correlation between patients with psoriasis and a past history of abuse, geographic distribution, emotional isolation, and vulnerability within the family. Ozden and colleagues[42] found that children with psoriasis were more likely to have a history of stressful life events, exposure to tobacco smoke at home, and a higher body mass index than controls.

The debilitating effects of psoriasis on patients' ability to function socially are comparable to those of other chronic conditions. As Gaikwad and colleagues[43] have shown, psoriasis affects patients' lives both at home and at work. Social functioning was affected in nearly half their study population, with reported decreased work efficiency in more than 50% and overall subjective distress in the workplace at 62.8%.[38] Nearly two-thirds reported problems relating to others at home, and approximately 20% reported impaired sexual functioning despite the absence of genital lesions.[43] These social findings were echoed by Evers and colleagues,[13] who reported that patients with psoriasis had the perception of a smaller social network, in addition to the social impairments shared with AD.

In a small study, Kleyn and colleagues[26] showed that patients with psoriasis have a decreased ability to recognize looks of disgust on the faces of others. On functional magnetic resonance imaging, patients with psoriasis showed a decreased response of the insular cortex compared with controls when viewing faces of disgust. However, control and experimental subjects did not differ in their insular response to fearful faces. The investigators postulate that this could be a developed coping mechanism of patients with psoriasis, or it could represent mere desensitization. This study is one of the first to show a functional connection between what the investigators call the "brain-skin axis" and could have powerful implications for further research if these results could be duplicated in a larger, statistically significant population.

In the case of acne, expected effects are similar if not more profound. Acne is primarily seen as a disease of adolescence, when much of one's personal and interpersonal identity is established. As Barankin mentions, acne affects one's self-image and therefore "assertiveness," both factors that are important in establishing friendships and dating. Dunn and colleagues[30] have shown how acne can negatively affect a teen's quality of life and an individual's social sensitivity, with women scoring higher and having poorer outcomes in social measures.

According to Niemeier and colleagues,[31] the psychosocial aspects of acne are profound. According to questionnaires, nearly 70% of patients with acne report feelings of psychosocial rejection; this seems more than just a subjective feeling, as "18–30-year-old acne patients are considerably more often unemployed than persons with healthy skin," according to the investigators. They continue by citing other research that demonstrates that positive attributes are ascribed to physically attractive strangers. Therefore, those with acne, it could be inferred, would suffer negative assumptions from strangers by virtue of their disfiguring disease.

## TREATMENT: GOALS AND RECOMMENDATIONS

It is hoped that this discussion has elucidated, at least partially, the interplay between dermatologic physical symptoms and emotional issues. Treatment, then, should include those things that take into account the emotional as well as the physical. However, what would such treatment look like, and what would the goals of a treatment program look like? Pharmacologic, nonpharmacologic, and psychiatric treatments must work together to manage the physical condition and the patient's experience.

Given inherent adolescent concerns about body image, it is important to maintain a positive and hopeful attitude toward improvement throughout treatment. Even in difficult-to-treat cases, reasonable hope should be brought forward by the dermatologist. For the adolescent, the difficulty of emotionally tolerating a body image situation can be mitigated by the physician by giving hope of improvement. Dermatologists and treating mental health professionals should routinely include life functioning screening questions. These might include inquiring about being a target of bullying, increasing isolation, and avoidance of social and extracurricular activities.

Stress reduction techniques could also be helpful. Hypnosis, biofeedback, and relaxation training have all been studied as adjunctive therapies for acne. These techniques prove especially helpful for excoriated acne. Furthermore, given the association between acne and depression and anxiety, physicians should be aware of current comorbid psychiatric conditions. Patients should be screened for these disorders and treated where necessary. As Dunn and colleagues[30] mention, a strong patient-physician relationship here is key.

Among pharmacologic options, isoretinoin has been shown to be effective in multiple studies for controlling acne. However, there has been some worry among patients with regard to increased depression with isoretinoin treatment. However, as Kaymack and colleagues[24] have shown, there is no increase in the number of depressive symptoms among those treated with isoretinoin compared with controls. On the contrary, successful treatment of a patient's acne with medication improved depressive and anxiety scores. There is persistent worry about increased depression in already depressed adolescents or those on antidepressant medication. Often, mental health professionals are asked to "clear" such an adolescent before treatment initiation. Rarely has this medication negatively affected a stable adolescent who is on antidepressant medication.

In the case of AD, treatment strategies are similar. As mentioned, stress can exacerbate AD. Kawana and Omi[9] from Japan studied the treatment of AD with the serotonin agonist tandospirone (5-HT$_{1A}$ agonist) and measured with the SCORAD index. During 4 weeks, those in the experimental group scored significantly better on the tension-anxiety portion than did controls. This result suggests that such medications can have a role in the treatment of AD by reducing stress and, hopefully, exacerbations of the disease. The investigators theorized that such strategies could work with patients with psoriasis as well, given the link between psoriasis and stress.

Another small Japanese study investigated the effect of showing children with AD humorous films before bedtime with promising results. As mentioned, children with AD have increased nighttime awakenings as a result of their disease. However, compared with controls, children with AD who were shown humorous films before bedtime showed reduced salivary ghrelin levels and reduced nighttime awakenings. Ghrelin, a hormone primarily involved in the regulation of appetite has also been shown to have effects on growth, stress, anxiety, and nighttime wakening. Therefore, a reduction in ghrelin levels could provide a link to a reduction in symptoms of AD, especially given ghrelin's involvement with IgE secretion. However, this link remains to be fully elucidated.

As has been demonstrated in many psychiatric conditions such as depression, anxiety, and somatization disorders, cognitive behavioral therapies (CBTs) hold considerable promise for being helpful with skin conditions such as AD. Several of the CBT techniques may be helpful. Traditional habit reversal involves actively performing behaviors (or active thoughts) that compete with persistent scratching. This approach may be combined with an "exposure" approach. Here the patient is encouraged create conditions in a therapy session that lead incrementally from mild to severe discomfort. The patient masters the discomfort with distraction, relaxation, or a competing activity until the impulse is attenuated and the coping skill learned. Good CBT therapists can be creative in the distractions and coping skills they use to bring relief. Discomfort followed by active, competing, and opposite behaviors that do not allow the scratching to occur is introduced. Examples would be systematic fist clenching or ball squeezing. Although there are few studies of these techniques in dermatologic conditions, CBT techniques probably hold the greatest promise of success. Psychologists who are expert at CBT can design protocols for this type of active behavior change. Clearly, more research is needed in this area of intervention.

Given the interplay between the psyche and the skin, many advocate for a multidisciplinary approach to care. According to Evers and colleagues,[13] "when examining factors contributing to psychological distress, approximately the same physical, psychological and social factors contributed to distress levels in patients with psoriasis and AD." Therefore, "patients with both psoriasis and AD could possibly benefit from multidisciplinary treatment options that focus on fatigue reduction...changing patients' pessimistic and helpless attitudes about their disease-...and promoting social support." The investigators go on to report that such care in screening and treatment could improve patients' quality of life through treatment of all facets of their disease.

The studies cited here generally have looked at skin conditions and interventions both medical and psychological at a particular slice of time, although many of the conditions are chronic in nature and do not become "cured" so much as "managed." The conditions can occur over a long period of months and years in a child and the family's life. It is worth commenting on the developmental and family dynamic complexities of a child with a chronic skin condition.

If a child has a chronic skin condition, there are medical visits for diagnosis and treatment to primary care pediatricians and dermatologists. Treatments that require a parent to perform therapeutic maneuvers to the child are prescribed, such as administering medication, topical and oral. The parent may be required to instruct or restrict the child in behaviors that would be out of their usual inclinations such as "no scratching," placing certain dressings or other skin barriers, or restricting sun exposure. The necessity of performing these activities to and with the child changes the nature of interaction in the parent-child relationship.

Emotional developmental markers such as the separation-individuation process has been well described (Mahler and Pine), and there is increasing knowledge of the variety of attachment and temperament styles. These developmental processes are not suspended during a period when a child is treated for a chronic illness but are clearly colored by the need for a parent to minister to the chronic skin condition. If a 3-year-old child is naturally going through some oppositionality related to the separation-individuation process and at the same time must have a topical cream applied several times a day and "not scratch," it is likely that a larger-than-usual amount of conflict will occur between the child and ministering parent. These interactions then become an unavoidable part of the developmental experience and change how future separation issues are perceived. Skilled child developmentalists who are also experienced in working at the medical-emotional interface might bring understanding, relief, and creative solutions to both parents and dermatologists navigating these complex waters. Keeping emotional development as on track as possible should be a goal of all clinicians working with children through difficult medical treatments.

The authors recommend that every dermatologist who treats children and adolescents develop a collaborative relationship with specific local mental heath professionals and not wait for a difficult situation to present itself for an emergent referral. These professionals would include a psychiatrist who can comfortably walk the line of the medical-psychiatric interface and a psychologist/therapist skilled in CBT techniques. Visits with the dermatologist should include some screening of the child's emotional state and functioning. Treatment of comorbid mood disorders, anxiety disorder, psychotic disorder, or attention-deficit/hyperactivity disorder might improve dermatologic outcomes and regimen compliance. If these disorders are suspected, the child should be referred to a psychiatrist for further evaluation. If life functioning erodes during the course of a treatment (school, socialization, extracurricular activities, isolation), a referral should be made to a mental health professional. A referral should also be made for patients not suspected of comorbid psychiatric conditions but who are not improving because of actions on their part. These might include scratching or noncompliance. Here would be a job for a CBT expert.

Sometimes families are so stressed, disorganized, or have such limited coping skills that improvements do not occur. A mental health evaluation of the family might assist in improving outcomes. If a parent is found to have a personality disorder by the psychiatrist/psychologist, the mental health professional may be invaluable in helping the dermatologist understand different ways to be effective in communicating with that parent, again improving dermatologic outcomes.

Dermatologists should become comfortable with recommending simple behavioral techniques. Although the dermatologist is not expected to have a full CBT palette of skills, simple behavioral suggestions may undo a need for a more costly and complicated mental health intervention. When making these suggestions, it is important to engage families as collaborators, as parents who know their particular child well might have clear knowledge of what works with particularly their child. Such collaboration may lead to a more targeted intervention and a better outcome. If scratching is heaviest in the 2 hours before bedtime, that would be the optimal time to use barrier techniques (gloves or mittens) and or distractions (video games, parent attention, and relaxation exercises).

Many skin diseases cannot be covered up and are so visible for all to see. Even a life-changing illness such as childhood diabetes is "invisible" to peers and peer parents unless an insulin injection is seen or an unexpected hypoglycemia or ketosis crisis occurs. Many of the skin diseases addressed here must be "worn on the outside" for the entire world to see. The fragile nature of child/adolescent self-esteem and identity is often tied to body issues, so the child with chronic skin disease inevitably suffers from these vulnerabilities. Body variation insults are a frequent method of bullying, and children with skin diseases must be protected.

Often, "skin-emotion specialists" take the form of a psychiatrist to aid dermatologists or primary care providers in the treatment of complex patients. Fried is a firm believer that psychocutaneous medicine has already come of age and that setting concrete observable goals is important. Doing so measures progress of therapy and encourages a sense of well-being and control for patients. Further, Fried advocates the alignment of dermatologists with "skin-emotion specialists," a euphemistic term for "psychiatrist, psychologist, social worker, biofeedback therapist, or other mental health or behavioral specialist," to fully address all aspects causing and exacerbating these conditions. This sentiment is echoed by Gaikwad and colleagues,[43] as well as others, who note

that a psychiatric liaison can not only help educate patients on their condition but also provide emotional support and guidance as necessary. Fried, quoting W. Mitchell Sams Jr, relays the following quote reminding that skin conditions are more than merely a physical ailment: "although the physician is a scientist and clinician, he or she is and must be something more. A doctor is a caretaker of the patient's person—a professional advisor, guiding the patient through some of life's most difficult journeys."

## REFERENCES

1. Al Shobaili HA. The impact of childhood atopic dermatitis on the patients' family. Pediatr Dermatol 2010;27:618–23.
2. Faught J, Bierl C, Barton B, et al. Stress in mothers of young children with eczema. Arch Dis Child 2007;92(8):683–6.
3. Fennessy M, Coupland S, Popay J, et al. The epidemiology and experience of atopic eczema during childhood: a discussion paper on the implications of current knowledge for health care, public health policy and research. J Epidemiol Community Health 2000;54:581–9.
4. Bockelbrink A, Heinrich J, Schäfer I, et al. Atopic eczema in children: another harmful sequel of divorce. Allergy 2006;61(12):1397–402.
5. Broom BC. A reappraisal of the role of 'mind body' factors in chronic urticaria. Postgrad Med J 2010; 86(1016):365–70.
6. Chung MC, Symons C, Gilliam J. Stress, psychiatric co-morbidity and coping in patients with chronic idiopathic urticaria. Psychol Health 2010;25(4):477–90.
7. Jafferany M, Stoep AV. Psychocutaneous disorders: a survey study of psychiatrists' awareness and treatment patterns. South Med J 2010;103(12):1199–203.
8. Jafferany M, Stoep AV. The knowledge, awareness, and practice patterns of dermatologists toward psychocutaneous disorders: results of a survey study. Int J Dermatol 2010;49:784–9.
9. Kawana S, Kato Y, Omi T. Efficacy of a 5-HT1a receptor agonist in atopic dermatitis. Clin Exp Dermatol 2010;35(8):835–40.
10. Fried R. Nonpharmacologic treatments in psychodermatology. Dermatol Clin 2002;20(1):177–85.
11. Czyzewski DI, Lopez M. Clinical psychology in the management of pediatric skin disease. Dermatol Clin 1998;16(3):619–29.
12. Barankin B, DeKoven J. Psychosocial effect of common skin diseases. Can Fam Physician 2002; 48:712–6.
13. Evers AW, Lu Y, Duller P. Common burden of chronic skin diseases? Contributors to psychological distress in adults with psoriasis and atopic dermatitis. Br J Dermatol 2005;152:1275–81.

14. Saunes M, Smidesang I, Holmen TL, et al. Atopic dermatitis in adolescent boys is associated with greater psychological morbidity compared with girls of the same age: the Young-HUNT study. Br J Dermatol 2007;156(2):283–8.

15. Schmitt J, Romanos M, Pfennig A, et al. Psychiatric comorbidity in adult eczema. Br J Dermatol 2009; 161(4):878–83.

16. Lee KH, Oh SH, Bae BG, et al. Association of stress with symptoms of atopic dermatitis. Acta Derm Venereol 2010;90(6):582–8.

17. Asfar FS, Isleten F, Sonmez N. Children with atopic dermatitis do not have more anxiety or different cortisol levels compared with normal children. J Cutan Med Surg 2010;14(1):13–8.

18. Bahmer JA, Kuhl J, Bahmer FA. How do personality systems interact in patients with psoriasis, atopic dermatitis and urticaria? Acta Derm Venereol 2007; 87(4):317–24.

19. Balkrishnan R, Housman TS, Grummer S, et al. The family impact of atopic dermatitis in children: the role of the parent caregiver. Pediatr Dermatol 2003; 20(1):5–10.

20. Basavaraj KH, Navya MA, Rashmi R. Stress and quality of life in psoriasis: an update. Int J Dermatol 2011;50:783–92.

21. Bilgic A, Bilgic Ö, Akış HK, et al. Psychiatric symptoms and health-related quality of life in children and adolescents with psoriasis. Pediatr Dermatol 2010;27(6):614–7.

22. Magin P, Adams J, Heading G, et al. The causes of acne: a qualitative study of patient perceptions of acne causation and their implications for acne care. Dermatol Nurs 2006;18(4):344–9.

23. Malhotra SK, Mehta V. Role of stressful life events in induction or exacerbation of psoriasis and chronic urticaria. Indian J Dermatol Venereol Leprol 2008; 74:594–9.

24. Kaymack Y, Taner E, Taner Y. Comparison of depression, anxiety and life quality in acne vulgaris patients who were treated with either isotretinoin or topical agents. Int J Dermatol 2009;48:41–6.

25. Kimata H. Viewing humorous film improves nighttime wakening in children with atopic dermatitis. Indian Pediatr 2007;44:281–5.

26. Kleyn CE, McKie S, Ross AR, et al. Diminished neural and cognitive responses to facial expressions of disgust in patients with psoriasis: a functional magnetic resonance imaging study. J Invest Dermatol 2009;129(11):2613–9.

27. Kotrulja L, Tadinac M, Jorkic-Begic N. A multivariate analysis of clinical severity, psychological distress and psychopathological traits in psoriatic patients. Acta Derm Venereol 2010;90:251–6.

28. Langan SM, Bourke JF, Silcocks P, et al. An exploratory prospective observational study of environmental factors exacerbating atopic eczema in children. Br J Dermatol 2006;154(5):979–80.

29. Sulzberger NB, Zaidens SH. Psychogenic factors in dermatologic disorders. Med Clin North Am 1948; 32:669–88.

30. Dunn LK, O'Neill JL, Feldman SR. Acne in adolescents: quality of life, self-esteem, mood, and psychological disorders. Dermatol Online J 2011; 17(1):1–11.

31. Niemeier V, Kupfer J, Gieler U. Acne vulgaris–psychosomatic aspects. J Dtsch Dermatol Ges 2006;4:1027–36 [in English, German].

32. Rapp DA, Brenes GA, Feldman SR, et al. Anger and acne: implications for quality of life, patient satisfaction and clinical care. Br J Dermatol 2004;151(1): 183–9.

33. Picardi A, Abeni D, Melchi CF, et al. Psychiatric morbidity in dermatological outpatients: an issue to be recognized. Br J Dermatol 2000;143:983–91.

34. Lorenz TH, Graham DT, Wolf S. The relation of life-stress and emotions to human sebum secretion and to the mechanism of acne vulgaris. J Lab Clin Med 1953;41:11–28.

35. Tom WL, Barrio VR. New insights into adolescent acne. Curr Opin Pediatr 2008;20(4):436–40.

36. Richards HL, Ray DW, Kirby B, et al. Response of the hypothalamic-pituitary-adrenal axis to psychological stress in patients with psoriasis. Br J Dermatol 2005;153(6):1114–20.

37. Evers AW, Verhoeven EW, Kraaimaat FW, et al. How stress gets under the skin: cortisol and stress reactivity in psoriasis. Br J Dermatol 2010;163(5): 986–91.

38. Heller MM, Lee ES, Yoo JY. Stress as an influencing factor in psoriasis. Skin Therapy Lett 2011;16:1–9.

39. Simonić E, Kaštelan M, Peternel S, et al. Childhood and adulthood traumatic experiences in patients with psoriasis. J Dermatol 2010;37(9):793–800.

40. Poot F, Antoine E, Gravellier M, et al. A case-control study on family dysfunction in patients with alopecia areata, psoriasis and atopic dermatitis. Acta Derm Venereol 2011;91:415–21.

41. Finzi A, Colombo D, Caputo A, et al. Psychological distress and coping strategies in patients with psoriasis: the PSYCHAE Study. J Eur Acad Dermatol Venereol 2007;21(9):1161–9.

42. Ozden MC, Tekin NS, Gurer MA. Environmental risk factors in pediatric psoriasis: a multicenter case–control study. Pediatr Dermatol 2011;28(3):306–12.

43. Gaikwad R, Deshpande S, Raje S, et al. Evaluation of functional impairment in psoriasis. Indian J Dermatol Venereol Leprol 2006;72:37–40.

# Index

Note: Page numbers of article titles are in **boldface** type.

Dermatol Clin 31 (2013) 357–362
http://dx.doi.org/10.1016/S0733-8635(13)00010-7
0733-8635/13/$ – see front matter © 2013 Elsevier Inc. All rights reserved.

derm.theclinics.com

# Moving?

## Make sure your subscription moves with you!

To notify us of your new address, find your **Clinics Account Number** (located on your mailing label above your name), and contact customer service at:

**Email: journalscustomerservice-usa@elsevier.com**

**800-654-2452** (subscribers in the U.S. & Canada)
**314-447-8871** (subscribers outside of the U.S. & Canada)

**Fax number: 314-447-8029**

**Elsevier Health Sciences Division**
**Subscription Customer Service**
**3251 Riverport Lane**
**Maryland Heights, MO 63043**

*To ensure uninterrupted delivery of your subscription, please notify us at least 4 weeks in advance of move.

# Moving?

## Make sure your subscription moves with you!

To notify us of your new address, find your Clinics Account Number (located on your mailing label above your name), and contact customer service at:

**Email: journalscustomerservice-usa@elsevier.com**

**800-654-2452** (subscribers in the U.S. & Canada)
**314-447-8871** (subscribers outside of the U.S. & Canada)

**Fax number: 314-447-8029**

**Elsevier Health Sciences Division**
**Subscription Customer Service**
**3251 Riverport Lane**
**Maryland Heights, MO 63043**

Printed and bound by CPI Group (UK) Ltd, Croydon, CR0 4YY

03/10/2024

01040347-0009